SCIENTIFIC
BASIS OF
ATHLETIC
CONDITIONING

SCIENTIFIC BASIS OF ATHLETIC CONDITIONING

CLAYNE R. JENSEN, P.E.D.
Professor and Dean
College of Physical Education
Brigham Young University
Provo, Utah

A. GARTH FISHER, Ph.D.
Director, Human Performance Research Center
Brigham Young University
Provo, Utah

SECOND EDITION

LEA & FEBIGER   *Philadelphia*

1979

Health Education,
Physical Education, and
Recreation

RUTH ABERNATHY, Ph.D., EDITORIAL ADVISER
Professor Emeritus, School of Physical and Health Education
University of Washington, Seattle, Washington, 98105

First Edition, 1972
  Reprinted, 1975
  Reprinted, 1977

Library of Congress Cataloging in Publication Data

Jensen, Clayne R.
  Scientific basis of athletic conditioning.

  (Health education; physical education; and recreation)
  Bibliography: p.
  Includes index.
  1. Sports—Physiological aspects. 2. Physical fitness. I. Fisher, A.
Garth, joint author. II. Title.
  RC1235.J46   1979   612'.044   78-8593
  ISBN 0-8121-0633-4

Published in Great Britain by Henry Kimpton Publishers, London

Printed in the United States of America

Print number: 4   3   2   1

Preface

It is claimed that Milo of Croton, the greatest athlete of the 6th century B.C., lifted a calf above his head every day until it was full grown. He became so strong that during his 24 years of competition he was never defeated and he was six times Olympic champion.

Other interesting accounts about athletic conditioning have been passed down through the ages. For example, Coroebus, a lowly cook of little native ability, trained so vigorously by running up and down hills that in the Olympics of 776 B.C. he won over the most noted Greek competitors. His event was the *stade* (from which came the word stadium), a 200-yard straight run. Polydamas of Thessaly, another great competitor, is said to have gained so much strength from lifting stones that he could kill a lion with his bare hands. Arrachian supposedly developed enough skill by wrestling beasts to win the Olympic pancratium (wrestling) crown five times before he was finally defeated and lay dead in the stadium.

Humans have consistently strived to run faster, jump higher, throw farther, and exhibit greater strength, endurance, and skill. We are naturally competitive and ambitious for excellence in athletic performance. As a result of practical experience, observation, and much scientific experimentation, old methods of conditioning, though fascinating and rich in tradition, have been discarded and replaced by new methods based on insight and understanding. For centuries, this evolution toward better methods of conditioning was slow, but in recent years the dramatic changes that have taken place have brought about some astounding results in performances.

These recent changes in conditioning methods are based on, and have been motivated by, an abundance of careful observation and scientific research. These procedures have produced valid and precise information about the relative effectiveness of different training methods. As a result, we currently know much more than ever before about the functioning of the body systems during training and competition, and how to develop strength, endurance, power, agility, speed, and athletic skills. We have learned much about the effects of diet, drugs, altitude, warm-up, and other influencing factors. In recent years we have gained new knowledge about almost every aspect of conditioning and performance.

Because of the great emphasis being placed on conditioning and performance, and because of the need to bring together the information available on the topic, this book was prepared. The book should be especially useful to coaches and teachers, and to upper division and graduate students majoring in physical education.

We express appreciation to Dr. Robert Conlee for his suggestions and comments during the preparation of the second edition, and to Dr. Philip Allsen for furnishing resource material.

Provo, Utah   CLAYNE R. JENSEN
                                                   A. GARTH FISHER

Contents

vii

PART I
THE PHYSIOLOGICAL BASIS
OF CONDITIONING

Excellent performances are directly dependent upon muscular function, and muscular function is strongly dependent upon other body systems. This section includes the pertinent information about muscular function and the systems that support it.

We assume that the reader has completed basic courses in human anatomy and physiology. Thus, Part I was written with that in mind. The content expands and further emphasizes selected information with great significance in athletic conditioning and performance.

Chapter 1 describes the role of energy and its production, as well as the meaning of energy measurements. In Chapter 2, the process of muscular contraction is discussed and the ultrastructure and architecture of muscle are described. Chapter 3 describes how the nervous system contributes to performance. Chapter 4 consists of the pertinent information about the involvement of the cardiovascular system in muscular work. Chapter 5 explains the role of the pulmonary system as it supports the oxidative process, and Chapter 6 explains both the acute and chronic adaptations to exercise of the various systems of the body.

Chapter 1
Energy and Metabolism

Metabolism is the process by which foods are broken down and converted into energy by the body. It involves numerous complex chemical reactions and processes. The purpose of this chapter is to investigate the pathways of metabolism and to discuss the significance of the metabolic processes to conditioning and performance.

THE BASIC SOURCE OF ENERGY

All energy as we know it comes from the sun. The sun loses mass in accordance with Albert Einstein's formula, $E = mc^2$, to produce energy which reaches the earth at a rate of about 2×10^{13} kilocalories (Kcal)/second.[3] The chloroplasts of plants provide chlorophyll, which uses some of this energy to break down water to hydrogen (H_2) and oxygen (O_2). Some of the hydrogen released from this breakdown goes through a respiratory chain and produces energy in the form of plant adenosine triphosphate (ATP). The rest of the hydrogen combines with carbon dioxide (CO_2) to form carbohydrates and release oxygen into the atmosphere. The plant carbohydrates have stored energy in their chemical bonds. It is this source, either directly or indirectly, that provides energy for man.

DIGESTION

The purpose of digestion is to break down large unabsorbable molecules of food to small molecules which can be absorbed through the intestinal walls and into the blood stream to be carried to the cells throughout the body. Only in the cells can the energy in the food be converted to ATP and be used by the body.

The three basic foods used by man can be classified into carbohydrates, fats, and protein. Carbohydrates enter the body at the mouth, where they are attacked by ptyalin which hydrolyzes the starches into maltose. There is little activity in the stomach toward carbohydrates, but in the small intestine they are worked on by several pancreatic amylases which break the particles into glucose, fructose, and galactose. In these forms, carbohydrates are absorbed through the intestinal walls into the portal vein, and through the sinusoids of the liver, where some are stored as glycogen to be released later as the body needs energy. The rest are transported directly to the cells of the body to be used as an immediate energy source.

Fats are not broken down much in either the mouth or the stomach. However, in the small intestine, bile from the liver emulsifies the fat molecules so that enzymes can act on their surfaces. Pancreatic lipases complete the process by breaking the emulsified fat into fatty acids, glycerol, and glycerides. Fat particles are carried from the intestines through the lymphatic system as chylomicrons and enter the blood stream near the heart.

There is little breakdown of protein in the mouth. However, in the stomach, the particles are hydrolyzed or broken apart at their peptide linkages by pepsin and gastricsin, enzymes that work well in the acidic environment of the stomach. The particles then pass into the small intestine where they are treated by chemicals from the pancreas and small intestine, and are broken into smaller units to yield amino acids and small polypeptides. The input of proteins is important because the body is unable to produce certain amino acids from other ingested food, so they must be provided from ingested protein to replace those used up by the body.

After the digested food particles have entered the blood, they are carried throughout the body to the cells where they are oxidized, and the energy released is converted to adenosine triphosphate (ATP). ATP is an essential chemical compound found in the cytoplasm of cells. It is composed of adenine, ribose, and three "high-energy" phosphate radicals (Fig. 1–1). The amount of energy stored in each of these bonds is approximately 8 Kcal, which is sufficient energy for almost any chemical reaction in the body. If the energy level of ATP is lower than that required by a chemical reaction, that chemical reaction cannot be energized by ATP.

ATP is the basic energy source for all activity and, when needed, is broken into adenosine diphosphate (ADP) and adenosine monophosphate (AMP), with the release of energy for muscular contraction. ADP

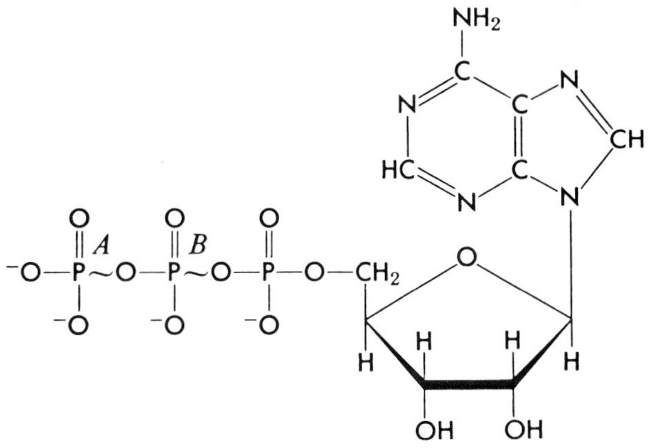

Adenosine triphosphate (ATP)

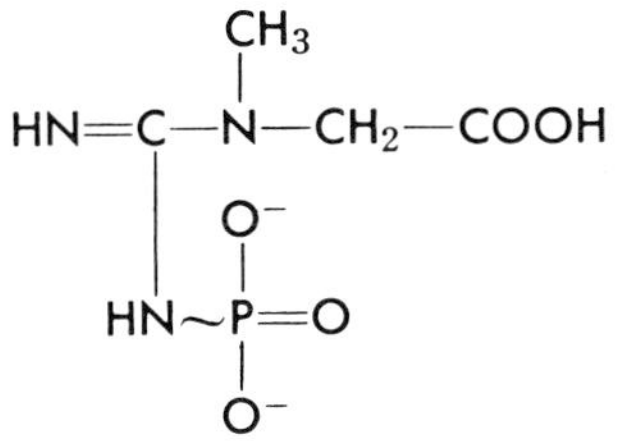

Creatine phosphate (CP)

Figure 1–1. Structural formulas of adenosine triphosphate and creatine phosphate.

and AMP are synthesized by the energy schemes in the body. Because of this relationship, ATP is sometimes referred to as the "energy currency" of the body.[10]

Another important chemical which provides stored energy is creatine phosphate (CP). The bond energy in CP is even higher than that in ATP. However, CP cannot be used directly by the cells as a source of energy, but it is used to synthesize ATP from ADP. Creatine phosphate is much more abundant in the cells than ATP and is used immediately to regenerate ATP during heavy work in order to keep the concentration of ATP at a constant level. For this reason, CP is sometimes referred to as an "ATP sparer." CP is important during muscular work because it can synthesize ADP to ATP much more quickly than the energy schemes to be discussed in the following sections.

PRODUCTION OF ENERGY IN THE BODY

After ingested foods are broken down by digestion, they are distributed to the cells of the body.

Carbohydrate Metabolism

The digestion of carbohydrates yields mostly glucose, with some fructose, and galactose. These small sugars are carried by the blood to all cells of the body to be used for energy. Immediately upon entering liver or muscle cells, the sugar molecules are captured through a process called *phosphorylation,* which means that a phosphate group is added to the sugar. This process is irreversible in muscle cells. Any sugar entering these cells is used immediately for energy or stored in the cell as glycogen. Muscles normally contain about 15 gm of glycogen/kilogram of wet muscle. This level can be raised dramatically by carbohydrate loading techniques to 35 or 40 gm/kilogram of wet tissue (see Chapter 15). Since the phosphorylated sugars cannot be released again into the blood stream, they will remain in the muscles until used.

Dephosphorylation of the glucose stored in the liver cells can be done by the enzyme glucose-6-phosphatase in the liver, so that it can be released again into the blood stream. This allows the body to maintain the blood sugar level at normal values between meals. Glucose, then, can be used immediately for energy, or it can be stored in the form of glycogen for future use.

GLYCOLYSIS. The most important pathway for metabolism of glucose is by glycolysis and the oxidation of the end products of glycolysis. The glycolytic energy scheme functions without oxygen and splits the glucose molecule to form two molecules of pyruvic acid. Energy is required in the initial stages of the pathway, but later, ATP is synthesized from the process for a net gain of two molecules of ATP for each molecule of glucose that starts through the cycle. Four hydrogen atoms also are released during the process. The fate of these atoms will be discussed later with other hydrogen atoms from the Krebs cycle.

During intense work, or when the body is unable to supply oxygen to the cell in sufficient quantity (such as in underwater swimming), the glycolytic pathway is able to supply energy for muscular contractions. However, this process is inefficient as compared to the oxidative pathways and yields a by-product called lactic acid, which is extremely detrimental to performance (Fig. 1–2).

It should be pointed out that lactic acid is pyruvic acid that has received two hydrogen atoms from the glycolytic pathway from the

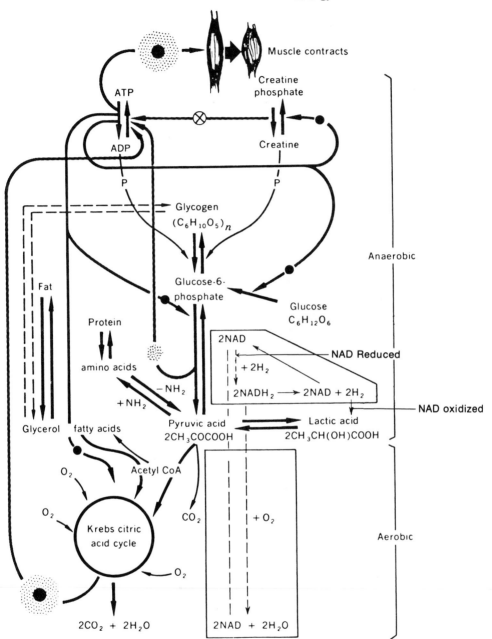

Figure 1–2.   Simplified schematic diagram showing energy liberation and transfer in the living cell. (From *Textbook of Work Physiology* by Astrand and Rodahl, page 14. Copyright © 1970 by McGraw-Hill, Inc. Used with permission of McGraw-Hill Book Company.)

hydrogen carrier nicotinamide adenine dinucleotide (NAD). In the presence of oxygen, NAD can carry hydrogen to the oxidative hydrogen-electron transport system where it is processed for energy. When insufficient oxygen is available, the NAD is forced to dump the hydrogen onto pyruvic acid, forming lactic acid. The lactic acid or lactate then diffuses into the blood stream and is carried away from the muscle cell, which allows the glycolytic process to continue. Of course, when high levels of blood lactate occur, the diffusion of lactate to the cell equals the diffusion away from the cell and no more hydrogen can be carried away. This results in a slowdown in the energy production of the glycolytic pathway, and work must slow down or stop. High levels of blood lactate are usually associated with high work intensity, where not enough oxygen is available to support the energy needs of the body. Of course, this process allows us to do high levels of work for a short period of time anaerobically. Without this capability, we would be limited to aerobic activities only.

KREBS CYCLE. If sufficient oxygen is available in the cell, lactic acid is not formed in large quantities, and decarboxylation (loss of a carbon as CO_2) of the pyruvate forms acetic acid. The two-carbon acetic acid is carried to the Krebs cycle by coenzyme A (CoA), which forms a compound with acetic acid called *acetyl CoA.* Upon arrival at the mitochondria, acetic acid is released, and coenzyme A returns for more. In the Krebs cycle, citric acid is joined to four-carbon oxaloacetic acid to form citric acid. This product is processed through a series of enzymes located on the cristae of the mitochondria. These enzymes are probably arranged in sequential order so the products of the reactions can be relayed from enzyme to enzyme as the chemical reactions occur which produce 2 more ATP molecules, 16 more hydrogen atoms, and some carbon dioxide. The 4 hydrogen atoms from glycolysis, the 4 from pyruvic acid breakdown, and the 16 from the Krebs cycle yield a total of 24 hydrogen atoms.

THE HYDROGEN-ELECTRON (H-E) TRANSPORT SYSTEM. After the hydrogen atoms have been released from the glycolytic pathway and the Krebs cycle, they must be oxidized to provide the rest of the energy gain from the breakdown. This is accomplished in the hydrogen-electron transport system, where a series of oxidative enzymes change hydrogen atoms to hydrogen ions, and dissolved oxygen to hydroxyl ions. These two products then combine to form the water of metabolism. The enzymes responsible for this process also are found in the mitochondria of the cell.

The role of oxygen cannot be overemphasized at this point. Oxygen must be present to receive the hydrogen ions produced by the cytochromes. Without O_2, this system will not function, and hydrogen atoms will be carried off and lactate will build up anaerobically.

It is in the hydrogen-electron transport system that the majority of the energy from the degradation of glucose is produced. Twenty of the 24 hydrogen atoms from glycolysis and the Krebs cycle yield energy at a ratio of 3 ATP molecules for each 2 hydrogen atoms entering the system. The other 4 hydrogen atoms enter the H-E transport system for a 1 ATP for 1 hydrogen exchange to yield 4 more ATP molecules. Thus, the total yield of this system is 34 ATP molecules. This, combined with the 2 molecules of ATP from the Krebs cycle and the 2 molecules of ATP from glycolysis, results in a net gain of 38 molecules of ATP for each molecule of glucose entering the system.

The net efficiency of the system is about 44%, since 1 mol of glucose contains 686 Kcal and yields 304 Kcal of energy stored as ATP (38 mol of ATP at 8 Kcal each). The energy not stored as ATP is released as heat.

Lipid Metabolism

Almost half of the calories ingested in the normal diet is from fat. In addition, some of the carbohydrate ingested is converted to triglycerides, and later used for energy. For this reason, the metabolism of fat is an important function in the body.

As mentioned previously, essentially all digested fats are converted into new molecules and are then transported up the thoracic duct and emptied into venous blood near the heart.

Most of the triglycerides in the chylomicrons are hydrolyzed into glycerol and fatty acids. The glycerol is metabolized in much the same way as is glucose. The fatty acids, combined with protein as lipoprotein, go to the various cells of the body where they can be oxidized for energy, or to the fat cells for storage. Some chylomicrons are absorbed directly into the liver where they are used for energy or are converted into other lipid substances.

The fatty acid molecule is usually a long chain containing 16 or more carbons. Two carbon segments are broken off the chain in a process called *beta oxidation* for degradation of fatty acids. The two carbon segments are carried to the Krebs cycle by acetyl CoA, just as acetic acid from glycolysis is carried, where they join with oxaloacetic acid and proceed through the oxidative enzymes of the Krebs cycle.

Four hydrogen atoms are released each time two carbon segments are broken off. If the fatty acid had 18 carbons (stearic acid), 32 hydrogen atoms would be released for each fatty acid molecule degraded. Eight more hydrogen atoms are released for each two-carbon segment, for an additional 72 hydrogen atoms. A total of 148 ATP molecules are formed from each 18-carbon fatty acid degraded. Two of these ATPs are needed for the reaction to occur, so the net gain is 146 ATPs.

It is interesting to note that the rate of free fatty acid turnover in the blood is extremely rapid. Half is replaced every 2 or 3 min. Normal fatty acid levels are about 150 mg/liter.

MEASUREMENT OF METABOLISM

Metabolism can be defined as the sum total of all the chemical reactions of the body. Metabolic rate is expressed in units of heat (calories). A calorie (cal) is the amount of heat needed to raise 1 gm of water 1° centigrade. The kilocalorie, or Calorie (with a capital "C"), is equal to 1000 cal, and is commonly used to express energy expenditure of the body.

Direct Calorimetry

Since the amount of heat released from the body is indicative of the metabolic rate, any means used to measure this output would be a good measurement of metabolism. To measure the amount of heat released from the body directly, a subject is placed in a large insulated chamber where the heat from the body warms the air of the chamber. The air in the chamber is kept at a constant temperature, however, and the warm air from the body is forced through pipes in a cool water bath. The rate of heat gain by the water bath is equal to the total heat output of the body.

This method has several disadvantages: (1) the equipment is expensive and difficult to use; (2) the equipment is inflexible and cannot be used except under ideal laboratory conditions; and (3) the test cannot be used as a maximal work test without much difficulty. For these reasons, other methods of calorimetry were developed.

Indirect Calorimetry

Since all of the metabolic processes of the body use oxygen and produce carbon dioxide, the energy production in the body is related directly to the quantity of these respiratory gases consumed and expelled. If these gases are collected and measured, an estimation of metabolic rate can be made. There are two basic ways in which these gases can be measured: closed-circuit calorimetry and open-circuit calorimetry.

CLOSED-CIRCUIT CALORIMETRY. The closed-circuit system is so named because the subject breathes directly into and out of a tank through a two-way valve with no access to outside air. The expired air passes through a container of soda lime, which absorbs all of the CO_2 produced. As the CO_2 is absorbed, the total volume of the tank decreases, and the amount of decrease is recorded on a revolving drum (Fig. 1–3). The problems with the closed-circuit system are that (1) the volume of the drum is usually too small to be used during any kind of exercise, (2) the resistance is too great, and (3) the accuracy is poor.

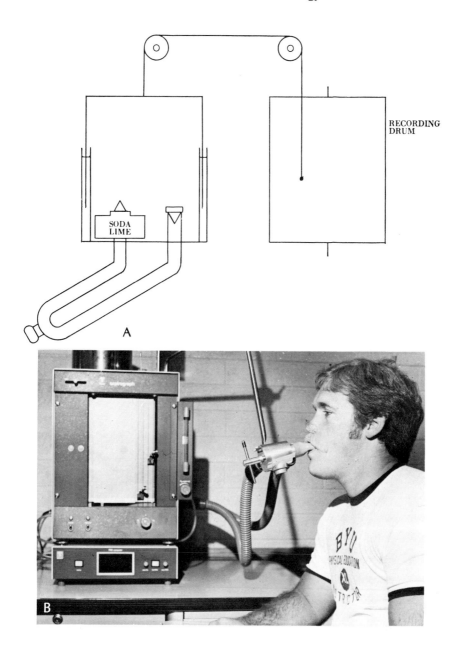

Figure 1–3.   A, Indirect closed-circuit calorimeter. B, Closed-circuit calorimeter in use.

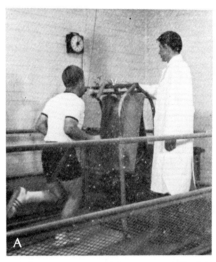

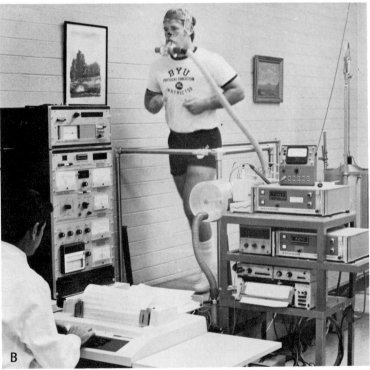

Figure 1–4.   A, Collection of expired air in Douglas bag. B, Open-circuit calorimeter with computer tie-in.

OPEN-CIRCUIT CALORIMETRY. Open-circuit calorimetry is the most commonly used method for determining metabolic cost during work. It is called open-circuit because the subject breathes room air and expires through a one-way, low-resistance type of valve into a volume-measuring device. Some laboratories collect expired air into Douglas bags or meteorological balloons, and measure the total volume later through a gasometer (Fig. 1–4A). Others use high-speed gasometers or pneumotachs for instantaneous volume determinations. Either system works well, but the instantaneous systems allow oxygen consumption calculations to be made during the test itself, and with computer tie-ins, allow complete metabolic evaluation during the test (Fig. 1–4B).

OXYGEN CONSUMPTION ($\dot{V}O_2$)

Oxygen is used by the cells of the body to produce energy for muscular contraction. In this section is a discussion of the theory behind oxygen consumption and the calculations needed to compute it.

Oxygen Consumption Theory

Oxygen consumption measurements are made to evaluate the energy used at any given work level. We must realize that oxygen consumption is equal to the amount of blood flowing past the tissues times the amount of oxygen removed from the blood or

$$\dot{V}O_2 = \dot{Q} \times \text{a-}\bar{v}\ O_2 \text{ diff.}$$

Q is a symbol used to describe the cardiac output, or total volume of blood pumped by the heart through the circulatory system. Since O_2 is carried by the blood, the more blood pumped, the more O_2 is available to the cells (see Chapter 4 for a more detailed discussion of cardiac output).

Arteriovenous difference (a-$\bar{v}$ O_2 diff.) refers to the amount of oxygen removed from the blood as it circulates through the body. The amount of oxygen removed is limited by the number of mitochondria and oxidative enzymes available to use the oxygen carried by the blood. The small "a" refers to arterial saturation and is usually about 20 ml of O_2/100 ml of blood or 200 ml of O_2/liter of blood. The small "v" with a line over it refers to the O_2 content of the mixed or average venous blood. This value is about 150 ml of O_2/liter of blood at rest, and decreases to 50 ml of O_2/liter of blood during work. The a-$\bar{v}$ O_2 diff. would then be 50 ml/liter at rest or 150 ml/liter during work.

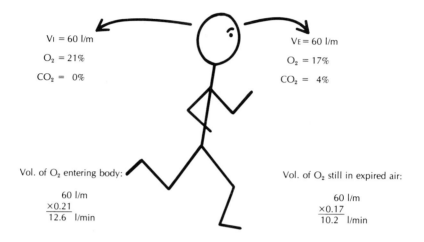

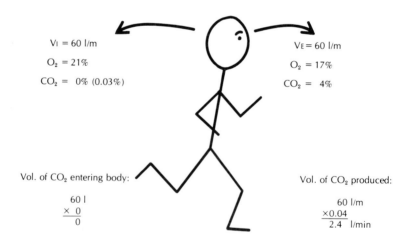

Figure 1–5. A, Calculation of oxygen consumption. B, Calculation of production of carbon dioxide.

Oxygen Consumption Calculations

In most open-circuit systems, only expired air is measured during the test. Since inspired and expired volumes are not usually the same, inspired volumes must be calculated before $\dot{V}O_2$ can be computed. Inspired volumes are calculated using the formula:

$$\dot{V}I = \frac{\dot{V}E \times N_2 \text{ in expired air}}{\% \ N_2 \text{ in inspired air}}$$

Percent nitrogen (N_2) in expired air is computed by subtracting the sum of the percent oxygen and percent carbon dioxide in the expired air from 100. The percent N_2 in the inspired air is always 0.7903.

To compute oxygen consumption, multiply the inspired volume (VI) by 21% (more exactly, 20.94%). This is the volume of oxygen that entered the body. Then, multiply the expired volume (VE) by the percent O_2 in the expired air and subtract this from the volume of inspired oxygen. For example, if VI = 60 l/minute, VE = 60 l/minute, and the percent O_2 in the expired air is 17, to compute oxygen consumption, first multiply 60 l by 0.21 (21%), which equals 12.6 l of oxygen going in. Next, multiply expired volume by 0.17 (17%), which equals 10.2 l of oxygen remaining in the expired air (Fig. 1–5A):

$$12.6 \ l - 10.2 \ l = 2.4 \ l/\text{minute } O_2 \text{ uptake}$$

Remember, the volume of expired air does not always equal the volume of inspired air. If the percent nitrogen is different, you must solve the equation for VI.

The volume of carbon dioxide can also be computed using the same technique. For example, if VI and VE are both 60 l/minute and the percent CO_2 in the expired air is 4.0, to determine the volume of CO_2 produced, multiply 60 l/minute by 0.04 (4%), which is 2.4 l in the expired air. Therefore, the volume of CO_2 produced (VCO_2) is 2.4 l/minute (Fig. 1–5B). (Since the percent CO_2 in the inspired air is only 0.03% [0.0003], we can ignore the inspired volume for this calculation, even though this small volume is computed in the laboratory.)

The Respiratory Quotient

The respiratory quotient (R) is defined as the volume of CO_2 produced divided by the volume of O_2 used (R = VCO_2/VO_2). This calculation is important in the determination of total caloric cost of work, since the number of calories is related to the amount of fat versus the amount of carbohydrate used by the body. (Although the R of protein is 0.8, it is well established that protein is not used as a fuel during muscular work in any appreciable extent when there is energy available from fats or carbohydrates.) The R for carbohydrates is 1.0, and for fats, 0.7. An R of 0.85 would indicate that both fats and carbohydrates are being used in equal portion, and that 4.862 cal are being used for each liter of oxygen consumed (Table 1–1). In the previous problem, the R is 1.0 (2.4 l/minute of $CO_2 \div$ 2.4 l/minute of O_2) and 5.05 cal are released for each liter of oxygen used.

Rs greater than 1.0 are often computed during maximal work. This indicates that the subject is working near or at maximal capacity and is hyperventilating. The hyperventilation causes an excess blow-off of

TABLE 1–1
Caloric Values for Nonprotein *R*

R.Q.	Calories/Liter O_2
0.707	4.686
0.71	4.690
0.72	4.702
0.73	4.714
0.74	4.727
0.75	4.739
0.76	4.751
0.77	4.764
0.78	4.776
0.79	4.788
0.80	4.801
0.81	4.813
0.82	4.825
0.83	4.838
0.84	4.850
0.85	4.862
0.86	4.875
0.87	4.887
0.88	4.899
0.89	4.911
0.90	4.924
0.91	4.936
0.92	4.948
0.93	4.961
0.94	4.973
0.95	4.985
0.96	4.998
0.97	5.010
0.98	5.022
0.99	5.035
1.00	5.047

Lusk, G.: *Science of Nutrition*, 4th ed. Philadelphia: W. B. Saunders Co., 1928, page 65.

CO_2 which yields a spurious R. This is one good indication that maximal oxygen uptake has been reached during a maximal or all-out test.

Maximal Oxygen Consumption

The term maximal oxygen consumption is often abbreviated $\dot{V}O_2$ max or max $\dot{V}O_2$, and refers to the maximal oxidative capacity during an all-out test of cardiovascular fitness. These tests normally begin at a low level of work on a treadmill, bicycle ergometer, or some other work task, and increase in regular increments until the subject can do no more work. Two criteria indicate that the subject has reached his maximal oxygen consumption: (1) oxygen consumption does not increase even though the work load increases, indicating the energy needed for the increased work load came from anaerobic sources, and (2) the R is above 1.0 at the end of the task, indicating that hyperventilation has occurred. Another good indication is a high level of blood lactate. However, this is not measured routinely in the average stress physiology laboratory.

There is much discussion as to the real meaning or values of the maximal oxygen uptake. Highly trained endurance athletes often have levels between 70 and 87 ml/kilogram/minute. (Note that the $\dot{V}O_2$ measured in liters/minute is converted to milliliters and divided by body weight in kilograms to standardize the value for body size.) Many untrained adults have values of only 20 to 30 ml/kilogram/minute, and there are all levels in between. Can one say that a person with 40 ml/kilogram/minute is more highly trained than one with 35 ml/kilogram/minute? Does a higher $\dot{V}O_2$ max mean that that person can run faster or longer than another? These questions and others of the same type must be answered with great care. True, the maximal oxygen consumption does indicate the maximal energy output by the aerobic processes and is indicative of the functional capacity of the circulatory system. However, there is much evidence to indicate that heredity and natural endowment play a large role in determining a person's maximal aerobic capacity, or $\dot{V}O_2$ max. Therefore, a person who has never trained at all may have a larger $\dot{V}O_2$ max than another who has trained daily for years. There is also a difference among persons in the percent of maximal capacity which can be used at a given distance, as well as in the basic efficiency of running. Therefore, it is difficult to determine who will perform best during any kind of race even if one person has a higher $\dot{V}O_2$ max than the other.

Another problem is related to the specificity of training. Someone who has trained aerobically in a swimming pool may not measure high in a test given on a treadmill and vice versa. It is interesting to note that Frank Shorter, one of America's best marathon runners, has a fairly low maximal oxygen consumption (around 70 ml/kilogram/minute) but routinely beats runners whose maximum may be in the 80s.

How can maximal oxygen consumption be used? In spite of the problem, it is still the best measure of functional oxidative capacity, and as such, indicates *potential* for events demanding great endurance. Figure 1–6 clearly shows that individuals participating in events related to endurance have higher max $\dot{V}O_2$ than those participating in

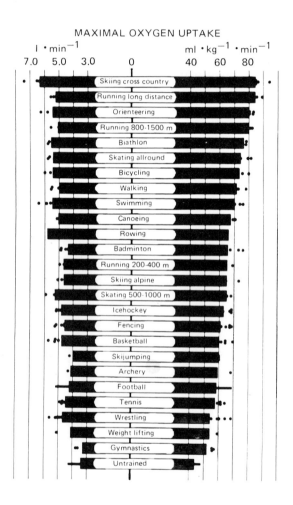

Figure 1–6.   Comparison of maximal oxygen uptake among various athletic events. (From *Textbook of Work Physiology* by Astrand and Rodahl, page 408. Copyright © 1977 by McGraw-Hill, Inc. Used with permission of McGraw-Hill Book Company.)

less demanding events. Max $\dot{V}O_2$ data also are used routinely in the evaluation of training programs used to develop endurance.

It should be pointed out that there is no significant difference between boys and girls in max $\dot{V}O_2$ before puberty, but after that, a woman's power is only about 70% to 75% that of men. Also, the maximal aerobic power decreases steadily with age, after about 25 yr. Of course, this decline can be slowed by consistent training. Many 65-year-olds have max $\dot{V}O_2$s as high or higher than those of many 25-year-olds.

METs

A MET is an expression of energy cost often used in cardiac rehabilitation programs and by members of the medical profession.

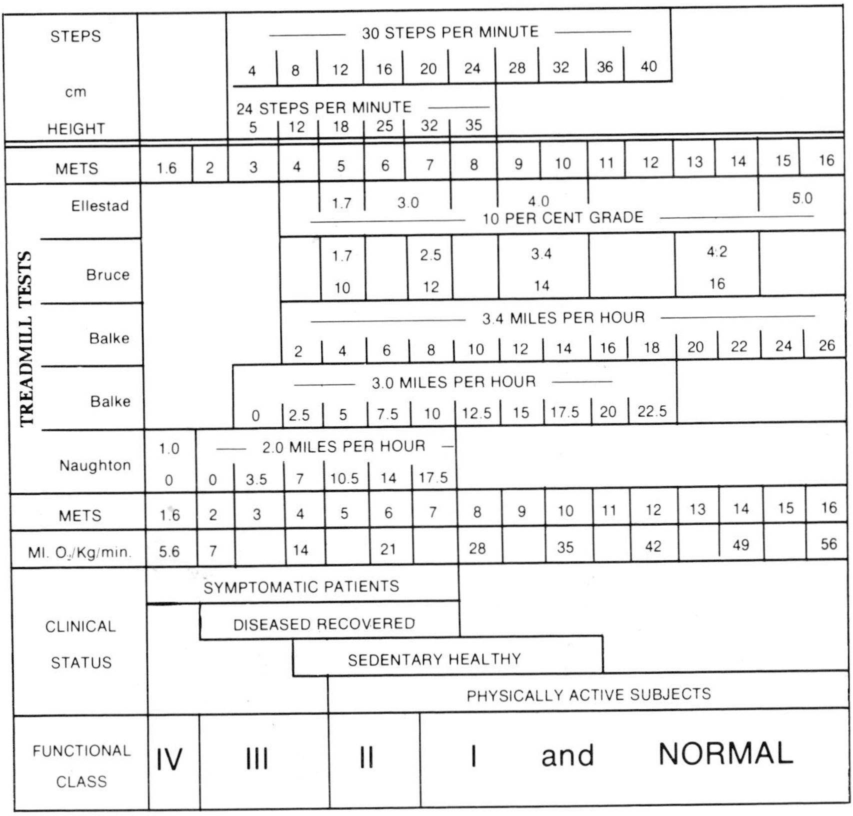

STEPS			30 STEPS PER MINUTE											
			4	8	12	16	20	24	28	32	36	40		
cm		24 STEPS PER MINUTE												
HEIGHT		5	12	18	25	32	35							

TREADMILL TESTS

METS	1.6	2	3	4	5	6	7	8	9	10	11	12	13	14	15	16
Ellestad			1.7		3.0				4.0						5.0	
									10 PER CENT GRADE							
Bruce			1.7		2.5		3.4					4.2				
			10		12		14					16				
Balke				3.4 MILES PER HOUR												
			2	4	6	8	10	12	14	16	18	20	22	24	26	
Balke			3.0 MILES PER HOUR													
		0	2.5	5	7.5	10	12.5	15	17.5	20	22.5					
Naughton	1.0		2.0 MILES PER HOUR													
	0	0	3.5	7	10.5	14	17.5									
METS	1.6	2	3	4	5	6	7	8	9	10	11	12	13	14	15	16
Ml. O_2/Kg/min.	5.6	7	14		21		28		35		42		49		56	

CLINICAL STATUS	
SYMPTOMATIC PATIENTS	
DISEASED RECOVERED	
SEDENTARY HEALTHY	
PHYSICALLY ACTIVE SUBJECTS	

FUNCTIONAL CLASS				
IV	III	II	I and	NORMAL

Figure 1–7. MET levels at various grades and speeds. (Fox, S.M., Naughton, J.P., and Haskell, W.L.: Physical Activity in the Prevention of Coronary Heart Disease. *Ann. Clin. Res.*, 3:424, 1971.)

One MET is equal to 3.5 ml/kilogram/minute of oxygen cost. Three METS would equal three times the resting cost or 10.5 ml/kilogram/minute. Several investigators have correlated the energy required to walk at various speeds and grades on a treadmill with oxygen cost or MET level (Fig. 1–7). Note that when walking on a horizontal surface, the MET level is equal to the speed in miles per hour (mph). At 3 mph, grade increases of 2.5% equal 1 MET increase in work, and at 3.4 mph, grade increases of 2% equal 1 MET increase in work.[1]

These relationships are helpful in evaluating work capacity when open-circuit calorimetry is not available or is not used during the evaluation. A subject can be stressed with increasing work loads to fatigue or some symptom-limited end point, and the final grade and speed can be used to predict maximal MET level or work capacity.

Approximate caloric cost can be computed from MET information by multiplying by weight (in kilograms) to get total oxygen cost and then multiplying by 5 (5 Kcal/liter) to get caloric cost.

PREDICTION OF ENERGY COSTS

There are several ways to predict the cost of various activities. Charts have been developed to predict the energy cost of recreational activities (Table 1–2), as well as of typical household and job-related activities (Table 1–3). These values are relatively accurate and can be used for normal caloric computations for weight control and other rough energy estimates. However, these values will vary because of body size and efficiency differences.

Equations have been developed for the more accurate prediction of energy cost in certain specific activities such as running, walking, and bicycling. These equations are more accurate than the chart values, and should be used if more accurate values are desired. The following equations were developed by a committee of the American College of Sports Medicine for use in exercise testing and prescription.[1] (Note: multiply miles/hour by the factor 26.82 to get meters/minute in the equations for walking and running.)

Walking

HORIZONTAL WALKING. Horizontal walking at speeds between 50 and 100 m/minute (1.9 and 3.7 mph or 3.0 and 6.0 km/hour).

$$\dot{V}O_2 \text{ (ml/kg-min)} = \text{speed (m/min)} \times 0.1 \text{ ml } O_2/\text{kg-min per m/min} + 1 \text{ MET (3.5 ml/kg-min)}$$

TABLE 1–2
Calories Expended in Various Sports Activities*

Activity	Cal/Min
Ping Pong—Table Tennis	4.9–7.0
Calisthenics	5.0
Rowing: Pleasure—Vigorous	5 –15
Cycling: 5–15 MPH (10 speed)	5 –12
Skating: Recreation—Vigorous	5 –15
Archery	5.2
Badminton: Recreational—Competitive	5.2–10
Basketball: Half—Full Court (more for fast break)	6 –9
Bowling (while active)	7.0
Tennis: Recreational—Competitive	7 –11
Water Skiing	8.0
Soccer	9.0
Snowshoeing (2.5 MPH)	9.0
Handball and Squash	10.0
Mountain Climbing	10.0
Judo and Karate	13.0
Football (while active)	13.3
Wrestling	14.4
Skiing: Moderate to Steep	8 –12
Downhill Racing	16.5
Cross-Country: 3–8 MPH	9 –17
Swimming: Pleasure	6.0
Crawl: 25–50 yds/min	6 –12.5
Butterfly: 50 yds/min	14.0
Backstroke: 25–50 yds/min	6 –12.5
Breaststroke: 25–50 yds/min	6 –12.5
Sidestroke: 40 yds/min	11.0
Dancing: Modern: Moderate—Vigorous	4.2– 5.7
Ballroom: Waltz—Rumba	5.7– 7.0
Square	7.7
Walking: Road—Field (3.5 MPH)	5.6
Snow: Hard—Soft (3.5–2.5 MPH)	10 –20
Uphill: 5–10—15% (3.5 MPH)	8–11 –15
Downhill: 5–10% (2.5 MPH)	3.6– 3.5
15–20% (2.5 MPH)	3.7– 4.3
Hiking: 40 lb. pack (3.0 MPH)	6.8
Running: 12 min mile (5 MPH)	10.0
8 min mile (7.5 MPH)	15.0
6 min mile (10 MPH)	20.0
5 min mile (12 MPH)	25.0

*Depends on efficiency and body size. Add 10% for each 15 lb above 150, subtract 10% for each 15 lb under 150, use activity pulse rate to confirm the caloric expenditures.

Sharkey, B. J.: *Physiological Fitness and Weight Control.* Missoula: Mountain Press Publishing Co., Inc., 1978, page 128.

TABLE 1–3
Calories Expended in Various Physical Activities*

Activity	Cal/Min
Standing, light activity	2.6
Washing and dressing	2.6
Washing and shaving	2.6
Driving a car	2.8
Washing clothes	3.1
Walking indoors	3.1
Shining shoes	3.2
Making bed	3.4
Dressing	3.4
Showering	3.4
Driving motorcycle	3.4
Metal working	3.5
House painting	3.5
Cleaning windows	3.7
Carpentry	3.8
Farming chores	3.8
Sweeping floors	3.9
Plastering walls	4.1
Truck and automobile repair	4.2
Ironing clothes	4.2
Farming, planting, hoeing, raking	4.7
Mixing cement	4.7
Mopping floors	4.9
Repaving roads	5.0
Gardening, weeding	5.6
Stacking lumber	5.8
Stone, masonry	6.3
Pick-and-shovel work	6.7
Farming, haying, plowing with horse	6.7
Shoveling (miners)	6.8
Walking downstairs	7.1
Chopping wood	7.5
Gardening, digging	8.6
Walking upstairs	10–18
Pool or Billiards	1.8
Canoeing: 2.5 MPH—4.0 MPH	3.0–7.0
Volleyball: Recreational—Comp	3.5–8.0
Golf: Foursome—Twosome	3.7–5.0
Horseshoes	3.8
Baseball (except pitcher)	4.7

*Depends on efficiency and body size. Add 10% for each 15 lb above 150, subtract 10% for each 15 lb under 150, use activity pulse rate to confirm the caloric expenditures.

Sharkey, B. J.: *Physiological Fitness and Weight Control.* Missoula: Mountain Press Publishing Co., Inc., 1978, page 129.

Example. Compute the values for $\dot{V}O_2$ and MET corresponding to a horizontal walking speed of 80 m/minute (3 mph or 4.8 km/hour).

$$\dot{V}O_2 = 80 \text{ m/min} + 0.1 \text{ ml/kg-min per m/min} + 3.5 \text{ ml/kg-min}$$
$$= 11.5 \text{ ml/kg-min}$$

$$\text{METS} = 11.5 \text{ ml/kg-min} \div 3.5 \text{ ml/kg-min} = 3.3$$

GRADE WALKING. Grade walking at speeds between 50 and 100 m/minute. This calculation is divided into two parts:
1. The horizontal speed component is calculated as described previously.
2. The vertical work component makes use of the relationship that 1 kilogram-meter (kg-m) of work requires 1.8 ml of oxygen. The additional vertical work equals percent grade (inches climbed per 100 inches traveled = percent grade) times walking speed, i.e., the actual vertical lift along the slope in meters/minute times body weight in kilograms.

$$\dot{V}O_2 \text{ (ml/kg-min)} = \text{percent grade (expressed as decimal fraction)} \times$$
$$\text{speed (m/min)} \times 1.8 \text{ ml/kg-m}$$

Example. Compute the $\dot{V}O_2$ and MET level for an individual walking at 90 m/minute (3.35 mph) up an incline of 13%.
First, compute the horizontal speed component:

$$\dot{V}O_2 = 90 \text{ m/min} \times 0.1 \text{ ml/kg-min per m/min} + 3.5 \text{ ml/kg-min}$$
$$= 12.5 \text{ ml/kg-min}$$

Then compute the vertical work component:

$$\dot{V}O_2 = 0.13 \times 90 \text{ m/min} \times 1.8 \text{ ml/kg-m} = 21.1$$

Combining horizontal and vertical work:

$$\dot{V}O_2 = 12.5 \text{ ml/kg-min} + 21.1 \text{ ml/kg-min} = 33.6 \text{ ml/kg-min}^*$$

$$\text{METS} = 33.6 \text{ ml/kg-min} \div 3.5 \text{ ml/kg-min} = 9.6$$

Running

HORIZONTAL RUNNING. Horizontal running for speeds exceeding 140 m/minute (5.2 mph or 8.4 km/hour).

*The total oxygen cost for grade walking is estimated by multiplying the $\dot{V}O_2$ ml/kg-min by kilograms of body weight.

$$\dot{V}_{O_2} \text{ (ml/kg-min)} = \text{speed (m/min)} \times 0.2 \text{ ml/kg-min per m/min} + 1 \text{ MET (3.5 ml/kg-min)}$$

Example. What $\dot{V}_{O_2}$ and MET value are required to run on the level at 200 m/minute (7.5 mph)?

$$\dot{V}_{O_2} = 200 \text{ m/min} \times 0.2 \text{ ml/kg-min per m/min} + 3.5 \text{ ml/kg-min}$$
$$= 43.5 \text{ ml/kg-min}$$

$$\text{METS} = 43.5 \text{ ml/kg-min} \div 3.5 \text{ ml/kg-min}$$

or

$$(43.5 \div 3.5) \text{ ml/kg-min} = 12.4$$

Note: For speeds in the units of ki' ɔmeters/hour (mph $\times$ 1.6 = km/hr), the MET requirement is approximate. ɔqual to the speed: 10 km/hr = 10 METS; 12 km/hr = 12 METS.

$$6 \text{ mph} = 1.6 \times 6 = 9.6 \text{ METS}$$

INCLINED RUNNING. Inclined running at speeds exceeding 140 m/minute. As in the energy expenditure calculation for percent grade, the calculation for running up a grade is divided into two components:
  1. Horizontal component—as discussed previously.
  2. Vertical work component is calculated by multiplying the percent grade (as a decimal fraction) times the speed (m/min) times 1.8 ml/kg-m.

$$\dot{V}_{O_2} = \text{speed (m/min)} \times \text{grade (expressed as a fraction)} \times 1.8 \text{ ml/kg-m}$$

Example. What are the $\dot{V}_{O_2}$ and MET level for running at 180 m/minute up a 5% grade?
  1. Horizontal speed component:

$$\dot{V}_{O_2} \text{ (ml/kg-min)} = 180 \text{ m/min} \times 0.2 \text{ ml/kg-min per m/min} + 1 \text{ MET (3.5 ml/kg-min)} = 39.5$$

  2. Vertical work component:

$$\dot{V}_{O_2} \text{ (ml/kg-min)} = 180 \text{ m/min} \times 0.05 \times 1.8 \text{ ml/kg-m} = 16.2$$

  3. Combining horizontal and vertical work:

$$\dot{V}_{O_2} = 39.5 \text{ ml/kg-min} + 16.2 \text{ ml/kg-min} = 55.7 \text{ ml/kg-min } \dot{V}_{O_2}$$

$$\text{METS} = 55.7 \text{ ml/kg-min} \div 3.5 \text{ ml/kg-min per MET} = 15.9$$

The total oxygen costs of grade running can be obtained by multiplying the $\dot{V}O_2$ in ml/kg-min by kilograms of body weight.

Cycling

BICYCLE ERGOMETER EXERCISE. The work associated with all modes of cycling, including bicycle ergometer exercise, is different from that induced by walking, running, or stepping, in that the body weight is supported by a seat. The work output for bicycle ergometer exercise is found by multiplying the force (kilograms of resistance) times the distance through which the force acts, i.e., the number of pedal revolutions times the distance traveled per pedal revolution. The oxygen uptake at any work rate is constant and independent of body weight. Consequently, a person weighing 60 kg will be at a higher work level than a 90-kg person when working at the same work rate.

The total work associated with bicycle ergometer exercise includes the load set on the ergometer, internal or friction work, and noncycling muscle involvement which counteracts the leg push. Consequently, there is an additional linear increase in energy demands with increasing work intensity. This additional work requires approximately 0.2 ml of O_2/kg-m and is added to the 1.8 ml of O_2/kg-m. Thus, in place of the constant 1.8 ml of O_2/kg-m used in prior examples, a new value of 2.0 ml of O_2/kg-m is used for cycling. Thus, the formula for estimating the O_2 demands for cycle ergometer work is:

$$\dot{V}O_2 \text{ (ml/min)} = \text{work rate (kg-m/min)} \times 2 \text{ ml } O_2\text{/kg-m} + \text{sitting } \dot{V}O_2 \text{ (300 ml/min)}$$

Example. What are the $\dot{V}O_2$ and MET level required to cycle at a work rate of 900 kg-m/minute for a 60-kg and a 90-kg person?

$$\dot{V}O_2 = 900 \text{ kg-m/min} \times 2.0 \text{ ml } O_2\text{/kg-m} + 300 \text{ ml/min} = 2100 \text{ ml/min}$$

For a 60-kg subject:

$$\begin{aligned} \text{METS} &= 2100 \text{ ml/min} \div 60 \text{ kg} \\ &= 35 \text{ ml/kg-min} \div 3.5 \text{ ml/kg-min per MET} \\ &= 10 \end{aligned}$$

For a 90-kg subject:

$$\begin{aligned} \text{METS} &= 2100 \text{ ml/min} \div 90 \text{ kg} \\ &= 23.3 \text{ ml/kg-min} \div 3.5 \text{ ml/kg-min per MET} \\ &= 6.7 \end{aligned}$$

This method provides reasonable estimates of the MET value up to approximately 1200 kg-m/minute.

OUTDOOR CYCLING. The energy requirement for bicycle riding varies with the type of bicycle (gears, tire size, and the like), and the cycling skill and the body weight of the individual. Rolling resistance and air resistance are a function of body size. However, the primary determinant is the speed of cycling. The energy requirement for horizontal bicycle riding can be estimated from the following regression equation.[1,5]

$$\dot{V}O_2 \text{ (ml/kg-min)} = 0.1 \text{ (m/min)} - 12$$

This relationship is useful for speeds from 15 km/hour (9.3 mph) to 32 km/hour (19.9 mph).

Example. What are the $\dot{V}O_2$ and MET value for a cycling speed of 250 m/minute (15 km/hour)?

$$\dot{V}O_2 \text{ (ml/kg-min)} = (250 \text{ m/min} \times 0.1) - 12 = 13$$

$$\text{METS} = 13 \text{ ml/kg-min} \div 3.5 \text{ ml/kg-min} = 3.7$$

Energy cost for highly trained athletes is slightly less than that for the average person. For this reason, the equation

$$\dot{V}O_2 \text{ (ml/kg-min)} = \text{speed (m/min)} \times 0.18 + 3.5$$

is more representative of actual cost of a distance runner. Using this information, you can predict the max $\dot{V}O_2$ required to run a marathon or some other race. For instance, the marathon is run at about 12 mph (26 miles in a little over 2 hours). The cost of running this rate is about 61.4 ml/kilogram/minute (321.84 m/min × 0.18 + 3.5). If an athlete can work at 80% of his maximum, his maximum needs to be about 76.7 ml/kilogram/minute (61.4/80% = x/100%). Using this kind of calculation you can predict the maximal capacity needed for any level of activity.

ANAEROBIC THRESHOLD

The anaerobic threshold is that point in exercise when the exercise is almost entirely aerobic (little lactate production), but if increased at all, would begin to cause the production of significant amounts of lactate. Exercise at this point and below may be classified as *steady-state exercise.* Athletes running long distances or subjects who work for long periods of time must work at or below the anaerobic threshold.

The anaerobic threshold is different for every person. Highly trained endurance athletes have higher anaerobic thresholds than do untrained or moderately trained subjects. Normally, highly trained athletes can work at 75% to 85% of their maximal $\dot{V}O_2$. Some highly trained endurance athletes can work at much higher levels than others. As mentioned previously, Frank Shorter has a fairly low maximal oxygen uptake for a world-class endurance athlete, but continually outruns opponents with higher values because of his ability to work at a high anaerobic threshold.

OXYGEN DEFICIT AND DEBT

During light work (below the anaerobic threshold), energy is produced almost entirely by oxidative, or aerobic, processes. During more severe work, anaerobic processes are required and play an increasingly prominent role as the severity of the work increases. The energy used beyond that supplied is called the O_2 *deficit*. Of course, blood lactate levels increase as the anaerobic processes become more prominent, and lactate levels in the blood can be measured following intense work as an index of the severity of the work (Fig. 1–8). Note that the highest

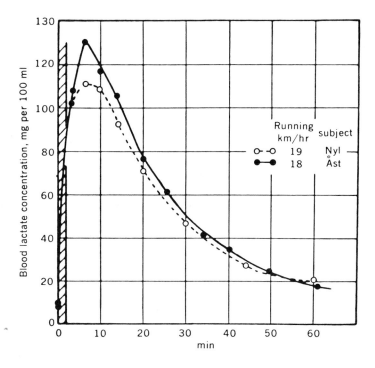

Figure 1–8. Blood lactate concentration after severe work of 2-min duration (shaded column) in two subjects. Peak values occur several minutes following the cessation of work. (From *Textbook of Work Physiology* by Astrand and Rodahl, page 308. Copyright © 1977 by McGraw-Hill, Inc. Used with permission of McGraw-Hill Book Company.)

levels are measured during the first 10 min of recovery and that it takes about an hour for the levels to return to normal.

It should be pointed out that the lag in peak lactate levels following exercise is because of the lag in diffusion of lactate from the muscles to the blood. Lactate levels measured directly in the muscle would be much higher than those measured in the blood.[2]

Most of the lactate produced by the muscles is either converted to blood glucose (10%) or oxidized directly for energy (75%).[5,6] Apparently, lactate removal is enhanced by light exercise rather than by complete rest following the work bout.

Oxygen debt is the oxygen consumption in excess of resting oxygen following a work bout and in highly trained athletes, the total value of this debt may reach 20 l or so during maximal exercise.

Several factors are involved in this "debt." First, the O_2 stores of the body must be refilled (blood and myoglobin). This accounts for about 1 l of oxygen. Elevated body temperature and epinephrine (Adrenalin) may account for another liter of debt. The increased cost of cardiac and respiratory function may consume an additional 0.5 l or so, and the refilling of the ATP-CP stores may require about 1.5 l. These factors may all be considered part of the alactacid portion of the debt, which probably totals about 4 l at maximum. It costs about another 16 l to convert the lactic acid portion of the debt back to energy. Since the total deficit is only about 8 l, the "interest" paid by the body is pretty high. Of course, we are happy to pay the interest when we need the energy for some high-intensity work, since oxygen can be supplied easily following the work.

FUEL FOR THE PRODUCTION OF ENERGY

In the past, it often has been assumed that the primary source of energy during exercise was carbohydrate and that fat was used only during rest and recovery. This idea came from the classic experiments which showed a large decrease in work capacity of subjects who worked after having consumed a high-fat diet. Using a standard work load which was essentially aerobic, subjects could work three times as long on a high-carbohydrate diet as they could on fat. It seems significant, however, that this load could be maintained for over an hour, with most of the energy coming from fat sources.[8]

The same subjects on normal balanced diets obtained 50% to 60% of their energy from fat. If the work was prolonged, the amount of energy supplied by fat increased significantly (up to 70%).

It seems clear that both fats and carbohydrates are essential, and that the proportion of each used during work depends upon the type of food eaten and the intensity and duration of the work. The higher the work level, the more dependent the body becomes on carbohydrate as an energy source. As work time increases, the more dependent the body is on fat.

Both carbohydrates and fats are stored by the body for use during activity. Fat is by far the most efficient fuel to store, having a high energy-to-weight value (9.1 Kcal/gram) and a storage form highly compatible with its storage function, that is, being easily mobilized and stored as a liquid droplet. The total amount of energy stored is also significantly greater in fats than in carbohydrates. For example, a 180-lb person who is only 15% fat has 27 lb of fat stores. Since each pound of fat contains 3500 Kcal, the total energy stored is nearly 95,000 Kcal.

Carbohydrates are stored primarily in the muscles or in the liver as glycogen. Muscle glycogen levels are normally about 15 gm/kilogram of wet muscle. Since muscle constitutes about 40% of the body weight, a 70-kg person would store about 420 gm of glycogen (28 kg of muscle at 15 gm/kilogram); therefore, 420 gm of glycogen yields about 1700 Kcal of energy stored in the muscle tissue. An additional 80 to 90 gm of glycogen is stored in the liver, and about 5 to 6 gm can be found in the blood. It is important to realize that the muscle glycogen cannot be released into the blood stream as can liver glycogen, since muscle does not contain the enzyme glucose-6-phosphatase. Therefore, the liver

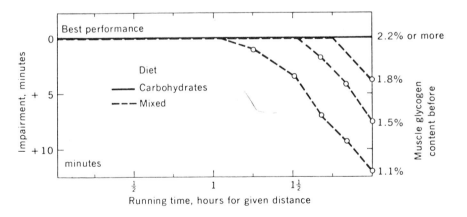

Figure 1–9. Schematic illustration of the importance of a high-glycogen content in the muscle before a 30-km race (running). The lower the initial glycogen store, the slower became the speed at the end of the race compared with the race performed when the muscle glycogen content was 2.2 g or more per 100 g muscle at the start of the race. For the first hour, however, no difference in speed was observed. (From *Textbook of Work Physiology* by Astrand and Rodahl, page 466. Copyright © 1970 by McGraw-Hill Inc. Used with permission of McGraw-Hill Book Company.)

stores are responsible for maintaining normal blood sugar levels, and may be depleted during exercise.

Glycogen is important to the performance of high level work, and its disappearance is usually associated with fatigue. In a study of long-distance running, it was discovered that subjects who were supersaturated with glycogen could maintain a race pace for a longer period of time than they could when they had consumed a normal diet before the race. Initial speed was not affected, but the time that speed could be maintained was greatly increased[2] (Fig. 1–9). The one drawback to glycogen supersaturation is the amount of water stored in the body with each gram of glycogen (2.7 gm of water/gram of glycogen).

A comparison of trained and untrained runners revealed that fat metabolism plays a greater role at a pace equal to 77% max $\dot{V}O_2$ in the trained than in the untrained, even though the actual glycogen used by each group was similar. The extra work capacity of the trained men was supported by an increased fat metabolism.[4]

It should be emphasized that the body also depends upon blood sugar levels for energy during work, and that the blood sugar is maintained under these circumstances by glycogenolysis (breakdown and release of liver glycogen), as well as by glyconeogenesis (the building of glucose by the liver from alanine, lactate, pyruvate, and glycerol).[4]

The fuel for energy during work, then, comes from a triphasic source in which muscle glycogen, blood glucose, and free fatty acids are used for the production of energy. In long moderate exercise, the fatty acids are used preferentially. In exhaustive work, the body apparently is much more dependent upon carbohydrate, and exhaustion coincides with depletion of the muscle glycogen stores.

SELECTED REFERENCES

1. American College of Sports Medicine: *Guide Lines for Graded Exercise Testing and Prescription.* Philadelphia: Lea & Febiger, 1975.
2. Astrand, P.-O., and Rodahl, K.: *Textbook of Work Physiology.* New York: McGraw-Hill Book Co., 1970.
3. Asimov, I.: *Life and Energy.* Garden City, N.Y.: Doubleday and Co., 1962.
4. Bleich, H. L., and Boro, E. S.: Fuel homeostasis in exercise. *N. Engl. J. Med.,* 293:1078–1084, 1975.
5. Brooke, G. A., Brauner, K. E., and Cassens, R. G.: Glycogen synthesis and metabolism of lactic acid after exercise. *Am. J. Physiol.,* 224:1162–1166, 1973.
6. Depocas, F., Minaire, Y., and Charonnet, J.: Rates of formation and oxidation of lactic acid in dogs at rest and during moderate exercise. *Can. J. Physiol. Pharmacol.,* 47:603–610, 1969.
7. DeVries, H. A.: *Physiology of Exercise for Physical Education and Athletics,* 2nd ed. Dubuque: Wm. C. Brown Co., 1974.
8. Christensen, E. H., and Hansen, O.: Arbeitsfähigheit und Ehrnährung. *Scand Arch. Physiol.,* 81:160, 1939.

 9. Falls, H. B. (Ed.): *Exercise Physiology.* New York: Academic Press, 1968.
10. Guyton, A. C.: *Textbook of Medical Physiology,* 4th ed. Philadelphia: W. B. Saunders Co., 1971.
11. Johnson, W. R. (Ed.): *Science and Medicine of Exercise and Sports.* New York: Harper & Row, 1960.
12. Jokl, E. (Gen. Ed.): Medicine and Sport. In *Biochemistry of Exercise.* J. R. Poortmans (Ed.) Vol. 1. Baltimore: University Park Press, 1968.
13. Karpovich, P. V., and Sinning. W. E.: *Physiology of Muscular Activity,* 7th ed. Philadelphia: W. B. Saunders Co., 1971.
14. Ricci, B.: *Physiological Basis of Human Performance.* Philadelphia: Lea & Febiger, 1967.
15. Ruch, R. C., and Patton, H. D.: *Physiology and Biophysics,* 19th ed. Philadelphia: W. B. Saunders Co., 1965.
16. White, A., Handler, P., and Smith, E. L.: *Principles of Biochemistry,* 4th ed. New York: McGraw-Hill Book Co., 1968.

Chapter 2
The Musculoskeletal System

Basic to the study of athletic conditioning and performance is an understanding of the musculoskeletal system, for this system is significantly involved in all motor movements. This chapter is a review of musculoskeletal structure and function. After reading it, the concepts of training presented in later chapters can be understood better and applied more effectively.

KINDS OF MUSCLES

There are two basic types of muscle in the human body from the structural point of view, *smooth* and *striated*. Striated muscle is further classified into *skeletal* and *cardiac* muscle. Thus, it can be said that three kinds of muscle exist: *smooth, cardiac,* and *skeletal.* All three kinds possess the basic characteristics of muscle tissue: *extensibility,* the ability to stretch; *elasticity,* the ability to return to normal length when the stretching force is removed; *excitability,* the ability to be excited by or respond to stimuli; and *contractility,* the ability to apply tension. The different kinds of muscle have some characteristics in common, but they also differ in several ways. For instance, the contractile process is essentially the same in each kind of muscle, but the speed of contraction, duration of contraction, and purposes served differ greatly. Each kind of muscle tissue as well as each individual muscle is especially suited in both structure and function to its particular task.

Smooth Muscle

Smooth muscle is located in the walls of the internal organs (viscera) other than the heart, such as the blood vessels, intestines, alimentary tract, and stomach. Like cardiac muscle, it contracts involuntarily. It is under the control of the involuntary portion of the nervous system, known as the autonomic system. Smooth muscle is characterized by smooth-appearing (nonstriated) muscle cells, which are slender and tapered toward both ends. The cells are much smaller than those found in most skeletal muscles. Even though smooth muscle is found in almost every internal organ, its specific characteristics and functions vary from one organ to another; for example: (1) smooth muscle around the pupil of the eye is somewhat different from that in the walls of the stomach and it performs different functions; (2) contraction of the smooth muscle which lines the hollow organs causes the organs to empty, as in that of the intestinal tract, where waves of contractions push the inner content onward; (3) when stronger contractions occur in the smooth muscle of the blood vessels, circulation is impeded and blood pressure rises.

Compared with skeletal muscle, smooth muscle possesses (1) greater extensibility, (2) greater sensitivity to temperature and chemical stimuli, (3) greater ability for sustained contraction, and (4) more sluggishness in its movements.

Cardiac Muscle

Cardiac muscle is the highly durable tissue that forms the walls and partitions of the heart. In adults it contracts rhythmically about 100,000 times each day (72 heartbeats a minute). Like all other muscle tissue, it is composed of thousands of fibers (cells). The most striking characteristics of its fibers are that (1) they are involuntary, meaning that normally we cannot willfully prevent them from contracting or cause them to contract; (2) they are striated, similar to skeletal muscle; and (3) they are syncytial—that is, they appear to be fused together. Recent discoveries have shown that the fibers are actually separate in structure but function as syncytia.

Physiologically, cardiac muscle differs from skeletal muscle in two ways: (1) Skeletal muscle contracts only when stimulated by nerve impulses, whereas cardiac muscle contracts consistently and rhythmically without receiving impulses from the nervous system. (2) Cardiac muscle remains depolarized longer following contraction (about 3/10 sec) compared to skeletal muscle (about 1/500 sec). (A more detailed discussion of cardiac muscle will be found in Chapter 4.)

In this chapter emphasis is placed on *skeletal muscle*, because this is the kind of muscle that we are the most concerned with in athletic conditioning and performance.

GROSS STRUCTURE OF SKELETAL MUSCLE

Because of our structure, we are able to accomplish a variety of performances that other forms of life cannot accomplish. But certain other species can perform practically every type of activity better than we can. Humans are highly versatile, but not highly specialized in gross motor performances. We can walk, run, hop, climb, jump, swing, throw objects, and manipulate implements. This great versatility is due primarily to the complexity and refinement of our muscular, skeletal, and nervous systems. The skeletal muscle system is the focal point in movement; the nervous system works through the muscle by providing impulses to control their contractions, and the skeletal system provides the levers against which the muscles apply force to cause bodily movement.

Muscles vary greatly in shape. Some are long and slender, whereas others are short, chubby, round, flat, or fan-shaped. Most muscles are *uniceps,* meaning that they taper into only one tendon at each end (one-headed). For example, the *brachioradialis* is a unicep muscle. A muscle is called a *biceps* (two-headed) muscle when it is divided at one end to form two tendons. The muscle in the front of the arm between the shoulder and elbow (biceps brachii) is an example of a biceps muscle. A *triceps* (three-headed) muscle is one that divides to form three tendons at one end, such as the triceps brachii muscle in the back of the upper arm.

The basic unit of skeletal muscle, as in any tissue, is the muscle cell or fiber, a long cylindrical structure containing numerous nuclei (Fig. 2–1). The nuclei are located immediately under the cell membrane (sarcolemma). The thickness of the cell varies from 10 to 100 microns, and the length varies from only a few centimeters (cm) to more than 30 cm. In some muscles, the fibers are shorter than the muscle as a whole, and must be connected to each other and to the bony surfaces they move with a network of tough connective tissue. The connective tissue around the cell, just outside the cell membrane, is called *endomysium.* Groups of muscle fibers are surrounded by a sheath of tissue called *perimysium.* These groups of fibers are known as fascicles and are visible to the eye.

The muscle as a whole is surrounded by a layer of connective tissue called *epimysium.* This connective tissue network binds together the single contractile units and groups of units, and it integrates their actions while allowing a certain degree of freedom and autonomy among the cells.

Each muscle fiber is innervated by a branch of a motor nerve and is fed by a rich network of capillaries, which surround the fiber in such a way that they can accommodate its changes in shape during contraction (Fig. 2–2).

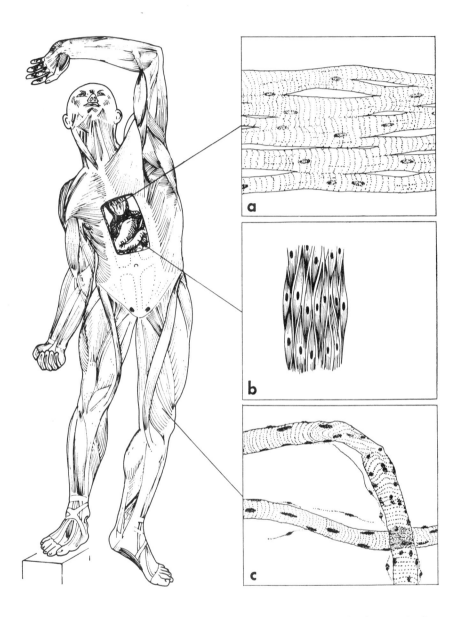

Figure 2–1.   The three different types of muscle tissue in the human body: a, cardiac; b, smooth; c, skeletal.

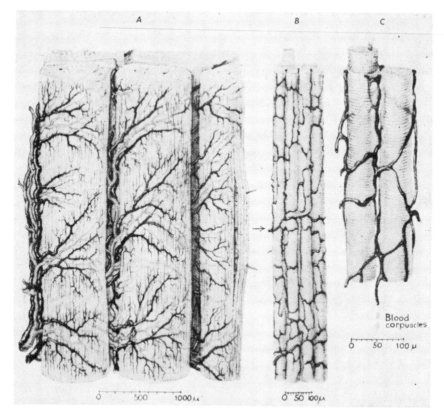

Figure 2–2. A, Drawing of the blood supply of muscle bundles in the human rectus abdominis muscle. B, The capillary network of muscle fibers; note thick loops crossing the fibers. C, The same at higher magnification showing red blood cells to establish scale. (Bloom, W., and Fawcett, D. W.: *A Textbook of Histology,* 9th ed. Philadelphia: W. B. Saunders Co., 1968.)

ULTRASTRUCTURE OF MUSCLE

A single muscle cell is surrounded by the sarcolemma, or cell membrane. (See Chapter 3 for a complete discussion of the cell membrane.) It also contains many small organelles, or subcellular components, which allow it to function as the contractile component of the system. Inside the cell is the cell fluid, or sarcoplasm, which provides the watery medium for the chemical processes of the cell. Each cell has many nuclei, all of which are near the outer edge, out of the way of the contractile mechanisms. There are numerous *mitochondria,* the cellular organelles responsible for producing oxidative energy for muscular contraction, as well as ribosomes (for the production of protein), fat droplets and glycogen (material used by the mitochondria to produce energy), myoglobin (a reddish oxygen-carrying compound much like hemoglobin in the blood), ATP and CP (high-energy phosphate molecules just waiting to be used), and hundreds of thin protein strands called *myofibrils*.

The muscle cell is also well endowed with *sarcoplasmic reticulum*, a netlike system of small tubes and vesicles surrounding the myofibrils, which give the interior components of the cell a communicative tie with the cell membrane (Fig. 2–3). The terminal cisternae are thought to store large quantities of calcium ion (Ca^{++}), a major ingredient of the contractile process. Although the entire function of the sarcoplasmic reticulum is not completely known, the transverse tubules (T tubules) are probably responsible for spreading the nervous impulse from the muscle cell membrane (sarcolemma) into the deep portion of the cell.

The myofibrils inside the cell are the source of the light and dark bands, which resulted in the term *striated* muscle as a name for skeletal muscle. The light areas are called *isotropic* (I) bands and the dark areas, *anisotropic* (A) bands. (These terms refer to the optical properties of the tissue.)

The I band is made up of a thin protein filament called *actin*, through which light passes freely. These filaments are anchored and stabilized by a protein structure called the Z *line*. The Z line is probably attached to the sarcolemma and may play a part in the transmission of impulses into the cell. From one Z line to the next is called a *sarcomere* (Fig. 2–4).

The A band is composed of the thick protein filament called *myosin*, as well as the interdigitating portion of actin. The myosin filaments are stabilized by a transverse protein located in the center called the M *line*. In the center of the A band is the H band, a slightly lighter area in the actin filament which widens or narrows as the muscle cell contracts or relaxes (Fig. 2–5).

The cross-sectional view of the actin and myosin filaments shows how they relate to each other in the muscle (Fig. 2–6). Notice that they make a hexagonal pattern with six actin filaments for each myosin filament, but that each actin filament is surrounded on three sides by a myosin filament.

It has been found that during contraction the length of the A band remains constant. The length of the I band, however, changes according to the change in length of the muscle. Since the A band consists primarily of the thick myosin filaments, it is assumed that these filaments remain a constant length. The H band varies with the increase or decrease of muscle length, and with the increase or decrease of the length of the I band, but the distance from the end of one H zone through the Z line to the end of the next H zone remains the same.

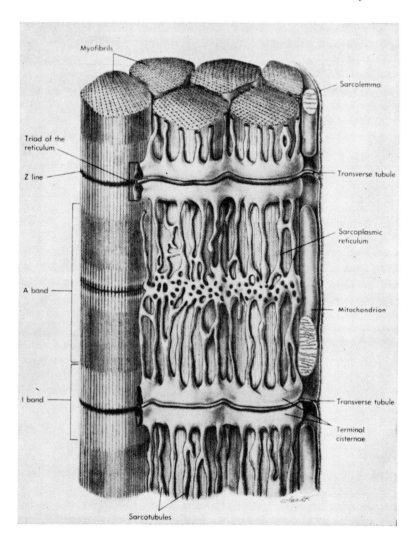

Figure 2–3. Sarcoplasmic reticulum. Schematic representation of the distribution of the sarcoplasmic reticulum around the myofibrils of skeletal muscle. The longitudinal sarcotubules are confluent with transverse elements called the terminal cisternae. A slender transverse tubule (T tubule) extending inward from the sarcolemma is flanked by two terminal cisternae to form the so-called triads of the reticulum. The location of these with respect to the cross-banded pattern of the myofibrils varies from species to species. In frog muscle, depicted here, the triads are at the Z line. In mammalian muscle there are two to each sarcomere, located at the A-I junctions. (Bloom, W., and Fawcett, D. W.: *A Textbook of Histology,* 9th ed. Philadelphia: W. B. Saunders Co., 1968.)

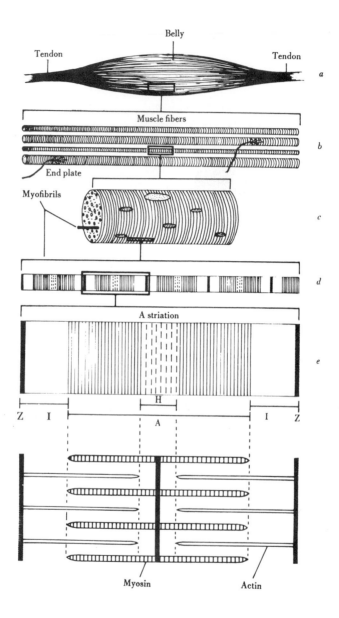

Figure 2–4. The details of the structure of skeletal muscle. (After Huxley, H. E.: The contractions of muscle. *Sci. Am.* 199:67, 1958. In Jensen, C. R., and Schultz, G. W.: *Applied Kinesiology.* New York: McGraw-Hill Book Co., 1970.)

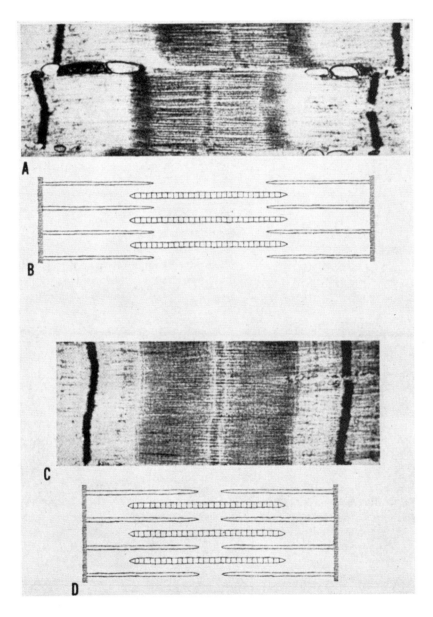

Figure 2–5. Band length changes in skeletal muscles. A, An electron micrograph showing two myofibrils in a stretched muscle. B, A drawing of the position of their filaments. The thick and thin filaments overlap only at their ends. C, A micrograph of a myofibril at its resting length. D, A drawing showing the position of the filaments. (Huxley, H. E.: The contraction of muscle. *Sci. Am.* 199:67, 1958.)

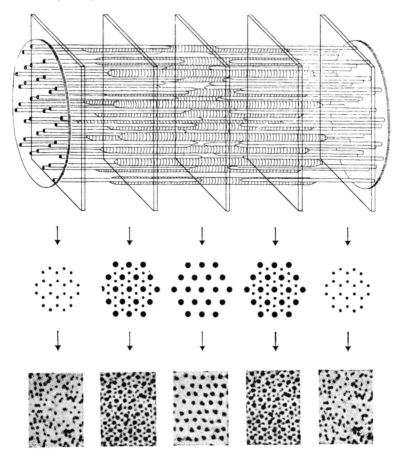

Figure 2–6. Transverse sections through a three-dimensional array of filaments in vertebrate striated muscle (top) show how the thick and thin filaments are arranged in a hexagonal pattern (middle). At bottom are electron micrographs of the corresponding sections. (Huxley, H. E.: The contraction of muscle. *Sci. Am. 199*:67, 1958.)

Because of this relationship, it has been concluded that when the muscle changes length the two sets of filaments (actin and myosin) slide past each other. When the muscle shortens greatly, the ends of the filaments meet, and heavy areas can be seen under an electron microscope.

Much is now known concerning the composition of the actin and myosin filaments, and this knowledge is helpful to the understanding of the contractile process.

A myosin molecule looks like a thin rod with two "heads" on one end. The molecules are arranged in the thick filament so that the heads are toward the two ends, which accounts for the bare zone in the center (Fig. 2–7). These protein heads are sometimes called *cross-bridges*.

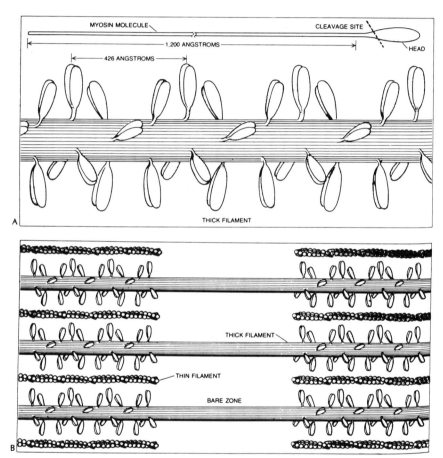

Figure 2–7. A, Thick filament is an assembly of myosin molecules, long rods with a double "head" at one end. The head has an active site where the chemical events involved in muscle contraction take place; purified heads are prepared for experiments by cleaving the molecule with an enzyme. In thick filaments myosins are bundled into a sheaf about 1.5 microns long with heads projecting in groups of three. Filament drawing includes pertinent aspects of a new model developed by John M. Squire of Imperial College London. B, Thick and thin filaments interdigitate in an orderly array to form a muscle fiber. Two sets of thin filaments extend toward each other from adjacent Z lines. They lie between, and partly overlap, a set of thick filaments. The combination accounts for the striated appearance of muscle. (From The cooperative action of muscle proteins by Murray and Weber, page 61. Copyright © 1974 by Scientific American, Inc. All rights reserved.)

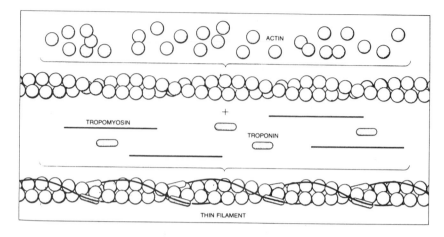

Figure 2–8. Thin filament is an assembly of actin, tropomyosin, and troponin molecules. The actins, present in the largest amount, are small spheroidal molecules that are linked to form a double helix. Tropomyosin, a long thin molecule, forms a continuous strand that sits on the string of actins alongside each groove of the double helix. A globular troponin molecule is affixed near one end of each tropomyosin. One tropomyosin extends over seven actin molecules and there are 300 to 400 actins in the micron-long filament. (From The cooperative action of muscle proteins by Murray and Weber, page 61. Copyright © 1974 by Scientific American, Inc. All rights reserved.)

There are three other major proteins involved in the contractile process and all are found in the thin filament. The *actin* molecules are small spherical particles arranged in the thin filament as a twisted double strand, each bead having a recognizable polarity, and each facing the same way. *Tropomyosin* molecules form a long thin thread on the surface of the actin strand. This strand lies near the groove between the paired strands. A *troponin* molecule is more globular than tropomyosin molecules and sits on the tropomyosin molecule a short distance from one end (Fig. 2–8). Note that the thin tropomyosin molecule extends over seven actin molecules with one troponin molecule on each tropomyosin. Each filament of actin contains 300 to 400 actin molecules and about 40 to 60 tropomyosins.[10]

MUSCLE CONTRACTION

The energy for muscular contraction is provided by the hydrolysis of ATP. ATP is thought to be bound to a particular site on the surface of the head region of the myosin molecule. The tendency is so great for this binding that almost every myosin head has an ATP bound during normal resting conditions. The "charged" myosin heads are not able to couple with the actin molecules in the absence of calcium.[10] In fact, the presence of ATP on the myosin cross-bridge actually inhibits any interaction of the two proteins.

When a signal to initiate contraction reaches a muscle cell, it causes a release of calcium into the fluid surrounding the filaments from the sarcoplasmic reticulum. The calcium is known to bind to the troponin. This action may cause the troponin to "twist" the tropomyosin strand physically, exposing the active sites of the actin molecules to the charged myosin heads. Although the charged myosin heads are fairly stable in the resting condition, they quickly link to the actin molecule when it is exposed, and swivel to a different angle, pulling the thin filaments toward the center with a concomitant splitting of the attached ATP. Apparently, the joining of the myosin head with the actin

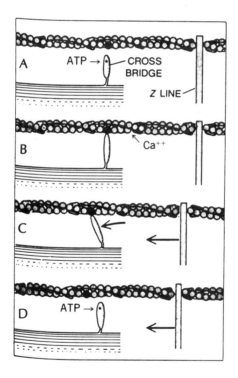

Figure 2–9. Summary of muscle contraction. A, Resting State—ATP is bound to myosin cross-bridges and interaction is inhibited. B, Calcium attached to troponin-tropomyosin "twisted" to uncover active site on actin. C, Myosin ATPase releases energy, myosin cross-bridge swivels, pulling actin toward center. D, New ATP bound to myosin cross-bridge–cross-bridge returns ready to attach again. (After Murray and Weber: The cooperative action of muscle proteins. *Sci. Am.*, 230:61, 1974.)

molecule activates an enzyme of the myosin filament called *adenosine triphosphatase* (ATPase). This enzyme is responsible for the splitting of ATP to ADP + Pi (inorganic phosphate) which releases the energy for the movement to occur.

The final stage of this reaction, the detachment of the cross-bridge, is reached only after a new ATP molecule has bound to the myosin head or cross-bridge. As long as calcium is present, and as long as there is ATP to bind to the myosin head, the cycle will continue. A single cycle of attachment, swiveling, and detachment by all cross-bridges of the fiber will shorten the muscle by about 1% of its total length (Fig. 2–9).

When the signal from the motor neuron ceases, calcium is quickly removed to the storage vesicles by a calcium "pump" situated in the membranes of the sarcoplasmic reticulum. The removal of calcium prevents the further cycling of cross-bridges, and the muscle relaxes.[7] Both the release and removal of calcium are fast processes, requiring only a fraction of a second.

If a muscle is triggered and no ATP is available following the initial contraction, a "rigor complex" is formed, since the detachment of the cross-bridge can occur only after a new ATP molecule is bound to the myosin head. This explains the rigor mortis of muscle occurring after death.[10]

Red and White Muscle Fibers

Classic experiments dealing with skeletal muscle fiber composition have identified two basic fiber types, white and red. Muscles in which white fibers predominate were shown to possess fast contraction times and contain low concentrations of myoglobin and oxidative enzymes. Muscles in which red fibers predominate often were shown to possess slow contraction times and contain high concentrations of myoglobin and oxidative enzymes. Because of these findings, white muscles in humans traditionally have been labeled as fast-twitch, low-oxidative, and red muscle, as slow-twitch, high-oxidative. Recently, several investigators have described a fast-twitch red fiber in man, which has many of the characteristics of white fibers, but is also fatigue resistant.

Other investigators, using small animals in their research, have classified muscles on the basis of their histochemical and biochemical properties as (1) fast-twitch, low-oxidative white fibers, (2) fast-twitch, high-oxidative red, and (3) slow-twitch, moderate-oxidative intermediate.[3] Studies of animal muscle fiber types have been important to the understanding of human muscle fibers, since animal fibers are much more heterogenous than human muscle fibers and lend themselves well to experimentation.

WHITE FAST-TWITCH FIBERS. A comparison of muscle types with regard to glycolytic enzymes shows that those enzymes associated with glycolysis (phosphorylase, alpha-glycerolphosphate, 3-phosphoglycer-aldehyde, pyruvate kinase, and lactate hydrogenase) had three to six times greater activity levels in the white fast-twitch fibers than in red. Phosphofructokinase (a glycolytic rate-limiting enzyme) also was much more evident in these muscles. A high glycolytic capacity is associated with anaerobic energy production, and rapid fatigue.

High levels of myosin ATPase activity also are found in the white fibers. There is a high correlation between the activity of this enzyme and the rate of speed with which a muscle will contract. Fibers with high levels of myosin ATPase are characterized by fast contraction times.

Motor units composed of white fast-twitch muscle fibers are inner-vated by motor neurons with large cell bodies which require a high threshold to initiate an impulse. The neural impulse for these fast-twitch units is generally transmitted down the axon more rapidly than the impulse for the slow-twitch units.

RED SLOW-TWITCH FIBERS. Whereas white muscle is characterized by a high glycolytic capacity, red muscle has been shown to be highly aerobic in nature and extremely fatigue resistant. This is due to the greater number of mitochondria found in this fiber type than in the other types and also its high oxidative enzyme activity. For instance, the enzyme activity of citrate synthase and malate dehydrogenase, two key enzymes of the citric acid cycle, is four times higher in red muscle than in white. Red muscle also has the increased capability to oxidize free fatty acids, as evidenced by the finding that carnityl palmityl transferase, a key enzyme in fatty acid metabolism, has an activity capacity in red muscle that is five times that found in white. Finally, cytochrome oxidase and succinate oxidase, enzymes which link elec-tron transport and oxygen utilization to ATP formation, are also found in greater abundance in the red muscle fiber than in the white.

These biochemical differences in fiber types are the basis for the functional use of these muscles during work. That is, the slowly contracting red fiber is preferentially used during low-intensity, long-duration work because of its aerobic nature. It should also be noted that these red fibers are innervated by nerves which respond to lower thresholds of stimulation than those to white fibers and would there-fore respond first to a call for mild work. With an increase in the intensity of work, the white fiber is recruited as the need for faster contractions arises.

TRAINING EFFECTS. Some studies have shown that prolonged treadmill running can result in as much as a twofold increase in the oxidative capacity of mixed skeletal muscle of rodents. This may lead to the conclusion that white fibers are changed to red fibers with training. Careful studies of identical amounts of red, white, and intermediate fibers in trained and sedentary pair-weighted rats showed, however, that skeletal muscle adapts to training as a result of a parallel shift in oxidative capacity of all three types of fibers and not as a result of a shift of one type into another.[6] This finding helps explain the observation that trained animals, at a given submaximal work level, have lower respiratory quotients, mobilize less glycogen, and get more energy from fat than their sedentary counterparts. The increase in capacity to oxidize fatty acids would naturally spare glycogen for more strenuous exercise intensities.

FIBER TYPES AND PERFORMANCE.   Although most persons have about as much red fiber as white, there is some evidence that outstanding performers have a high percentage of whichever fiber type would be advantageous to their event. Counselman reported that a world-class sprinter on his swimming team had 70% white fiber and 30% red as compared to a distance swimmer on the same team who had 91% red and only 9% white.[3] Researchers at Ball State University found the same trend. Track sprinters had up to 92% white fiber as compared to the distance runners who had as much as 90% red.

Because training does not appreciably alter the fiber type ratios, one must conclude that elite athletes were genetically endowed with an abundance of one particular fiber, and were then fortunate to gravitate to an activity for which they were exceptionally equipped.

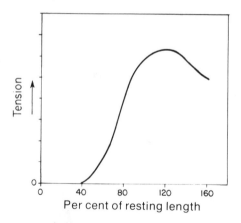

Figure 2–10.   Relationship between tension developed during contraction and muscle length in an isolated muscle. Outside the body, the muscle is strongest at resting length (100%). (Mathews, K. D., and Fox, E. L.: *The Physiological Basis of Physical Education and Athletics.* Philadelphia: W. B. Saunders Co., 1976, page 123.)

Effect of Speed of Contraction and Length of Muscle on Tension

It is generally known that as the speed of shortening increases, the tension exerted by a muscle decreases. This can be explained by assuming that the cross-bridges form their attachments at a given rate. There is only a certain period of time available for a bridge to become attached as the actin filaments slide past. Therefore, if the speed of contraction were increased, the number of effective bridges would be decreased and the tension would decrease.[7]

The amount of tension a muscle can exert is related to the length of the muscle as it contracts. This phenomenon can be explained by referring to the principles of contraction discussed previously. A shortened muscle loses tension because of the "bare" zone in the center of the myosin molecule. This area is devoid of cross-bridges. No tension would be applied to the actin filament pulled into area in the shortened muscle. Muscle that is lengthened to such a point that the overlap between actin and myosin is reduced would also decrease the number of cross-bridge attachments, and decreased tension would result. The length-tension relationship is shown in Figure 2–10.

Types of Contraction

The term *contraction* means that a muscle responds to a stimulus. When a muscle responds, tension develops, pulling toward the muscle's middle. Muscle can contract in different ways.

CONCENTRIC CONTRACTION. When muscles develop tension sufficient to move a body segment, the muscles shorten and the body segment moves. The muscles are then said to have contracted *concentrically*. (This is a form of isotonic or dynamic contraction.) For example, in a pull-up, the biceps brachii and other muscles contract, causing the elbows to bend and drawing the shoulders close to the hands. In vigorous motor movements, such as in athletics, most of the apparent contractions are *concentric*, but many of the less apparent contractions are either eccentric or static in nature.

ECCENTRIC CONTRACTION. A muscle contracts *eccentrically* when it applies tension, but the external resistance dominates, thus causing the muscle to lengthen instead of shorten. (This also is a form of isotonic contraction.) Eccentric contractions are demonstrated by moving slowly from a standing to a squatting position. To allow this movement, the leg extensor muscles must lengthen while contracting (applying tension) to control the body's weight. Eccentric contraction also is demonstrated in the actions of the biceps when the body is lowered from a pull-up position, and in the actions of the triceps in lowering the body from the push-up position.

In all eccentric contractions, the movement is directly opposite the action ordinarily assigned to the muscle. In lowering from the pull-up, the movement is elbow extension, but the active muscles are the elbow flexors. Eccentric contractions are common in wrestling and football, in which force applied by the opponent often causes muscles to lengthen while in contraction, and in gymnastics, in which the body, in arm-supported positions, is often lowered slowly. When the body lands, or when a heavy object is received, the muscles contract eccentrically to absorb the shock of the force. It should be noted that the lengthening of a muscle in a relaxed condition (no tension) owing to contraction of opposite muscles is not considered eccentric contraction.

ISOMETRIC (STATIC) CONTRACTION. A muscle contracts isometrically when it attempts to shorten (applies tension) but does not overcome the resistance; therefore, shortening of the muscle and movement of the body segment fail to occur. Isometric contraction occurs when a person pushes or pulls against a fixed object, or when the muscular tension equals the opposing force. Such contractions are used frequently in stabilizing the body or portions of the body during performance.

Gradations of Muscle Contraction

Everyday experiences show us that the same muscles contract with various gradations of force according to the requirements of a particular act. The leg extensor muscles are able to contract with just enough force to support the weight of the body, or they can contract with much more force, as when they project the body into the air. In the different motor performances, it is essential that a particular muscle or group of muscles contract with various degrees of force at different times. This is controlled by two important variables.

The first variable is the *number of motor units* contracting at once. (See Chapter 3 for the explanation of a motor unit.) When a weak contraction is desired, only a few units are activated. When a maximal contraction is needed, as many motor units as possible are contracted simultaneously. Gradations of muscle contractions between minimal and maximal can be obtained by varying the number of contracting units. The number of motor units that are contracted depends on the number of motor neurons that are activated by the stimuli emanating primarily from the brain and being distributed throughout the central nervous system.

The second variable which influences force of contraction is the *summation wave*. Impulses can be sent to the muscle fibers in slow succession, causing the fibers to contract and allowing sufficient time to relax between impulses. If the impulses are close enough, further contraction will occur before the shortening from the previous contraction can allow return to resting length. Therefore, each succeeding

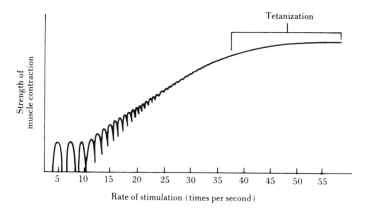

Figure 2–11. Wave summation, showing progressive summation of successive contractions as the rate of stimulation is increased. Tetanization occurs when the rate of stimulation reaches approximately 35 per second, and maximum force of contraction occurs at approximately 50 per second for large skeletal muscles. (After Arthur C. Guyton, *Functions of the Human Body*, 2nd ed., W. B. Saunders Company, Philadelphia, 1965. From *Applied Kinesiology: The Scientific Study of Human Performance* by Jensen and Schultz, page 20. Copyright ©1977 by McGraw-Hill, Inc. Used with permission of McGraw-Hill Book Company.)

contraction will add to the force of the previous contraction. This process is limited, finally, because the actin filaments are physically incapable of sliding any further. Figure 2–11 illustrates the buildup of the contractile force as the rate of impulses per second (frequency) increases. In large skeletal muscles, when the rate of impulses reaches about 35 per second, the muscle tetanizes, meaning that the responses to individual impulses are no longer detectable, and the contraction becomes smooth and continuous. Maximal contractile force occurs at about 50 impulses per second in large muscles. However, in smaller muscles which cause highly precise and rapid movements, such as those controlling the eyelid, maximal contraction comes at 400 to 600 impulses per second. Tetanization produces about three to four times the contractile force that occurs from a single nerve impulse. By varying the frequency of impulses to the motor unit, the amount of force can be varied to any amount between that produced by the single impulse (muscle twitch) and maximal contraction.

SELECTED REFERENCES

1. Astrand, P. O., and Rodahl, K.: *Textbook of Work Physiology*. New York: McGraw-Hill Book Co., 1970.

2. Barnard, R. J., Edgerton, V. R., Furukawa, T., and Peter, J. B.: Histochemical, biochemical, and contractile properties of red, white, and intermediate fibers. *Am. J. Physiol., 220*:410–415, 1971.
3. Counselman, J. E.: The importance of speed in exercise. *Athletic Journal, 56*:72–75, 1976.
4. Etemadi, A. A., and Hosseini, F.: Frequency and size of muscle fibers in athletic body build. *Anat. Rec., 162*:269, 1968.
5. Guyton, A. C.: *Textbook of Medical Physiology*, 3rd ed. Philadelphia: W. B. Saunders Co., 1966.
6. Holloszy, J. O.: Adaptations of muscular tissue to training. *Prog. Cardiovasc. Dis., 18*:445–458, 1976.
7. Huxley, H. E.: The contraction of muscle. *Sci. Am., 199*:67, 1958.
8. Jensen, C. R., and Schultz, G. W.: *Applied Kinesiology*, 2nd ed. New York; McGraw-Hill Book Co., 1977.
9. Murray, J. M., and Weber, A.: The cooperative action of muscle proteins. *Sci. Am., 230*:58–71, 1974.

Chapter 3
The Nervous System

This chapter emphasizes the aspects of the nervous system that relate to motor performance. Through his nervous system, a person is able to interpret and respond to the events of his environment and to coordinate the functions of his organs and muscles to accomplish the various tasks of life. In essence, the purpose of the nervous system is communication.

All body movements, both external and internal, are coordinated by nerve impulses. Without nerve impulses the skeletal muscles are unable to contract; consequently, the organism is unable to function or even survive.

From the standpoint of function, the nervous system is divided into two parts: autonomic system and voluntary system. The *autonomic system* is responsible for the automatic functions of the organs. While this system is of utmost importance to the functions of life, it is only of secondary importance in the preparation for athletic performance. The *voluntary system* is the part of the nervous system over which we can exercise conscious control, but which often operates below the conscious level. This is the portion of the system that controls the skeletal muscles.

Structurally, the voluntary system is divided into the *central nervous system* (CNS) and the *peripheral nervous system* (PNS). The CNS includes only the brain and spinal cord, and the PNS includes all of the other nerve tissue in the voluntary system. The tissue of the PNS is distributed in all areas of the body and connects with the CNS at various levels along the spinal column.

NEURONS

Cells in the nervous system are called neurons. Structurally, these cells are unique compared to other cells of the body. They are large cells with long extensions, called axons or dendrites, extending from the central portion or *cell body,* which contains the nucleus and other cell organelles. The dendrites receive messages from other neurons or from peripheral sensory receptors. The axons receive information from the cell body and transmit it to other neurons or muscle fibers (Fig. 3–1).

Neurons exhibit the properties of *excitability* and *conductivity.* When a cell has excitability, it will respond to a stimulus, and if it passes the response to other cells, it has conductivity. To understand

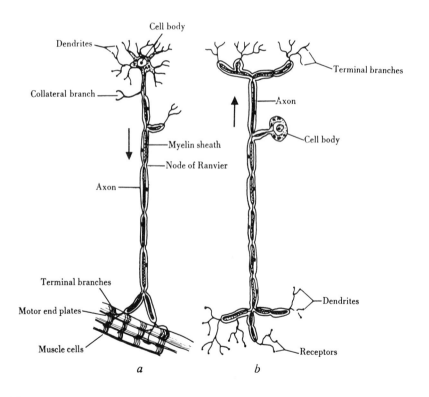

Figure 3–1.   Types of spinal neurons: a, motor; b, sensory. (Jensen, C. R., and Schultz, G. W.: *Applied Kinesiology.* New York: McGraw-Hill Book Co., 1970.)

how neurons respond to a stimulus and then conduct that response to other cells, one must understand something about the cell membrane.

The Cell Membrane

A single neuron (or muscle cell for that matter) has a membrane surrounding its cytoplasm which controls the passage of material into and out of the cell. It is thin (70 to 90 angstroms) and elastic, and is composed of protein (about 50% to 70% by weight) and lipid molecules. For years, this structure has been visualized as a lipid bilayer covered on both sides by a layer of unfolded protein (Fig. 3–2). This model postulated that the lipid molecules were lined up in a polar fashion on the inside, with an unfolded layer of protein on the outside. Protein-lined pores were thought to be present throughout the membrane to allow small molecules (such as water or urea) to pass through.

A more likely model has been postulated by Singer.[11] He visualized large, globular proteins possessing one hydrophobic and one hy-

CELL MEMBRANE

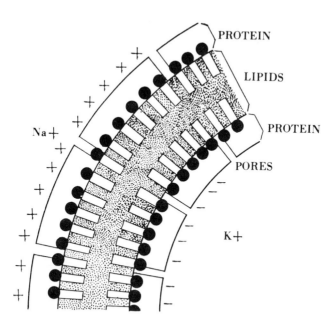

Figure 3–2. Early (Danielli) model of membrane structure visualized "unrolled" protein covering both sides of lipid bilayer, with hydrophobic amino acid residues interacting with similar lipid chains; hydrophilic residues were thought to form "pores" for molecular transport.

drophilic end (just as the membrane lipid molecules) embedded in the lipid bilayers of the membrane (Fig. 3–3). Some proteins were thought to be large enough to span the entire membrane. If they spanned the membrane, they would have two hydrophilic ends, and could conceivably be organized in such a way that a channel was formed through the protein (Fig. 3–4), which could be involved in active transport of material into and out of the cell (Fig. 3–5).

There is an electrical potential across the membrane of muscle and nerve cells which is a result of the difference in the amount of sodium ion (Na+) and potassium ion (K+) on each side of the membrane. This potential gives the cell the capacity to become *excited*.

It seems obvious that the concentration of ions inside and outside the cell membrane would remain equal unless some force upsets the equilibrium. In the cell there is such a force called the *sodium pump*, which pumps large quantities of sodium ions (cations) out of the cell into the fluid surrounding the cell. This is an *active transport* mechanism, which means that it works against the concentration gradient of

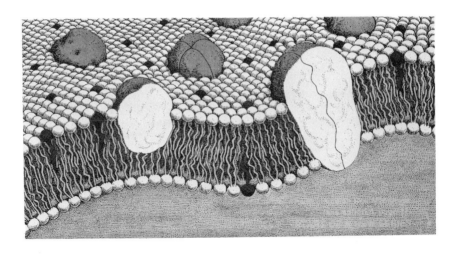

Figure 3–3. Current (Singer) membrane model sees proteins as predominantly globular (dark gray) and amphipathic, with their hydrophilic ends protruding from the membrane and their hydrophobic ends embedded in the bilayer of lipids (light gray) and cholesterol (black). The proteins make up the membrane's "active sites"; some of them are simply embedded on one side or the other, whereas others pass entirely through the bilayer. Some of the latter presumably contain transport pores. (Singer, S. J.: Architecture and Topography of Biological Membranes. In *Cell Membranes, Biochemistry, Cell Biology and Pathology.* G. Weissman and R. Clairborne (Eds.). New York: H. P. Publishing Co., Inc., 1975, page 37. Reprinted with permission from *Hospital Practice,* Vol. 8, No. 5.)

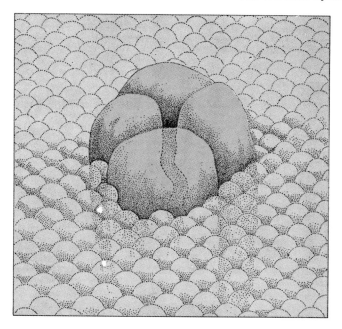

Figure 3–4. Water-filled channels for transport of specific ions and hydrophilic molecules through membrane may be formed by groupings of four (or more) protein subunits, as schematized above. Such a channel, about 10 Å across, is known to exist between the subunits of the hemoglobin molecule, though the protein is, of course, not found in membranes. (Singer, S. J.: Architecture and Topography of Biological Membranes. In *Cell Membranes, Biochemistry, Cell Biology and Pathology*. G. Weissman and R. Clairborne (Eds.). New York: H. P. Publishing Co., Inc., 1975, page 42. Reprinted with permission from *Hospital Practice*, Vol. 8, No. 5.)

the cell, and it requires energy to function. At the same time, it also pumps potassium ions into the cell. However, since the cell membrane is at least 100 times more permeable to potassium than to sodium, most of the potassium ions tend to diffuse out of the cell because of the concentration gradient. This tendency is counteracted by the −75 to −85 millivolts (mV) membrane potential created by the sodium pump where the negative charge inside the cell tends to attract the positive potassium ion. Therefore, potassium ions remain in the cell primarily as a result of the negative charge in the cell and partially from the potassium pump mechanism. As long as the membrane of a nerve or muscle fiber remains undisturbed, *resting potential* exists. However, when something changes the permeability of the membrane to sodium, a rapid change in membrane potential, called *action potential*, occurs.

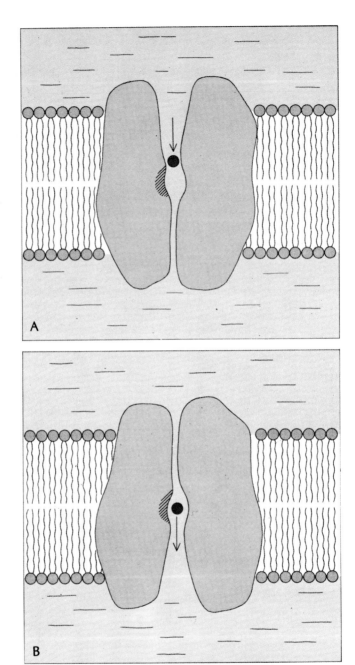

Figure 3–5. A, Active transport of molecule through membrane protein channel is visualized two-dimensionally. Molecule impinges on active site (shaded) of protein. B, Then some energy-yielding enzyme reaction triggers shift in subunit configuration that "squeezes" the molecule through the membrane. (Singer, S. J.: Architecture and Topography of Biological Membranes. In *Cell Membranes, Biochemistry, Cell Biology and Pathology.* G. Weismann and R. Clairborne (Eds.). New York: H. P. Publishing Co., Inc., 1975, page 43. Reprinted with permission from *Hospital Practice*, Vol. 8, No. 5.)

The action potential can be caused by electrical stimulation, chemical stimulation, mechanical damage, and heat and cold.

The first part of the action potential is called *depolarization*. This is thought to be associated with the loosening of calcium ions from the interior of the membrane. When the calcium ions are dislodged, they can no longer effectively resist sodium and, therefore, sodium ions rush into the membrane in ever-increasing numbers, and this dislodges still more of the calcium ions. So much sodium rushes into the cell that the potential actually reverses (Fig. 3–6). This is called *reverse potential*. As more and more sodium ions enter the cell, their positive charges repel additional flow. The calcium binds back to the pores in the interior of the membrane, and the *action potential* ceases.

Meanwhile, the cell membrane becomes *repolarized*. Potassium ions respond to the inflow of sodium ions by leaving the site of high sodium concentration. The outflow of potassium is the most important mechanism for the repolarization process. The return of the membrane to a *resting potential* is caused almost entirely by the outflow of potassium

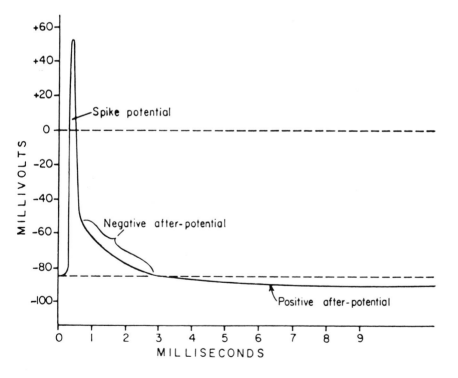

Figure 3–6. The action potential, showing the initial spike followed by a negative after potential and a positive after potential. (Guyton, A. C.: *Textbook of Medical Physiology*, 3rd ed. Philadelphia: W. B. Saunders Co., 1966.)

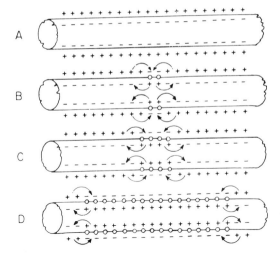

Figure 3–7. Propagation of action potential along a conductive fiber. (Guyton, A. C.: Textbook of Medical Physiology, 3rd ed. Philadelphia: W. B. Saunders Co., 1966.)

ions and not by the sodium pump, which would be much too slow to repolarize the membrane at the required speed. Of course, as soon as possible, the sodium pump expels the sodium ions, and the potassium ions are exchanged to the inside of the membrane once again.

In muscle cells this action potential triggers the contraction mechanism so that the muscle fiber contracts. In nerve cells the action potential causes a propagation impulse to travel down the nerve cell to transmit information to other body parts. Apparently, the action potential at a particular point along the membrane causes an increased permeability to sodium in adjacent sections of the membrane, and the action potential spreads in all directions like circles in water caused when a rock is thrown into it (Fig. 3–7). This transmission of the depolarization process along a nerve or muscle fiber is called an *impulse*.

Each muscle or nerve fiber has its own *threshold* of excitation. This refers to the amount of stimulation necessary to cause the membrane to depolarize. It should be obvious, however, that once the membrane depolarizes, the depolarization process will travel over the entire membrane. This is referred to as the *all-or-none law* and it applies to all nerve and muscle fibers. To state the all-or-none law another way, it means that if a fiber responds to a stimulus it responds completely; otherwise it does not respond at all.

Types of Neurons

Three types of neurons are important for motor activity: *sensory, motor,* and *interneurons.* Sensory and motor neurons relay messages to and from the central nervous system, respectively, whereas interneurons relay messages within the central nervous system. If a sensory neuron receives a stimulus (sight, noise, pain), the information usually terminates in a specialized area of the brain where it is interpreted. On the other hand, a stimulus may originate in the brain, travel down a descending tract to an interneuron, which stimulates a motor neuron, and then to several or many muscle cells, causing them to contract. Some sensory impulses may travel to the spinal cord and, once there, may transfer to motor neurons and arrive at the muscle without any brain involvement (a reflex arc).

SENSORY NEURONS. Sensory neurons are responsible for passing information to the CNS from the periphery of the body. Information passes up the dendrite to the cell body, located in the dorsal root ganglion, and into the spinal cord to terminate on a motor neuron or an interneuron.

MOTOR NEURONS. Special attention is devoted to motor neurons because they carry impulses to muscles. The motor neuron, like other cells, is surrounded by a cell membrane. The potential difference between the inside and outside of the cell membrane of a typical motor neuron has been measured at about -80 mV. When the membrane potential is reduced to a critical value (about -60 mV), the sodium ions rush through the membrane and it becomes *depolarized*. The critical point at which the cell depolarizes is called the *threshold*.

The axons of motor neurons are surrounded by a special cell called a *Schwann cell*. The Schwann cell wraps itself around the axon, forcing its cytoplasm into the outside wrapping (Fig. 3–8). The internal wrappings, containing little cytoplasm, are called the *myelin sheath*. These wrappings electrically insulate the axon and enhance impulse conduction. Even axons that are not myelinated are partially covered by Schwann cells. The sheath of Schwann and the myelin sheath are interrupted at regular intervals by structures called *nodes of Ranvier*, which are small uninsulated areas almost 500 times as permeable as are the membranes of some unmyelinated fibers. Since the myelin sheath is an excellent insulator which prevents almost all flow of ions from the cell membrane, the depolarization of myelinated fibers occurs at the nodes of Ranvier, instead of continuously along the entire fiber. This conduction from node to node is thought to be the explanation for the high transmission rate of myelinated fibers, and probably conserves energy for the axon since only the nodes need to depolarize. It is this property which allows information to be transmitted the length of the axon at the speed of up to 100 m/second.

The rate of impulse conduction is related to the size of the axon, the thickness of the myelin sheath, and the distance between the nodes of Ranvier. If the impulses jump from node to node, it is called *saltatory conduction*.

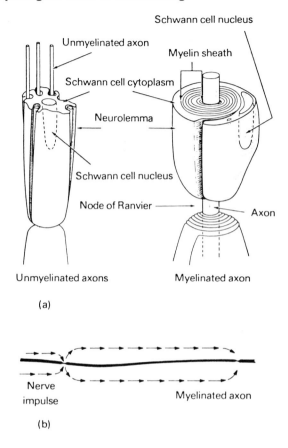

(a)

(b)

Figure 3–8.   A, Diagram of unmyelinated and myelinated nerves. B, Saltatory nerve impulse between nodes on axon drawn in elongated position.
(Reprinted from *The Biology of Physical Activity* by D. W. Edington and V. R.
Edgerton. Copyright © 1976 by Houghton Mifflin Company. Used by permission of the publisher.)

INTERNEURONS. All sensory and motor nerve cells in the body can
be classified functionally as excitatory neurons. However, in the gray
matter of the spinal cord, there are short neurons, called *interneurons,*
which can be either excitatory or inhibitory. Some of these neurons,
when excited, liberate a chemical that excites other nerve cells by
depolarizing the membrane. Others inhibit nerve cell transmission by
hyperpolarizing the cell membrane. The obvious importance of an
interneuron system which can inhibit as well as excite is that information from other areas can be modified to suit the needs of the organism,
by either passing it along the pathways or stopping it from being

transmitted. For example, the inhibition or blocking of nerve impulses to those muscles in opposition (antagonistic) to a desired movement is of utmost importance to the efficiency and speed of that movement. The process of inhibiting contractions is mostly automatic and is done at the subconscious level. However, it also can be done consciously to some extent. Ordinarily, with additional practice of a movement the inhibition of the antagonistic muscles becomes quicker and more complete, and the movement becomes more efficient and effective. Thus, the nervous system can either excite or inhibit muscle activity, depending on information received from the higher centers or from receptor organs.

SPINAL NERVES

Extending from the spinal cord are 21 pairs of large nerves, called *spinal nerves*. Each one is about the size of a pencil and contains thousands of individual axons. The axons in a spinal nerve vary in length, with long axons being several feet and the shorter ones hardly measurable. The larger axons are capable of conducting over 2000 impulses/second.

There is a tendency to confuse the term "nerve" with "neuron" or "nerve fiber." *Neurons* are the basic cells in the nervous system and include the axon, the cell body, and the dendrites. *Nerves* are groups of neurons or nerve fibers.

The cell bodies of motor neurons are located in the anterior horn of the spinal cord, and their axons group together and extend, via the

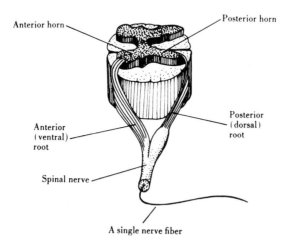

Figure 3–9. Motor and sensory nerves in spinal cord. (Jensen, C. R., and Schultz, G. W.: *Applied Kinesiology.* New York: McGraw-Hill Book Co., 1970.)

spinal nerves, to the muscle fibers. Sensory neuron cell bodies are located near the posterior side of the spinal cord in the *dorsal root ganglion*. However, their axons originate in specialized sensory receptors through the body and carry information up the spinal nerves to the spinal cord.

Thus, the spinal nerves are groups of axons from both motor and sensory neurons which function much like a cross-country telephone cable, with messages traveling both ways in the communication process (Fig. 3–9).

NEURAL JUNCTIONS

This section is a discussion of the nerve-nerve and the nerve-muscle junctions.

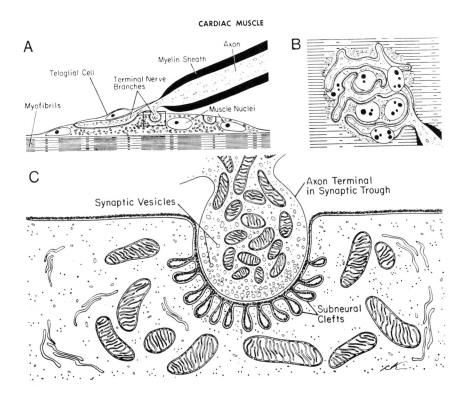

Figure 3–10. Schematic representations of the motor end plate as seen by light and electron microscopy. A, End plate as seen in histological sections in the long axis of the muscle fiber; B, as seen in surface view with the light microscope; C, as seen in an electron micrograph of an area such as that in the rectangle on A. (Bloom, W., and Fawcett, D. W.: *A Textbook of Histology*, 9th ed. Philadelphia: W. B. Saunders Co., 1968.)

Motor End Plate

The branches of the nerve fiber contact the muscle fibers at motor end plates (Fig. 3–10). These small knoblike processes containing vesicles of acetylcholine (ACh) fit into depressions on the muscle sarcoplasm called *synaptic troughs*. When impulses arrive at the end plate, the vesicles release their ACh, and depolarization of the membrane occurs. Another chemical, cholinesterase, functions to inactivate ACh almost immediately so that the membrane can again repolarize.

Synapses

A synapse is a junction between two or more neurons. These junctions operate much like the motor end plates, with a release of a chemical which causes depolarization of the fiber to which the message is being passed. Information is passed from one neuron to another via the synapse that connects them (Fig. 3–11).

The body is able to regulate the activity of motor neurons by the amount of chemical released at the synapses. For instance, if enough of the vesicles at the end of one neuron release their chemical, the membrane potential of the connecting neurons will be reduced to a critical value, and depolarization will occur. However, sometimes the

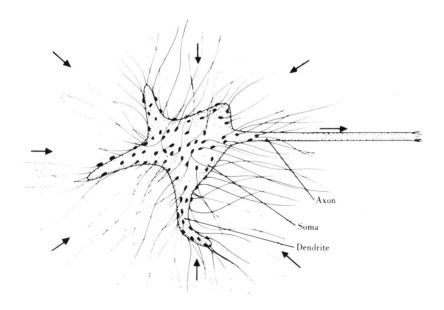

Figure 3–11. A typical synapse, showing hundreds of terminals that originate in other neurons. (Jenson, C. R., and Schultz, G. W.: *Applied Kinesiology.* New York: McGraw-Hill Book Co., 1970.)

amount of chemical liberated is insufficient to cause depolarization, but it does lower the membrane potential. This is called *facilitation,* and it prepares the neuron to fire more readily if a second volley of impulses arrives while the membrane is still facilitated. If this occurs because of repeated impulse volleys from the same synapse, it is called *temporal summation.* If several synapses are in proximity to each other, their combined effort is called *spatial summation.* Acetylcholine has been identified as the transmitter substance in some synapses. Located close to synapses is a supply of the enzyme cholinesterase which inactivates ACh to allow the membrane potential to be restored quickly (repolarized).

MOTOR UNITS

The motor unit is defined as an *alpha-motoneuron* (referring to size) and all of the skeletal muscle fibers that are innervated by that motoneuron. The cell body is located in the anterior root of the spinal cord, and is controlled by thousands of direct and indirect neural connections from interneurons, sensory neurons, and descending tract neurons. A long axon extends from the cell body to the muscle, where it branches to innervate 10 to 1000 individual muscle fibers. The number of fibers innervated by the motor neuron depends upon the quality of movement expected of the muscle. Usually, muscle groups required for highly refined movements have fewer muscle fibers than those from which gross movement is expected. All muscle fibers in the specific motor unit contract when the motor neuron associated with that motor unit depolarizes (all-or-none contraction sequence). The muscle fibers of motor units overlap each other and are scattered throughout the muscle among fibers from other motor units.

Motor units differ in several important ways: (1) *Speed.* Motor units containing fast-twitch fibers reach peak tension almost twice as fast as do motor units containing slow-twitch fibers (see Chapter 2). The neural pathways are larger to the fast-twitch fibers than to the slow-twitch fibers, and the conduction is faster. (2) *Force.* The motor units containing fast-twitch fibers not only have larger neural connections, but also produce the highest force of contraction. Motor units containing fast-twitch oxidative fibers contract with less force than those containing fast-twitch glycolytic fibers. (3) *Endurance.* The slow-twitch oxidative motor units are much more resistant to fatigue than are motor units containing the fast-twitch muscle fibers.[3,4]

CONTROL OF MOTOR ACTIVITY

In addition to the transmission of impulses across motor neurons, motor activity is dependent upon (1) the coordination of impulses from sensory organs through the body, and (2) information from the higher centers where memories of previous experience are stored and conscious movements are initiated.

Sensory Information

Much information comes to the motor neuron from sensory organs by way of the sensory nerves. Sensory organs are located in and around the muscles, in the skin, and in various other kinds of tissue. One of the most important sensory organs is the *muscle spindle*.

THE MUSCLE SPINDLE. Each spindle consists of a connective tissue sheath containing several *intrafusal* muscle fibers and is large enough to be visible to the naked eye. There are more spindles in the antigravity, predominantly slow-twitch muscles than in the faster muscles of movement.

The muscle fibers in the sheath have a central, heavily nucleated area called the *nuclear bag*, which has lost its striations and is unable to contract. Whenever the muscle is stretched, the nuclear bag is stretched, and nerve endings, found entwined around the nuclear center of the spindle, called *annulospiral endings*, are excited (Fig. 3–12). From these nerve endings come large A (alpha) nerve fibers which carry information concerning the stretch of the spindle to the dorsal root (sensory portion) of the spinal cord. On each side of the annulospiral endings are *flower-spray receptors*, which transmit on smaller nerve fibers than the A fibers used by the annulospiral endings. The function of the flower-spray receptors is thought to be the same as that of the annulospiral endings, except that a much greater stretch is required to excite these receptors.

After entering the dorsal root of the spinal cord, the impulses from the spindle travel to the ventral root, and connect *monosynaptically* with a motor neuron which innervates muscle cells surrounding the spindle. These muscle cells then contract to decrease the length of the spindle. When the original length is established, the nuclear bag is no longer stretched, and annulospiral endings are then quiet.

The spindle, as described previously, functions to measure muscle length, the amount of stretch applied to the muscle, and the rate at which the stretch is applied.

In addition to giving the body information about length and stretch of a muscle, the spindle also may be involved in movement through the gamma motor system. The gamma motor fibers are located in the anterior horn of the spinal cord and end only on the contractile portion of the intrafusal fibers within the muscle spindle. Stimulation of the gamma efferent fibers causes the intrafusal fibers in the spindle to contract, stretching the nuclear bag, and evoking a contraction of the extrafusal fibers near the spindle through a reflex, or feedback, action. This mechanism is called a *servomechanism*, and it allows an arm or a leg to be contracted to a predetermined length in a coordinated movement. This response is quite apparent to anyone who has lifted an empty can that he thought was full, or tried to pick up a small bottle of mercury without knowing what was in the bottle. The gamma servo system helps us apply the correct amount of force to pick up an object

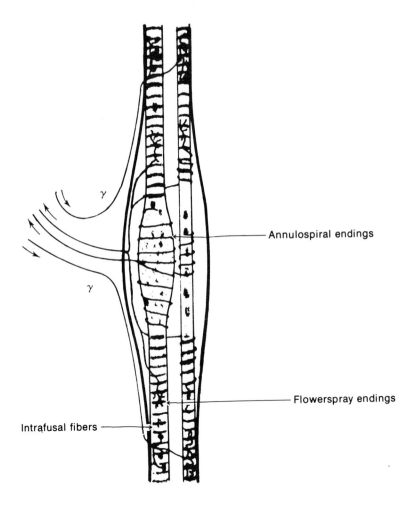

Figure 3–12. Diagram of a muscle spindle. In the middle it has a nonstriated region supplied by so-called annulospiral afferent nerve fibers. There is a second type of afferent nerve fibers, called flower-spray endings, mainly localized at the ends of the muscle spindle. The polar region of the muscle spindle with intrafusal muscle fibers is supplied by gamma (γ) motor efferents. The muscle spindles are arranged parallel to the extrafusal muscle fibers. (Astrand, P.-O., and Rodahl, K.: *Textbook of Work Physiology.* New York: McGraw-Hill Book Co., 1970.)

based on past experience. When the object is not the same as predicted, the muscles overreact or under react.

Although much information is yet to be gathered concerning this second role, it is known that the muscle spindles are important for the execution of well-coordinated movement.

The muscle spindle can be tested easily by tapping the patellar tendon. The tap on this tendon stretches the spindles of the quadriceps muscle, which excites the annulospiral endings and sends a signal through the spinal cord and back to the muscle fibers around the spindles. The knee jerk is a result of the muscle's contracting in response to this stimulus.

GOLGI TENDON APPARATUS. Another important sensory organ is the Golgi tendon apparatus. It lies between the fibers of a tendon and is excited by high tension on the tendon. Its function is to detect too much load on the muscle and to protect the muscle from injury. Excitation of this organ sends a signal on a large A fiber to an inhibitory interneuron, which inhibits the contraction of the muscle being stretched.

PACINIAN CORPUSCLES. Pacinian corpuscles are fat, biscuitlike organs which sense pressure of the tendons across joints. They make it possible to detect the position of body parts without looking at them. They are essential to most motor activity and can be tested easily by touching the fingertips together with the eyes closed.

Higher Centers

Most of the cranial cavity is occupied by the largest section of the brain called the *cerebrum*. The surface portion of the cerebrum is known as the *cortex* (cerebral cortex). The cerebral cortex appears to be the seat of voluntary movement. It orders gross muscular actions, but relies on lower levels of the CNS to control the details.

The cortex is responsible for *consciousness, perception, memory* (including the memories of movement patterns), *interpretation,* and *reasoning.* A combination of these functions results in what is known as *judgment.* The exact response is probably based upon the success or failure of similar actions in the past; successful actions tend to be repeated, and failures tend to be rejected. The more extensive and well established its store of memories, the faster and more accurate will be its responses in terms of muscular actions. If the particular situation at hand is a near duplicate of successfully handled situations of the past, the response will probably nearly duplicate past responses. But if the problem is unique or only rarely experienced, the chances of responding quickly and correctly are considerably lessened. In the latter case, the judgment of how to respond will be based on the most nearly related experiences.

All these factors indicate that children should be provided with opportunities for experience in a great variety of basic movement patterns before their interests become too specialized. Otherwise, overall skill development will be limited. Extensive experience in motor movements will undoubtedly cause development of the nervous system (both central and peripheral), which will result in increased success in a variety of motor movement patterns (skills). The parts of the cerebral cortex directly concerned with motor movements are the *sensory cortex, motor cortex,* and *premotor cortex* (Fig. 3–13).

The *sensory cortex* is the terminating area for most of the afferent (sensory) information coming from the various sensory receptors. Interpretation of the sensory impulses takes place in this area. On the basis of the interpretation action is initiated.

The *motor cortex* provides stimulation to individual muscles and to small muscle groups. A single shock of near-threshold level from an electrode in the motor cortex area usually elicits a discrete motor movement such as a flick of the finger or a deviation of the lip. The muscle groups of the body are represented in this area according to the discreteness of the movement required. The thumb and forefingers, lips, vocal cords, and the like, have large representation, whereas the areas for postural muscle activities are relatively small. A large shock in this area, however, may result in a coordinated movement to place the limb to a fixed "final position." Changing the position of the electrode minutely could cause the limb to change to another "final position,"

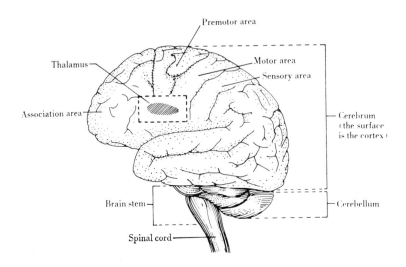

Figure 3–13. Parts of the CNS which have major functions in the control of skeletal muscle action. (Jensen, C. R., and Schultz, G. W.: *Applied Kinesiology.* New York: McGraw-Hill Book Co., 1970.)

demonstrating that the motor cortex does have a coordination function as well as single response functions.[7]

The premotor cortex produces impulses for complicated patterns of movement (complex coordinations). It has been found that loss of function in this area of the brain destroys the sequence and timing of complex movement patterns. Many coordinations are basically repetitious, so the performance of the premotor area is not as complex as it might seem. But it is still the key area of the brain so far as motor performance is concerned.

The most important differences between the motor cortex and the premotor cortex are the functional differences. When first learning a skill in which conscious attention must be given to each action, the motor cortex has the greatest involvement. As the skill progresses, the origin of the movements very likely shifts to the premotor cortex. However, the motor cortex still acts as a relay station, with fibers passing through it from the premotor cortex.

The interior of the cerebrum is composed mostly of white matter which links the cerebrum to all the levels of the spinal cord. This white matter provides fast and often direct impulse conduction from the highest centers of the central nervous system to the various junctions in the spinal cord, and vice versa. The nerve fibers composing the white matter are bundled together according to common functions; the bundles are called nerve tracts. The afferent (sensory) bundles are ascending tracts and transmit sensory impulses to be interpreted in the sensory cortex. The efferent (motor) bundles are descending tracts which conduct impulses from the highest centers to the motor nerves.

In addition to the white matter in the interior of the cerebrum, several clusters of gray matter, called nuclei, are present. Little is known about the functions of some of these clusters. However, the largest and probably the most important to motor movement is the thalamus. The thalamus serves as an important relay center for both motor and sensory impulses. It has extensive connections with the cortex.

The cerebellum is not in the main line of impulse travel between the cerebral cortex and the spinal cord, but it is tied to the main tracts through a series of collateral nerve endings. As far as motor performance is concerned, the function of the cerebellum is to modify motor impulses and thereby contribute to the perfection of the desired movements. An individual with a malfunction of the cerebellum will not have the ability to refine a movement nor will he be able to make needed adjustments as the movement progresses. He will exhibit extreme inaccuracy, overcompensation, and a marked jerkiness in movement. In fact, the cerebellum can predict from the present state of the muscles and joints what will occur as the movement progresses, and distribute signals that prevent errors in the movement pattern.

The *brain stem* is the direct connection between the brain and the spinal cord, and thus impulses pass through it in both directions. The functions of the brain stem are more directly concerned with autonomic responses than with responses involving the voluntary nervous system. Part of the stem (the *medulla* and the *pons*) governs the rates of respiration and heart beat. Some authorities think inhibitory impulses originate in the cerebrum, but most neural experts claim they originate in the brain stem. The inhibitory impulses produce conditions that make it necessary for more facilitative impulses to arrive in order to excite a neuron in the spinal cord. If this phenomenon did not exist with a normal degree of efficiency, we would experience unwanted contractions, and perhaps the inability to stop contractions short of complete fatigue.

Thus, motor activity is influenced by the sum of all of the information reaching the motor neuron from both the higher centers and the sensory organs. The descending impulses from the higher centers of the brain, including those voluntarily evoked, are modified on the basis of information from the receptor organs because of the many possible alternatives available through the synaptic system of interneurons within the spinal cord. This coordination of motor information makes possible the movement pattern associated with athletic performance.

AUTONOMIC NERVOUS SYSTEM

The autonomic nervous system is involved in a major way with many of the responses the body makes during exercise. There are two major divisions: the sympathetic and the parasympathetic, which generally have antagonistic functional effects.

Autonomically, the neurons of the sympathetic system exit the spinal cord between the first thoracic and the second lumbar vertebras and synapse at that point (the sympathetic ganglia) with the postganglionic fibers. The postganglionic fibers then travel to the organs being affected.

The parasympathetic fibers exit the spinal cord and travel to the walls of the affected organ or area before synapsing with the postganglionic fibers.

The preganglionic fibers of both systems secrete acetylcholine (ACh) as the transmitter substance. The postganglionic fibers of the parasympathetic system are cholinergic (that is, they also secrete ACh), whereas the postganglionic fibers from the sympathetic system are usually adrenergic and secrete norepinephrine.

Some of the most important actions of the autonomic system are associated with the heart and circulatory system. These actions will be discussed in detail in later chapters.

SELECTED REFERENCES

1. Astrand, P.-O., and Rodahl, K.: *Textbook of Work Physiology.* New York: McGraw-Hill Book Co., 1970.
2. Bloom, W., and Fawcett, D. W.: *A Textbook of Histology,* 9th ed. Philadelphia: W. B. Saunders Co., 1968.
3. Buchthal, F., and Schmalbruch, H.: Contraction times and fiber types in intact human muscle. *Acta Physiol. Scand., 79:*435–452, 1970.
4. Burke, R. E., and Edgerton, V. R.: Motor unit properties and selective involvement in movement. In *Exercise and Sports Science Review.* J. Wilmore and J. Keogh (Eds.). New York: Academic Press, 1975.
5. DeVries, H. A.: *Physiology of Exercise for Physical Education and Athletics,* 2nd ed. Dubuque: Wm. C. Brown Co., 1974.
6. Edington, D. W., and Edgerton, V. R.: *The Biology of Physical Activity.* Boston: Houghton Mifflin Co., 1976.
7. Guyton, A. C.: *Textbook of Medical Physiology,* 4th ed. Philadelphia: W. B. Saunders Co., 1971.
8. Jensen, C. R., and Schultz, G. W.: *Applied Kinesiology,* 2nd ed. New York: McGraw-Hill Book Co., 1977.
9. Karpovich, P. V., and Sinning, W. E.: *Physiology of Muscular Activity,* 7th ed. Philadelphia: W. B. Saunders Co., 1971.
10. Ricci, B.: *Physiological Basis of Human Performance.* Philadelphia: Lea & Febiger, 1967.
11. Singer, S. J.: Architecture and topography of biological membranes. In *Cell Membranes, Biochemistry, Cell Biology and Pathology.* G. Weissman and R. Clairborne (Eds.). New York: H. P. Publishing Co. Inc., 1975.

Chapter 4
Cardiovascular Function

The amount of work a person can do is limited largely by his cardiovascular system, for this system provides oxygen and nutrients to the cells of the body and carries away the waste products. The purpose of this chapter is to discuss the several components of the cardiovascular system in terms of their importance to conditioning and performance.

CARDIAC MUSCLE

The heart is the "pump of life" for all body tissues. In the absence of the consistent beating of the heart, body cells cease to function and die. The heart is composed of a unique kind of tissue known as *cardiac muscle*. Although striated, cardiac muscle is different in many respects from skeletal muscle. Early physiologists thought that cardiac muscle was syncytial, that is, a mass of protoplasm that acted as a unit with numerous nuclei. The muscle is not syncytial in structure (even thought it appears to function as two syncytia), but it is made up of separate muscle fibers joined by surface connections called *intercalated discs*. These discs run transversely across the fibers, and are areas of low electrical resistance which allow the rapid spread of excitation from cell to cell. Another difference in cardiac muscle is the location of the nuclei. They are deep within the interior of the fiber instead of beneath the sarcolemma as in skeletal muscle. Also, the fibers of cardiac muscle are shaped differently from fibers in other muscle. The fibers are not simple cylindrical units, but they bifurcate and connect with adjoining fibers to form complex three-dimensional networks (see Fig. 2–1a).

One of the most interesting characteristics of cardiac muscle is its ability to beat rhythmically without external stimuli of any kind. The part of the heart with the most rapid inherent rhythm causes depolarization throughout the rest of the heart. In man, this is the *sinoatrial node (SA node)*, which is commonly called the *pacemaker* of the heart. The SA node is composed of a small mass of specialized myocardial tissue embedded in the atrial mass near the entrance of the superior vena cava. The spontaneous signal which originates in the SA node spreads in all directions at about 1 m/second throughout the right and left atria. This wave of excitation is delayed at the atrioventricular (AV) node for about 0.08 to 0.12 sec to allow the ventricles to fill, then proceeds through the *bundle of His* where it is carried into the left and right bundle branches (Fig. 4–1). These branches are composed of specialized cardiac muscle called *Purkinje's fibers*, which carry the depolarization wave to the interior of the ventricular chambers at about 4 to 5 m/second. The endocardial surfaces are excited rapidly and are the first to contract, but the excitation spreads rapidly to the epicardial surfaces and yields a more or less simultaneous contraction of the ventricular muscle.

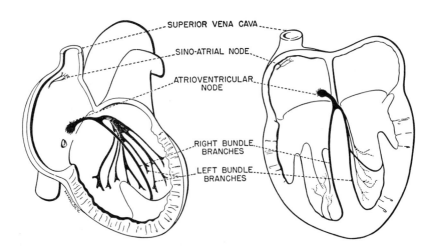

Figure 4–1. Conduction system of the heart. The sinoatrial node is the normal pacemaker of the heart. No specialized conduction system has been described in the atria. The AV node, common bundle, and bundle branches conduct the wave of excitation from the atrium to the ventricular myocardium. (Rushmer, R. F.: *Structure and Function of the Cardiovascular System*, 2nd ed. Philadelphia: W. B. Saunders Co., 1976, page 87.)

If a section of heart muscle is removed from an animal and cut into pieces, each piece will have its own inherent rhythm. As a result of certain pathological conditions, other areas of the heart sometimes become more excitable than the pacemaker and drive the cardiac system at a different rate or with a poor rhythm. Warming of the pacemaker of the heart will increase the rate of depolarization of the entire heart muscle, whereas cooling of the pacemaker will cause an opposite effect.

Cardiac muscle also is different from skeletal muscle in that each cell

POTENTIALS IN SINGLE MYOCARDIAL FIBERS

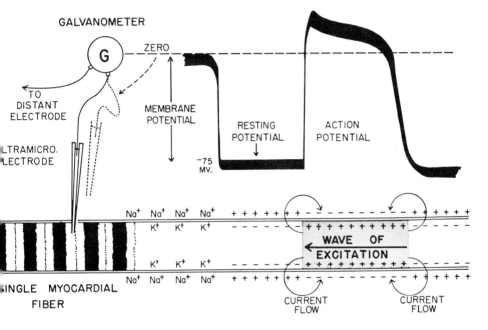

Figure 4–2. Potentials between the inside and outside of myocardial cells can be measured directly with an ultramicroscopic electrode consisting of a thin glass tube drawn out to a very fine tip (less than 0.5 μm) and filled with a solution of potassium chloride. The potential difference recorded when the electrode is inserted into the cell amounts to about 75 mV. This potential is due to a difference between the concentrations of ions (mainly Na^+ and K^+) inside and outside of the cell, so that the inside of the cell is negative (−) in relation to the outside. As a wave of excitation passes over the fiber, an action potential is recorded; the potential rapidly approaches zero and overshoots (reversed polarity of the membrane). The resting potential is restored gradually at first and then rapidly during the later stages of the repolarization process. (Rushmer, R. F.: *Structure and Function of the Cardiovascular System*, 2nd ed. Philadelphia: W. B. Saunders Co., 1976, page 283.)

is able to increase its contractile force. Skeletal muscle contracts in accordance with the all-or-none law, and increased force of contraction occurs primarily as a result of increasing the number of motor units (and therefore the number of cells) that contract at any given time. However, since each cardiac muscle cell contracts each time the heart beats, it is important to have the capability of increasing the force of contraction of each cell. The increase in contractile force is related to an increased calcium flux through the cardiac muscle cell membrane. There is no doubt that calcium is the coupler in both skeletal and cardiac muscle. There are major differences, however, in the way that calcium is handled by the two tissues. For example, perfusion of heart muscle with solutions containing zero calcium results in immediate decreases in tension. In skeletal muscle, the same decreases in tension take 20 min or more. In any case, the location of the calcium coupler in heart is more superficial on the cell and calcium is much more rapidly exchangeable than in skeletal muscle. This concept has been poorly understood for years, but explains the increased inotropic effect (force of contraction) which is observed during exercise and following the administration of drugs such as digoxin or epinephrine (Adrenalin).[3]

The action potential of cardiac muscle is also different from that of skeletal muscle (Fig. 4-2). Note the plateau on the cardiac muscle potential. This long refractory period protects the heart from premature contraction and will not allow the heart to tetanize under normal situations. Although tetany is a normal phenomenon in skeletal muscle, the heart would be unable to pump if it were tetanized.

CARDIAC CYCLE

The cardiac cycle is helpful to an understanding of heart functions. The vertical lines in Figure 4-3 help relate the electrical activity, the sound recordings, and the pressure changes that occur during a complete cycle of contraction. Notice that the first and second heart sounds are related to the closure of the atrioventricular (AV) valves and the aortic and pulmonic valves. Remember that smooth flowing blood makes no sound. As the valves close, turbulence is created, which results in the "lubb-dupp" heard through a stethoscope. The phonocardiogram merely records the sound of that turbulence related to the valve closures.

The valves themselves respond to the changes in pressure within the heart. As the ventricles relax, the AV valves open and allow the blood in the atria to pour in. This yields the rapid and slow filling phases of the volume curve shown in Figure 4-3. As the ventricles contract, the pressure rise forces the AV valves to close (yielding heart sound 1) and directs the flow to the aorta or pulmonary artery. However, no flow can occur into these major arteries until the ventricles overcome the

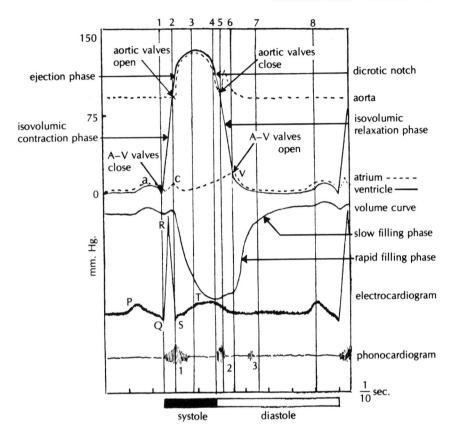

Figure 4–3. The cardiac cycle. Superimposed curves of ventricular, auricular, and aortic pressures, together with a ventricular volume curve, an electrocardiogram, and a phonocardiogram. (Best, C. H., and Taylor, N. B.: *The Physiological Basis of Medical Practice*, 3rd ed. Baltimore: Williams & Wilkins, 1943.)

pressure in these systems. Figure 4–3 also shows the pressures in the left heart. Note that no flow occurs until the ventricle exerts about 80 mm Hg of pressure, which is the systemic pressure of the aorta. The contraction phase from zero pressure to systemic pressure is called the *isometric* or, more properly, the *isovolumic contraction phase* of the heart. The same phenomenon would be observed in the right heart, except the systemic pressure would be only 18 to 20 mm Hg.

When ventricular pressure reaches and slightly exceeds systemic pressure, the aortic (and pulmonic) valve opens and blood pours rapidly into the system. This phase is called the *ejection phase*. At rest, the pressure in the left heart reaches about 120 mm Hg, which is the systolic blood pressure. This pressure may rise to 200 mm Hg during heavy work. As the ventricles relax, the pressure decreases rapidly, and the aortic or pulmonic valves close as systemic pressure returns. The isovolumic relaxation phase follows the closure of the aortic or pulmonic valves and is terminated as the AV valves open once again to fill the relaxed ventricle.

Note the dicrotic notch as the aortic valve closes (Fig. 4–3). This is associated with the rebound action of blood in the aorta. Astrand refers to the aorta as a "windkessel vessel" because of its ability to distend as it fills with blood and then to propel the blood into the arterial tree after the aortic valve closes.[2] This action keeps the hydraulic energy level near the heart continuously high instead of permitting great variations in pressure which would occur if the tube were rigid.

The third heart sound is associated with the rapid filling phase of the ventricle immediately following AV valve opening. The ventricle fills rapidly after emptying. Increasing the heart rate has little effect on filling even at the high heart rates associated with exercise.

It should be noted that the atria have little effect on ventricular filling during rest. However, during work, atrial contraction does aid the filling process.

An electrocardiogram is the recording of electrical activity of the heart during the cycle. The P wave is associated with atrial contraction. The QRS complex is indicative of the large ventricular contraction and hides the repolarization of the atria. The T wave is ventricular repolarization. Knowing how each wave is associated with a contractile process will help to clarify the activity of the cardiac cycle, and these relationships should be studied until they are understood.

CARDIAC FUNCTION

Many attempts have been made to assess cardiac function. Starling and associates subjected the exposed heart of an anesthetized dog to various volume and pressure manipulations.[9] These studies resulted in what has commonly been referred to as "Starling's law of the heart." According to Starling, the normal response to either a greater volume load or a greater pressure load is an increase in both the diastolic and systolic ventricular volumes. Although many of his ideas are sound, the idea that the heart gets larger and larger as stroke volume increases is probably incorrect. Later investigators, using sophisticated equipment for measuring heart size during work, have found no such increase. Apparently, hearts exposed under the conditions of Starling's experiments tend to decrease drastically in size. Pressure and volume manipulations in these preparations caused an increase in size out of proportion to those of intact hearts.

It is now clear that the ventricles normally are maximally distended in the resting recumbent person and in the person who is exercising. Quiet standing decreases the distention of the ventricles.[10] Of course, the size variations are related to the volume of blood returned to the heart (venous return), which is maximal during supine rest and during exercise.

Sarnoff and Mitchell performed experiments that led to "cardiac function curves."[12] These curves showed the "length-tension" or "pressure-volume" relationship of cardiac muscle under various conditions of filling and state of myocardial contraction. These relationships also have been studied by using samples of myocardium, particularly papillary muscles, in which the fibers are nearly parallel in orientation and are more easily studied. Although these curves may not completely represent the functional characteristics of myocardium, they are extremely helpful to an understanding of this function.

Figure 4–4 shows a simple cardiac function curve. Notice that muscle performance is altered (1) by change in initial muscle length and (2) by changes in the contractile state of the muscle. The initial length of the fibers is a product of increased or decreased venous return, which yields a larger or smaller volume as plotted on the passive pressure-volume line. The amount of blood returned is designated A (small return), B, and C (large venous return). Notice that the increased venous return causes the line to rise, indicating an increase

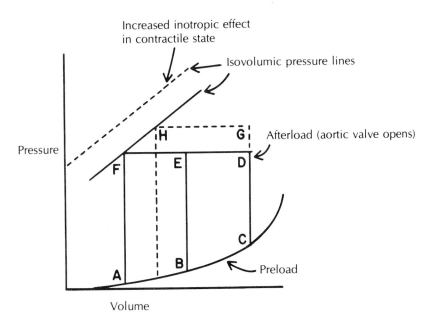

Figure 4–4.   Cardiac function curve. (See text for discussion.)

in passive pressure with the increased filling. The isovolumic pressure line represents the force of myocardial contraction. It is plotted by filling the ventricle to some given volume, clamping the aorta, and plotting the pressure (isometric) exerted by the myocardium under that condition. Of course, with the aorta clamped, no flow occurs and the pressure rise is plotted for each increasing volume to form the isovolumic pressure line. If the muscle contracts with more force, a new isovolumic pressure line would result, which would be above the old line.

Cardiac performance can be plotted on the cardiac function curve using the following terms;

1. Preload—initial length of the fibers as a result of venous return.
2. Afterload—the load that the heart works against. This is the pressure in the aorta and is the point at which the aortic valve opens.
3. Contractile state—the vigor of the cardiac contraction, which depends on calcium flux within the individual cardiac fibers.

With a large venous return (preload) to point C, the heart contracts. The pressure in the heart rises until the aortic valve opens. At this point, the blood flows into the aorta and continues to flow until the isovolumic pressure line is reached (point F) and pressure returns to point A, where filling once again commences. If the subject were to stand, the venous return would be decreased (say, to point B). At the same aortic pressure, the pressure would rise to point E, and a decreased volume (point E to point F) would result. An increase in aortic pressure (point G) would also decrease the amount of blood pushed out, since the volume would flow only to point H.

This curve explains why stroke volume, or the amount of blood pumped each beat, decreases with standing and increases with exercise. With exercise, the isovolumic pressure line rises because of the increased force of contraction caused by sympathetic activity. At any given venous return, the stroke volume increases because the emptying continues until the new isovolumic pressure line is reached.

CARDIAC OUTPUT

Cardiac output is the amount of blood ejected by one ventricle in 1 min, and can be abbreviated as C.O. or $\dot{Q}$. (The dot over the "Q" is a shorthand way of indicating a *unit time* function and is placed over many symbols relating to physiology.) Normal cardiac output at rest is about 5 l/minute (for adults), and can increase to 40 l/minute in well-trained athletes during intensive work. The amount of blood that can be expelled is probably the most important limiting factor in heavy work.

Cardiac output is the result of two factors: *heart rate* (the number of times the heart beats each minute) and *stroke volume* (the amount of blood ejected from the heart each time it beats). Because of the importance of these two factors to performance, they will be discussed separately.

HEART RATE. The natural rhythm of the SA node is influenced by the balance between the slowing effect of the parasympathetic (vagus) nerve and the accelerating effects of the sympathetic (accelerator) nerves. The parasympathetic nerves are distributed mainly to the pacemaker, the AV bundle, and the atria.

Stimulation of the *parasympathetic (vagus) nerve* to the heart causes a release of acetylcholine (ACh) from the nerve endings. Acetylcholine has two major effects on the heart muscle: (1) it decreases the depolarization sequence of the pacemaker, and (2) it slows the transmission velocity of the delay circuit around the AV bundle, which slows the impulse into the ventricles. The result is a slower heart rate, but there is little effect upon the strength of the beats.

Stimulation of the *sympathetic (accelerator) nerves* to the heart releases norepinephrine at the nerve endings. The sympathetic nerves on the right side of the heart apparently converge on the SA node to act on the pacemaker, while the sympathetic nerves on the left are more widely distributed to the atrial and ventricular myocardium. The effects of this stimulation tend to (1) increase the discharge at the pacemaker, and (2) increase the excitability of the cardiac muscle, which increases the force of contraction of the whole heart.

The heart rate tends to be kept in correct balance by the constant slowing effects of the parasympathetic nervous system and the accelerating effects of the sympathetic nervous system. If both sets of nerves are cut, the heart rate increases. In cardiac transplant patients in whom nervous influences are not a factor, the resting heart rate is about 100 beats/minute.

There are areas in the medulla of the brain with a profound effect upon cardiac function. The areas that cause an increase in function are referred to as *cardioaccelerator centers,* and those causing a decrease in function are *cardioinhibitory centers.* Reciprocal innervation between these areas provides a means whereby excitation of one set of fibers results in inhibition of the other. These areas are affected by a number of sources classified as either *pressor* or *depressor.* Some of the pressors are described below: (1) Higher centers in the CNS have powerful effects on cardiovascular function, as evidenced by the great increase in heart rate during frightening experiences or before an athletic contest. (2) Stimulation of the adrenal medulla causes a release of the hormones norepinephrine and epinephrine into the blood stream. The effects of these hormones are almost the same as direct sympathetic stimulation (acceleration), except the effects last much longer. (3) There is some evidence that heart rate is increased by the movement of the legs or arms, possibly through muscle spindle excitation. (4) Impulses arising in the *carotid body* and *aortic body* as a result of decreased pH or increased P_{CO_2} cause an increase in heart rate.

The main source of depressor activity results from stretch receptors in the aortic arch and the carotid sinus, which are sensitive to increased pressure in the arterial system. The feedback from these receptors tends to decrease heart rate.

It should be pointed out that the heart is able to adjust to increased activity without the help of innervation through intrinsic autoregulation. Donald et al.[4] found that denervated dogs had almost no change in capacity to do work. Heart transplant patients who are also denervated are able to increase their heart rates by 50% or so during exercise stress tests, going from a resting heart rate of about 100 beats/minute to about 150 beats/minute. It is postulated that the increased stretch of the fibers owing to higher pressure of returning blood could cause an increased membrane permeability and, therefore, an increase in the depolarization rate of the membrane.

STROKE VOLUME.   The amount of blood forced out one ventricle with each beat of the heart is the stroke volume. The stroke volume varies within certain limits, and the variations relate to such things as changes in body position and work load. The amount of blood forced out of the ventricle during work is, of course, limited by the size of the ventricle. The left ventricle of a normal subject contains about 75 ml (± 15 ml)/square meter of body surface area at the end of diastole (filling).[10]

The smallest stroke volume probably occurs in an erect, standing position. This is also the position in which the heart functions at its smallest size. The heart probably functions at its greatest size during supine rest and during work. However, greatest stroke volume occurs during work because of the increased vigor and strength of the ventricular contraction, which yields a more complete emptying of the ventricle. The fact that increased power of contraction is the most important adjustment mechanism for increased stroke volume rather than increased size was graphically shown by Rushmer, who found that the size of a dog's ventricle was not increased during work.[11] Changes in ventricular dimensions are difficult to monitor in man during exercise. However, when silver-tantalum clips were attached to the walls of the right and left ventricles to measure changes in ventricular length, high speed x-ray photographs showed no increase in these dimensions during exercise.[10]

Prior to exercise, the stroke volume of most subjects is between 50% and 75% of the maximum they can reach. As exercise begins, stroke volume increases and continues to increase with increasing work loads

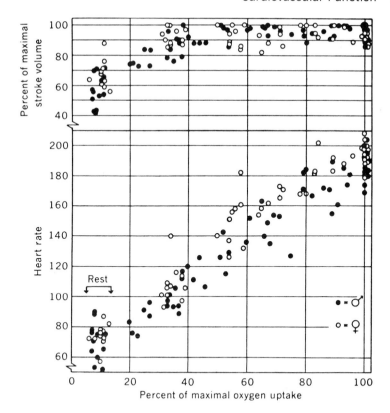

Figure 4–5. Stroke volume in percent of the individual's maximum, and heart rate at rest and during exercise. The oxygen uptake on the abscissa is expressed in percent of the subject's maximum. Circled dot at "100 percent" represents 11 of the 23 subjects. Measurements were made with the subjects in the sitting position. (From *Textbook of Work Physiology* by Astrand and Rodahl. Copyright © 1970 by McGraw-Hill, Inc. Used with permission of McGraw-Hill Book Company.)

until the work reaches about 40% of the maximum the subject can reach (Fig. 4–5). At this point, with a heart rate of about 110 to 120 beats/minute, the stroke volume is maximal and does not increase further as work continues to increase. Even though the systolic filling time decreases significantly, there is no tendency for a decrease in stroke volume at maximal work.

What causes the changes in stroke volume? Four factors are routinely listed: (1) effective filling pressure, (2) distensibility of the ventricles, (3) contractility, and (4) the systemic pressure.

Filling pressure and distensibility of the ventricles are related to Starling's law. There is no doubt that cardiac muscle demonstrates a length-tension relationship which makes the muscles more efficient with the increased tension of returning blood. Asmussen and Christensen elevated the legs of their subjects for about 10 min and then put pressure cuffs around the thighs to maintain a large venous return to the heart.[1] Even though the heart rate was decreased, the cardiac output was about 30% higher because of the increased efficiency of the heart. The effects of decreased volume of blood returned to the heart can be seen easily by performing Valsalva's maneuver, such as lifting a heavy weight while holding the breath. Because of the decreased volume of blood returning to the heart, the heart rate increases rapidly to maintain cardiac output. Conversely, recovery can be hastened after exercise by lying down or by moving around to aid the venous system to return the blood to the heart.

Contractility is the change in ventricular performance which causes the ventricles to produce more force per unit of time (dp/dt). Fortunately, increased force is a routine adjustment with increased heart rate as a response to appropriate stimulation. In addition to causing the ventricles to empty more completely, this factor also yields greater time for diastolic filling because the systolic stroke is completed much more quickly.

The importance of systemic pressure is obvious. If systemic pressure were increased to equal contraction pressure, no blood could leave the heart. Endurance athletes often experience a decrease in systemic pressure during high work levels. This decrease, along with the increase in contractile strength of the ventricle, allows a large stroke volume adjustment.

The role of stroke volume in the performance of endurance activities cannot be overstressed. There is a clear relationship between maximal aerobic work and cardiac output. What many persons fail to realize is that, to a large extent, stroke volume determines the limits of cardiac output, because almost everyone has about the same heart rate parameters. Thus, stroke volume is the primary difference between a person with great cardiac output and one with only average output (Fig. 4–6).

CALCULATION OF CARDIAC OUTPUT. Cardiac output can be calculated using either the direct Fick method or the dye method. Both methods involve advanced laboratory techniques, but the principles should be understood by each student.

Fick Method. Catheters must be inserted into the heart to sample both arterial and venous blood. At the same time, expired air is collected and analyzed to measure oxygen consumption ($\dot{V}O_2$). Cardiac output is computed using the formula:

$$\dot{Q} = \dot{V}O_2 \div a\text{–}v\ O_2\ \text{diff.}$$

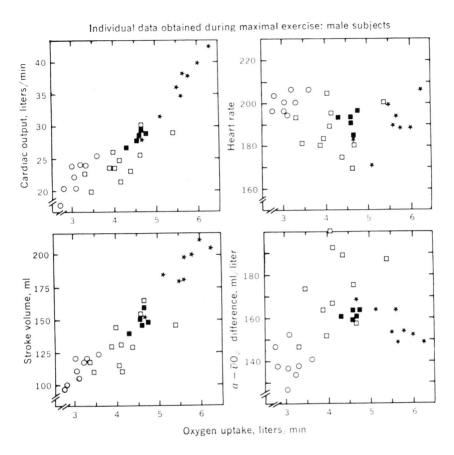

Figure 4–6. Cardiac output, heart rate, stroke volume, and arteriovenous oxygen difference during maximal exercise in relation to maximal oxygen uptake in top athletes who were very successful in endurance events (stars), well-trained but less successful athletes (filled squares), and 25-year-old habitually sedentary subjects (unfilled circles). (Astrand, P.-O., and Rodahl, K.: *Textbook of Work Physiology.* New York: McGraw-Hill Book Co., 1970.)

For example, if $\dot{V}O_2$ is measured at 250 ml/minute and the difference between the oxygen content of arterial and venous blood is 50 ml/liter, the cardiac output would be 5 l/minute (250 ml/min ÷ 50 ml/l = 5 l/min).

Dye Method. A quantity of dye is injected into a vein as near to the heart as possible. Samples are drawn from a systemic artery, and the concentration of the dye in the arterial blood is plotted on a curve (Fig. 4–7). Notice that the dye begins to be recirculated before the dye curve

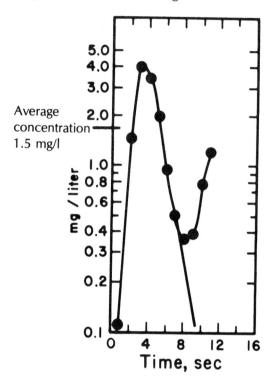

Figure 4–7.   Dye concentration curve for measuring cardiac output.

reaches zero, so the curve must be extrapolated to zero by the researcher. Cardiac output is computed from Figure 4–7 using the formula:

$$\dot{Q} = \frac{I}{C \times t}$$

where I is the amount of dye injected, in milligrams; C is the average concentration of dye; and t is the time it takes for the dye to pass through the artery. Assume that 5 mg of dye were used and that the average concentration is 1.5 mg/liter. Compute cardiac output with the dye curve extrapolated to 10 sec.

$$\dot{Q} = \frac{5 \text{ mg}}{\dfrac{1.5 \text{ mg}}{1} \times \dfrac{10}{60}}$$

Remember that the time should be expressed in number of seconds over 60 so that the answer will be in liters/minute. Rearranging the formula:

$$\dot{Q} = 5 \text{ mg} \times \frac{1}{1.5 \text{ mg}} \times \frac{60}{10} = 20 \text{ l/min cardiac output}$$

This would be a typical dye dilution curve during work.

CIRCULATION

One of the important factors in the ability to do intense work is the amount of blood circulated past the cells. The factors that affect circulation are discussed in this section.

Vascular System

Blood vessels can be classified as arteries, arterioles, capillaries, venules, and veins. True capillaries are thin-walled endothelial tubes with no muscle or fibrous tissue. The rest of the vessels also have an internal endothelial layer but are reinforced by networks of elastic fibers, smooth muscle, fibroblasts, and collagenous fibers to a varying extent, depending upon the size and function of the vessel.

Arteries are large vessels that carry blood away from the heart and act as pressure tanks or "windkessel vessels" during the systolic ejection phase. They have large diameters and low resistance, with the ability to absorb the great increases in pressure near the heart, and then to convert these pressures to continuous flow throughout the system.

Arterioles are small vessels between the arteries and capillaries. They have a high resistance to flow, which causes a large drop in pressure at this location in the system. Much of the control of blood flow to the various tissues is brought about by adjustments in the diameters of the arterioles. It is important that constriction of one arteriolar tree is balanced by the relaxation of another.

Capillaries are the "nuts-and-bolts" structure of the vascular system. True capillaries are only about 1 mm long and hardly large enough for red blood cells to pass through. The capillary wall is composed of thin endothelial cells with no muscle or elastic fibers. This structure is important because it is through the walls of the capillaries that diffusion occurs to feed the cells and to remove waste materials from them. Capillaries are often arranged in parallel-coupled circuits with preferential channels from which other capillaries branch. The branching capillaries may have a group of muscle fibers forming precapillary *sphincters* at the origin of the capillary. These sphincters are controlled by the metabolic activity of the cells they feed and not by nervous information from the brain. Other capillary beds may have no preferen-

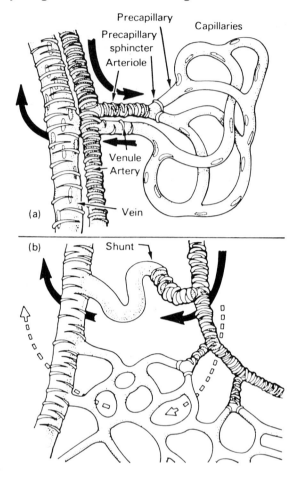

Figure 4–8.   Precapillary sphincter regulating capillary flow or shunting. (Elias, H., and Pauly, J. E.: *Human Microanatomy.* Philadelphia: F. A. Davis, 1966, pp. 114, 126.)

tial channels nor precapillary sphincters. Still other tissue areas are supplied by arteriovenous shunts which bypass capillary beds until the tissues in the bed need supply (Fig. 4–8).

Venules (small veins) connect the capillaries to the larger veins. Blood entering the venules is used blood, high in carbon dioxide and low in oxygen, which is being returned to the heart.

Veins are the larger vessels that carry the blood from venules to the heart. In progressing back to the heart, the *veins* gradually increase in caliber and their walls become thicker.

There are more veins and venules than arteries and arterioles, and the veins and venules are larger than their counterparts. For this reason, more than 60% of the blood is normally contained in the veins and venules during rest.

Valves are found in most veins of the extremities to aid the return of blood to the heart. As the veins are compressed by the muscles, the blood is forced toward the heart and is prevented by the valves from draining back.

Blood and Body Fluids

The body contains a great deal of water. The purpose of this water is to provide a fluid medium for the processes that must be carried on to maintain life. The relationship between total water and lean body tissue is quite constant, with total water being about 72% of the total lean body mass (there are techniques using this relationship for determining total lean body mass).

The body's water can be divided into three different areas: (1) intracellular fluid, which includes all fluid within the cells; (2) interstitial fluid, which includes all fluid outside of the cells, but not in the blood vessels; and (3) intravascular fluid, which is the fluid within the vascular system itself.

Extracellular fluid is all fluid outside of the cells (both interstitial and intravascular) and is similar to sea water in composition, although much weaker in concentration. The fluid inside the cells is quite different from the fluid outside the cells in terms of ionic concentration. This difference was discussed in Chapter 3 under membrane potential, and is the result of the active work of the cell membrane to maintain a resting membrane potential.

The purpose of blood is to carry nutrients and oxygen to the cells, and to remove waste products and carbon dioxide from them. There is approximately 5 to 6 l of blood in average size men and about 4 to 4.5 l of blood in average size women. The red blood cells (RBCs) carry hemoglobin (Hb), an iron-containing protein which can carry oxygen and carbon dioxide in a loose, reversible chemical combination. Normal Hb levels are 15.8 gm/100 ml of blood in men and about 14 gm/100 ml of blood in women. Each gram of Hb can carry about 1.34 ml of oxygen. It is easy to see that men do have an advantage in the amount of oxygen carried per 100 ml of blood (21.17 ml O_2 for men; 18.76 ml O_2 for women). This increased volume of oxygen is a significant factor in oxidative energy production and cannot be ignored.

There are about 5.6 million RBCs/cubic millimeter in man and about 4.8 million RBCs/cubic millimeter in women. The RBC-fluid ratio, or percent RBC, is called hematocrit (Hct). Men normally have hematocrit levels of 44 to 48, and women, of 39 to 45. Low Hct levels would

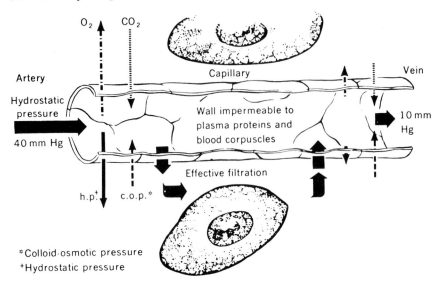

Figure 4–9. Movement of fluid out of the capillary due to hydrostatic pressure as balanced by movement of fluid in the opposite direction due to colloid-osmotic pressure. (From *Textbook of Work Physiology* by Astrand and Rodahl, page 157. Copyright © 1977 by McGraw-Hill, Inc. Used with permission of McGraw-Hill Book Company.)

decrease the work capacity of a person. High levels of Htc are often found in subjects acclimatized to high altitude, in whom increases in the percent RBC are common.

It should be mentioned that the total fluid in the vascular beds is maintained by the osmotic pressure of the plasma proteins, which tend to balance the filtration pressure of the fluid in the vessels from the pressure within the vessel (Fig. 4–9). Notice that the hydrostatic pressure is greater than the osmotic pressure at the proximal end, but less than the osmotic pressure at the distal end. It is easy to understand tissue edema caused by heart failure in terms of this concept. For instance, if the left heart is unable to maintain its pump responsibilities, the pressure at the distal end of the pulmonary capillaries rises, which causes a net outflow of fluid. This tissue fluid results in pulmonary edema.

Physics of Blood Flow

The often-used analogy of the circulatory system resembling a system of water pipes is meaningful but somewhat misleading. Water pipes act as passive carriers of fluid, whereas the blood vessels are active participants in the adjustments made by the body under various circumstances. Without the adjustments made by the blood vessels to direct blood to areas of increased need, athletes would be unable to exercise.

Blood flows through the vessels as a result of a pressure gradient. If two garden hoses were hooked together and attached to separate taps, no flow would occur. Only when there is a pressure difference is there a flow of fluid. In the circulatory system, the point of highest pressure occurs in the left ventricle (usually about 120 mm Hg at rest), and the difference between this pressure and the pressure at the right atrium (between 0 and 5 mm Hg at rest) causes blood to flow throughout the body.

Since the circulatory system is a *closed* system, the same volume of blood must pass through the various sections of the system per unit of time. Thus, the velocity of the blood at a particular point depends on the total cross-sectional area of the vascular system at that point. The capillary system is about 700 times as large in total cross-sectional area as is the aorta. Therefore, the blood velocity is much slower in the capillary beds than in the aorta. Of course, this is important to the system because of the need for diffusion of gases between the capillaries and the cells. The formula which explains this relationship is:

$$\text{Velocity of flow} = \frac{\text{Blood flow}}{\text{Diameter}^2 \text{ (cross-sectional area)}}$$

The resistance to blood flow results from the friction between the blood and the vessel walls. The nearer the blood is to the center of the vessel, the less resistance it encounters and the faster it flows. This flow pattern is referred to as *laminar flow*. Because of this phenomenon, the *radius* of the vessel is of great importance to the volume of blood which can flow through the vessel. The resistance to flow of the vessel is related to the radius to the fourth power. This means that a reduction of the radius to one-half its original size would decrease the volume of flow to one-sixteenth the original flow if all other factors remain constant. This helps to explain how the body is able to direct blood from one area to another with only a small change in vessel size.

The theory of *hemodynamics*, the factors that affect blood flow, is summarized by the Poiseuille-Hagen formula:

$$F = \Delta P \times \frac{\pi}{8} \times \frac{1}{n} \times \frac{r^4}{l}$$

This formula states that the blood flow (F) is proportional to the force or pressure difference (ΔP) and vessel radius to the fourth power, and inversely proportional to the viscosity or thickness of the blood (n) and the length of the vessel (l). Since we can do little about vessel length or blood viscosity, it is easy to see that pressure change and vessel size are by far the most important factors for increasing flow.

Systemic Pressure

As mentioned previously, the pressure within the left ventricle varies from zero to about 120 mm Hg each cardiac cycle. Because of the nature of the large arterial vessels, pressure is maintained within the arterial system without such a drastic change (Fig. 4–10). Normal systemic pressure at rest is 120/80 mm Hg. This means that the heart is exerting enough pressure to push a column of mercury 120 mm up an evacuated

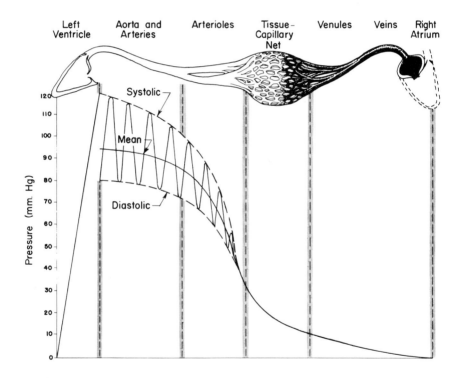

Figure 4–10. Blood pressure differential along the systemic vascular tree. Blood always flows from an area of high pressure to one of low pressure. Note also that the pressure (and thus the flow of blood) fluctuates in the arteries and arterioles, but that it is steady in the capillaries. Systolic pressure is the highest pressure obtained, diastolic the lowest; the average of the two is the mean arterial pressure. (Mathews, K. D., and Fox, E. L.: *The Physiological Basis of Physical Education and Athletics.* Philadelphia: W. B. Saunders Co., 1976, page 242.)

tube and that the residual pressure in the vessel would push that same column 80 mm up the tube. This pressure is measured on the upper arm using a sphygmomanometer or pressure cuff at the same level as the heart. The cuff is inflated until the flow of blood through the artery is stopped (usually to 180 mm or so). The pressure is then slowly released until the pumping pressure of the heart equals the constrictive pressure of the cuff. When this occurs, the blood flow through the tightly constricted vessel can be heard with a stethoscope. As the pressure is further decreased, the sound of the blood flow changes to a low, quiet thump, and finally disappears. Remember that blood flowing through a vessel cannot normally be heard unless the vessel wall is constricted to cause a disruption of the smooth flow of the vessel. The disappearance of sound is commonly called *diastolic pressure*.

During exercise, the systolic pressure rises with work at about 10 mm Hg per MET increase (see Chapter 1 for a discussion of MET). The diastolic pressure usually stays about the same or decreases with work as the vessels open in the active muscles. An increase in diastolic pressure would indicate maladjustment to exercise, and levels of 100 mm Hg would be ground for stopping an exercise test.

The peripheral resistance to flow is decreased during work as the muscle capillary beds open, but the elevated cardiac output causes the blood pressure to rise. This relationship is expressed in the formula:

$$R = P/F$$

where R is resistance units, P is the pressure pushing the blood, and F equals the flow of blood in liters per minute. Resistance at rest is equal to about 20 resistance units (100 mm mean pressure/5 l/min Q) but decreases during work to 6 or so (120 mm mean pressure/20 l/min Q).

Measuring blood pressure during work is difficult, especially in running subjects. Exercise blood pressure can be measured in walking subjects after a little practice, and older subjects who are poorly conditioned or postcardiac patients must be monitored during graded exercise stress tests. Sometimes the diastolic sounds can be heard all the way down to zero during an exercise or in recovery. This is caused by the rebound action of the blood in the vessel and is not necessarily a cause for alarm. This blood pressure is usually recorded as 180/90–0, indicating a systolic pressure of 180 mm, the change in sound from bright to dull at 90 mm, and that the dull sound could be heard all the way to zero.

Arterial blood pressure is significantly higher in arm exercise than in leg work because the cardiac output is forced into the smaller muscle beds of the arms instead of those of the legs. This is why it is dangerous for cardiac patients to shovel snow or do other work that requires use of their arms only. There is also a powerful cardiovascular reflex associated with sustained static muscle contraction. This pressor response is largely independent of the muscle bulk involved, and is just as strong with arm-muscle work as with leg-muscle work, if the same percent of maximum force is used. This reflex is most often noticed in cardiac patients who carry a suitcase (sustained contraction in the forearm) and causes a significant increase in blood pressure and heart rate. It also increases the myocardial oxygen need, which may lead to angina (chest pain) or other cardiac aberrations.

Hydrostatic pressure, or the pressure of the blood because of gravity, is an important consideration in exercise. When a normal man is standing, the column of blood from the heart to the feet exerts about 85 to 100 mm pressure. This pressure, plus the pressure of the heart, will yield measured pressures of 175 to 200 mm Hg at the ankle. Luckily, the veins of the legs with their one-way valves are able to act as a pump when squeezed rhythmically by the muscles of the legs. After only one or two steps this muscle pump mechanism significantly decreases the blood pressure in the ankles to about 90 to 100 mm Hg. This mechanism is important in several ways. (1) It drastically lowers the venous and capillary pressures, reducing the effective filtration pressure. (2) It reduces the volume of blood within the veins of the leg and allows that blood to be used by the body. (3) It accelerates the flow of blood back to the heart, which helps maintain venous return and allows stroke volume to be maintained. The pump is so effective that the venous abdominal pressure has been measured at about 22 mm Hg during exertion.[9] It has been calculated that at least 30% of the total systemic circulatory work during running must be done by the pumping action of the musculature in the legs. Understanding this concept helps explain why it is so necessary to cool off slowly following heavy work, and why persons who stop suddenly or who stand for long periods without moving may faint from lack of blood to the brain.

Control of Circulation

Since there is potentially much more room in the circulatory system than there is blood in the system, some control must be exerted to direct blood to areas of need and to reduce its flow to other areas.

The major control of blood flow is under the direction of the sympathetic nervous system, which has both cholinergic vasodilator fibers and adrenergic vasoconstrictor fibers. The arterioles feeding skeletal muscles are under the control of sympathetic vasodilator fibers which release acetylcholine (ACh) and allow the smooth muscle of the vessels to dilate. The arterioles to the skin and gut are under the control of adrenergic sympathetic fibers which restrict the flow of blood to these areas, so that increased supply is available to the muscles.

Capillaries in the muscle tissue open in response to local metabolic demand of the cells, to allow blood to flow freely into the areas of greatest need. It should be remembered that active dilation cannot occur. The pressure of the blood in the system opens vessels that are relaxed.

The regulation of circulation during exercise is a complex series of events. The changes that must occur are initiated from the brain and affect many functions. The increase in sympathetic activity probably reciprocally decreases parasympathetic activity which allows the heart (pump) to increase both rate and force. The skeletal muscles also begin to receive a larger share of the circulation because of their innervation with sympathetic cholinergic vasodilator fibers, which opens the vessels near the increasingly active muscle cells. The capillary beds open in response to the increased metabolic activity and allow an increased flow of blood past each cell. At the same time, the flow of blood to the gut and other organs is decreased by the action of the sympathetic adrenergic vasoconstrictor fibers, and the veins constrict and increase their pumping action owing to the contraction of the working muscles, which increases venous return. Later, as heat is produced, the vessels of the skin open and blood flow increases to that area to aid the cooling process. Through this series of actions, the cardiac output is increased and the circulation is adjusted to pump the blood where it is needed most.

SELECTED REFERENCES

1. Asmussen, E., and Christensen, E. H.: Einfluss der Blutverteilung auf den Kreislanf bei Korperlicker Arbeit. *Skand. Arch. Physiol.*, 82:185, 1939.
2. Astrand, P.-O., and Rodahl, K.: *Textbook of Work Physiology.* New York: McGraw-Hill Book Co., 1970.
3. Berne, R. M., and Leng, M. N.: *Cardiovascular Physiology*, 2nd ed. St. Louis: C. V. Mosby Co., 1972.
4. DeVries, H. A.: *Physiology of Exercise for Physical Education and Athletics*, 2nd ed. Dubuque: Wm. C. Brown Co., 1974.
5. Donald, D. E., et al.: Effect of cardiac denervation on the maximal capacity for exercise in the racing greyhound. *J. Appl. Physiol.*, 19:849, 1964.
6. Guyton, A. C.: *Textbook of Medical Physiology*, 4th ed. Philadelphia: W. B. Saunders Co., 1971.
7. Karpovich, P. V., and Sinning, N. E.: *Physiology of Muscular Activity*, 7th ed. Philadelphia: W. B. Saunders Co., 1971.
8. Morehouse, L. E., and Miller, A. T.: *Physiology of Exercise*, 7th ed. St. Louis: C. V. Mosby Co., 1976.
9. Patterson, S. W., Piper, H., and Starling, E. H.: The regulation of the heartbeat. *J. Physiol.* (Lond.), 48:465, 1914.
10. Rushmer, R. F.: *Structure and Function of the Cardiovascular System*, 2nd ed. Philadelphia: W. B. Saunders Co., 1976.
11. Rushmer, R. F., Smith, D. A., Jr., and Franklin, D. L.: Mechanisms of cardiac control in exercise. *Circ. Res.*, 7:605, 1959.

12. Sarnoff, S. J., and Mitchell, J. H.: The control of the function of the heart. In *Handbook of Physiology*, section 2, *Circulation*, Vol. I. W. H. Hamilton and P. Dow (Eds.). Washington, D.C.: American Physiological Society, 1962.
13. Scheuer, J., and Tipton, C. M.: Cardiovascular adaptation to physical training. *Am. Rev. Physiol.*, 39:221–225, 1977.

Chapter 5
Pulmonary Function

No matter how well the blood is circulated past the cells, there must be some mechanism for the blood to load up with oxygen and get rid of carbon dioxide. Otherwise, the blood flow would be practically useless. Total respiration involves three different exchanges of gases: the exchange of air into and out of the lungs (ventilation), the exchange of gases between the lungs and the blood, and the exchange of gases between the blood and the various tissues of the body.

VENTILATION

Ventilation is the exchange of air into and out of the lungs. Air enters the mouth and nose and goes through the pharynx, larynx, and trachea into the bronchial tree. The bronchial tree branches dichotomously into bronchioles, terminal bronchioles, respiratory bronchioles, alveolar ducts, and alveolar sacs (Fig. 5–1). The first 16 branches are primarily conducting pathways, covered by a tough, continuous cartilaginous material which is supported by connective tissue and elastic fibers. The inner surface is made up of ciliated cells with goblet cells interspersed at regular intervals. As the bronchioles divide into ducts, they lose the cartilage, the ciliated cells, and the goblet cells.

The blood vessels into the lungs generally follow the respiratory ducts and terminate at the alveoli in a dense network of capillaries. The small separation between the air and the blood at the alveoli is only the distance of the capillary endothelial cells, the alveolar epithelium, and a small interstitial space (Fig. 5–2).

99

The air is saturated with water, and adjusted to body temperature by the mucous membranes of the mouth, nose, and pharynx, regardless of how hot or cold, dry or humid it may be. Particles in the air are caught by the mucus and removed from the airways by the beat of the cilia. As the air is expelled, the respiratory tract recovers some of the heat and moisture, but the moisture loss can be seen easily on a cold day.

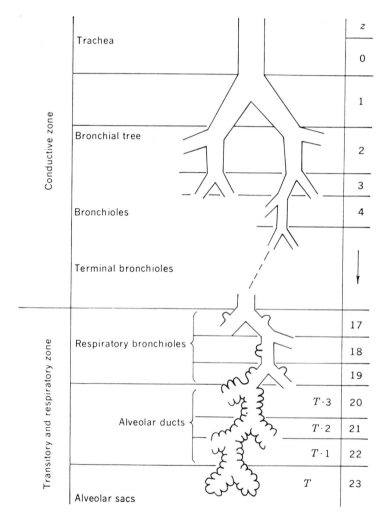

Figure 5–1.   General architecture of conductive and transitory airways. z designates the order of generations of branching; T, the terminal generation. (Astrand, P.-O., and Rodahl, K.: *Textbook of Work Physiology.* New York: McGraw-Hill Book Co., 1970.)

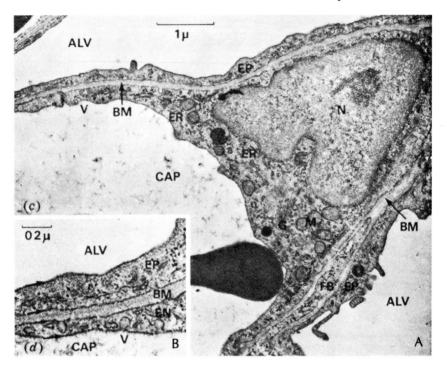

Figure 5–2. Electron micrographs of alveolar-capillary interface. A, Magnification ×23,500. Alveolus, ALV; basal membranes, BM; capillary, CAP; endoplasmic reticulum, EP; nucleus, N; pinocytotic vesicle, V. B, Magnification ×59,000 of the thin portion of air-blood barrier with four membranes. (From *Textbook of Work Physiology*, 2nd ed., by Astrand and Rodahl, p. 215. Copyright © 1977 by McGraw-Hill, Inc. Used with permission of McGraw-Hill Book Company.)

Air is pulled into the lungs by the contraction of the diaphragm and intercostal muscles. The diaphragm descends 1 to 10 cm, depending on the level of work. The intercostal muscles are brought into play more extensively as the volume of respiraton increases. They raise the rib cage to create additional volume in the lung area. The lungs maintain their position in the rib cage because of the pleural surfaces on the outside of the lungs and on the inside of the thoracic cavity. These two surfaces are held together by a fluid surface which allows a sliding action much like that of two wet panes of glass. The inspiratory phase is the active phase, whereas the expiratory phase is largely due to the elastic recoil of the diaphragm and intercostal muscles as they return to their resting positions.

During the inspiratory phase the alveolar ducts enlarge in both width and length, which has been calculated to result in a 70% increase in alveolar area.

During exercise the depth of breathing is greatly increased by use of the additional muscles. During inspiration, greater volume is obtained because of activity of the scaleni and the sternocleidomastoid muscles as they help lift the ribs. During expiration, the abdominal muscles aid the internal intercostals.

Volumes and Capacities

The various volumes and capacities of the lungs are shown in Figure 5–3. To do away with ambiguity, these terms were standardized in 1950 by a group of American physiologists. All volumes and capacities can be measured easily with a respirometer except residual volume.

The *tidal volume* (VT) is the normal volume of air moved in and out of the lungs. This volume can be expanded during exercise by using the *inspiratory reserve* volume (IRV) and the *expiratory reserve* volume (ERV) of the lungs.

Note that *capacities* are derived from two or more volumes or a combination of volumes and capacities, and can be expressed "algebraically" as follows:

$$FRC = RV + ERV$$
$$IC = VT + IRV$$
$$VC = IRV + VT + ERV$$
$$TLC = FRV + VT + ERV + RV$$

where FRC = functional residual capacity; IC = inspiratory capacity; VC = vital capacity; and TLC = total lung capacity.

Residual volume (RV) is the air remaining in the lungs after maximal expiration. Since this volume of air cannot be measured using normal expiration techniques, physiologists have derived other ways to measure this volume. The *nitrogen washout* technique is used most commonly in respiratory physiology laboratories and is probably the most accurate method. In this method, the subject begins to breathe pure oxygen at end VT for about 6 min (or longer with pulmonary disease) to "wash out" the nitrogen (N_2) in the lungs. All expired air (N_2 and O_2) is collected.

The volume of expired air is measured, and the percent of nitrogen is determined. From these data, the volume of N_2 can be determined. Since the volume of N_2 was 79% of the total volume in the lungs at the start of the washout, the total volume in the lungs can be calculated.

A sample problem may help. A subject breathes O_2 for 6 min. A total of 29 l of air is collected, of which 7% is N_2. What was the volume of air

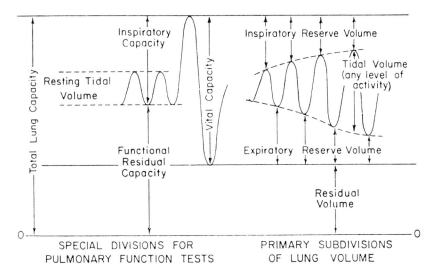

Figure 5–3. Lung volumes and capacities. (Ricci, B.: *Physiological Basis of Human Performance.* Philadelphia: Lea & Febiger, 1967.)

in the lungs (FRC) when he started breathing O_2? The total volume of N_2 is 7% of 29 l, or 2.03 l. This represents 79% of the total volume in lungs. A simple ratio equation can be used to solve for total volume:

$$2.03 \text{ l}/0.79 = x/100 = 2.56 \text{ l FRC.}$$

Another technique often used to determine residual volume or functional residual capacity (FRC) is *helium dilution.* At end tidal volume, a subject begins breathing a mixture of air containing a known percent of helium (He). The amount of dilution (or decrease in percent of He) can be used to calculate FRC. The formula is:

$$FRC = Vs \times (He_1 - He_2)/He_2$$

where Vs is the volume of the measurement system (spirometer), He_1 is the original percent of helium, and He_2 is the percent of helium after the subject has completely diluted the system. Vs = ml of He added/ He_1. Compute FRC if 600 ml of helium is added to the system and He_1 is 10% and He_2 is 8%.

$$Vs = 600/0.10 = 6000 \text{ ml}$$

$$FRC = 6000 \times 2/8 = 1500 \text{ ml}$$

Lung volumes and capacities are normally adjusted to body temperature, ambient pressure, and saturated with water at body temperature (BTPS).

It should be pointed out that *vital capacity* (the maximal amount of air that can be exchanged in one respiration) is not highly related to the ability to do work and cannot be used as a fitness evaluation. However, an oxygen uptake of 4.0 l/minute or more does require a vital capacity of at least 4.5 l.[1] Vital capacity is closely related to age and body height.

Pulmonary Ventilation during Work

Pulmonary ventilation is often abbreviated by the symbol $\dot{V}E$ (volume of expired air per minute).

$$\dot{V}E = VT \times f$$

where f is frequency of breathing. During rest, VT is about 500 ml and f is usually about 10 to 15/minute ($\dot{V}E = 5-7.5$ l/min). During work, the tidal volume increases to about 1/2 VC and f increases to 45 or 50/minute. For a person whose VC is 6 l, the VT would be about 3 l/breath, and with an f of 50, would yield 150 l/min of $\dot{V}E$.

$\dot{V}E$ increases fairly linearly with increased work until maximal work, at which point most subjects begin to hyperventilate, and the amount of air moved increases much more rapidly than the oxygen consumption (Fig. 5–4). Most subjects breathe 20 to 25 l of air for each liter of oxygen consumed at moderate work loads and increase to 30 to 35 l of air/liter of oxygen at maximal work.

The cost of breathing at rest is 1% to 3% (1.0 ml of O_2/liter of ventilation). At maximal work, the cost may be as high as 10%.[1] However, this high respiratory cost is not thought to limit work capacity to any marked degree.

$\dot{V}E$ during work is normally measured by collecting expired air into Douglas bags or meteorological balloons, or by measuring directly through a high-speed gasometer or pneumotach. In either case, it is important to use a low-resistance valve and large tubing to decrease the internal resistance to breathing as much as possible. Measurements of expired air are always corrected to standard conditions (STPD).

There seems to be a nice reserve capacity to support almost any work level, since $\dot{V}E$ can be increased even at maximal work. Patients who have had one lung removed can still supply enough air for normal exercise and many of them exercise on a regular basis.

Regulation of Ventilation

Since the basic purpose of ventilation is to provide oxygen and to discharge carbon dioxide, it would seem logical to find that these two

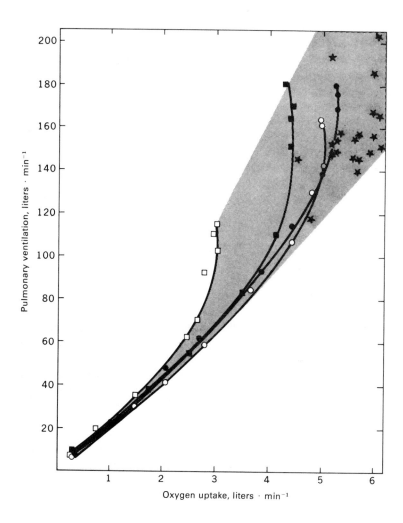

Figure 5–4. Pulmonary ventilation at rest and during exercise (running or cycling). Four individual curves are presented. Several work loads gave the same maximal oxygen uptake. Work time for 2 to 6 min. Stars denote individual values for top athletes measured when maximal oxygen uptake was attained. (Data from Saltin and P.-O. Astrand, 1967.) Individuals with maximal oxygen uptake of 3 l/min or higher usually fall within the shadowed area. Note the wide scattering at high oxygen uptakes. (From *Textbook of Work Physiology*; 2nd ed., by Astrand and Rodahl, page 229. Copyright © 1977 by McGraw-Hill, Inc. Used with permission of McGraw-Hill Book Company.)

gases play a major role in the regulation of breathing. This is actually the case. A change in the partial pressure of oxygen and carbon dioxide does, in fact, have an effect on the rate and depth of breathing. However, numerous other factors affect respiration in man, such as nervousness, heat, epinephrine, and the like. None of the theories about the control of respiration fully explains how respiration is varied to meet the demands of differing metabolic rates.

The respiratory control center is located in the medulla oblongata, and to some extent, in the lower part of the pons. There seem to be areas of the medulla that are specific to inspiration and expiration, but the neurons intermingle so much that the specific control centers are not clearly defined. The respiratory center has a basic rhythmicity which has been difficult to explain. However, it is partly explained by the fact that there is a reciprocal pathway between the fibers of inspiration and expiration which inhibit each other so that the circuits cannot oscillate simultaneously.

The inspiratory center inhibits itself by discharging impulses to the *pneumotaxic center* in the pons, which in turn dampens the activity of an *apneustic center* which would normally stimulate the inspiratory center by spontaneous activity.[1] The apneustic center is also inhibited by information from stretch receptors in the lungs when these tissues are stretched by inspiration. Respiratory muscles also contain stretch receptors which may inhibit inspiration.

Carbon dioxide and hydrogen ions (H^+) have a direct effect upon the respiratory neurons in the medulla. An increase of either in the tissue fluids of the respiratory center greatly increases the rate and depth of respiration. An increase in the concentration of hydrogen ions in the cerebrospinal fluid has almost the same effect. However, this occurs as a result of high blood carbon dioxide not of high blood hydrogen ion concentration. This is because the cerebrospinal-blood barrier is almost impermeable to hydrogen ions but not to carbon dioxide. When carbon dioxide diffuses into the cerebrospinal fluid, it causes the formation of carbonic acid, which in turn raises the hydrogen ion concentration. Therefore, this mechanism is more sensitive to blood carbon dioxide concentrations than to blood hydrogen ion concentrations.[6]

Besides the direct effect of hydrogen and carbon dioxide on the respiratory neurons, there is an effect through *chemoreceptors* located near the carotid and aortic bodies of the large arteries of the neck. Changes in blood hydrogen ion concentration and carbon dioxide excite these chemoreceptors and indirectly increase respiratory activity. However, the *direct* effect of hydrogen ion and carbon dioxide on the respiratory neurons is so great that the indirect effect through the chemoreceptors is probably not too important. The chemoreceptors are important as far as oxygen supply is concerned. Oxygen lack has almost no direct effect on the respiratory centers, but when the partial pressure of oxygen falls below normal, the chemoreceptors are strongly stimulated, and this increases the rate and depth of breathing.

There is some evidence to indicate that increased activity of the sympathetic nervous system during exercise may decrease the blood flow to chemoreceptors which simulates anoxia or oxygen lack. The respiratory centers are also affected by signals from other parts of the nervous system. There are stretch receptors in the lung which transmit information through the vagus nerves to inhibit inspiration when the lungs are inflated (Hering-Breuer reflex). This reflex also works in reverse to cause inspiration when no signals are generated from the stretch receptors.

Temperature increases also affect rate and depth of respiration. The increase in temperature with exercise may help in the final regulation of respiration.

There may be an effect through the muscle proprioceptors on the respiratory center. DeVries suggests that the afferent impulses from proprioceptors in moving limbs may be a factor in the adjustment of the respiratory system to exercise, with the changes in carbon dioxide and hydrogen acting to stabilize the rate and depth.[4]

How do all the aforementioned factors work to increase the volume of air moved during exercise? This is still an unanswered question. There must be "feed forward" mechanisms which begin the increase in respiratory activity and "feed backward" mechanisms to adjust the rate and depth of respiration to match the need.* Astrand found that ventilatory increases with different work loads were similar for the first 20 sec.[1] Only after enough time for blood to circulate back to the sensory system did the ventilation response match the need. This suggests that the initial trigger, or feed forward, mechanisms are tied to the activity and could include such stimuli as increased muscle spindle activity, and central nervous system activity from the motor cortex. The actual regulation of the respiratory volume then takes place through the feedback systems which include CO_2 production (decreased pH, increased H^+ concentration), and perhaps a decrease in blood flow to the chemoreceptors in the carotid and aortic bodies by sympathetic activity.

PROPERTIES OF GASES THAT INFLUENCE RESPIRATION

To understand the process of gas exchange from the air to the blood, it is necessary to understand a little about the nature of gases. A gas has no definite shape or volume, and it exerts a pressure that depends upon

* ACSM Symposium: Respiratory Control During Exercise. Chicago, 1977.

the activity and number of molecules in its volume. Gases move from place to place by diffusion, and the cause of diffusion is the pressure gradient. Unlike liquids, gases can be compressed into smaller volumes with a corresponding increase in pressure. If gas is heated, the activity of the molecules increases, and increased pressure results. The laws that explain these relationships in gases are as follows;

Boyle's Law

With a constant temperature, the volume of a gas varies inversely with its pressure. A gas volume would increase if taken from sea level to a high altitude where the atmospheric pressure is reduced.

Charles' Law

With a constant pressure, the volume of gas varies directly with absolute temperature (Kelvin scale), 1/273 its volume for each degree centigrade. The volume of a gas increases if the gas is warmed and decreases if it is cooled.

Dalton's Law (Law of Partial Pressure)

In a mixture of gases, each gas exerts a pressure according to its concentration. This law explains the relative partial pressures of the various atmospheric gases. For instance, if the total atmospheric pressure was 760 mm Hg, the partial pressure of oxygen would be approximately 159 mm Hg because the atmosphere is 20.94% oxygen. Therefore, $20.94 \times 760 = 159.14$.

The percentage of nitrogen (N_2) in atmospheric air is 79.03; the percentage of oxygen (O_2), 20.94; and the percentage of carbon dioxide (CO_2), about 0.03. The partial pressure exerted by any of these gases can be computed easily by multiplying these percentages by the total pressure at the altitude for which the computations are desired. Even though the total pressure decreases with altitude, the percentage of each of the respiratory gases in atmospheric air remains the same.

EXCHANGE OF GASES INTO AND OUT OF THE BLOOD

When atmospheric air enters the lungs, it is completely saturated with water in the form of vapor, which contributes to the total pressure of the gas. Since the water vapor pressure at 37° C (body temperature) is 47 mm Hg, to determine partial pressure it is necessary to subtract this pressure from the total gas pressure before multiplying by the percentage of a respiratory gas. For instance, if the total atmospheric pressure was 760 mm Hg, the partial pressure of oxygen in the trachea would be decreased to about 149 mm Hg, because the total pressure would be reduced by the water vapor pressure. Therefore, $(760 - 47) \times 20.94 = 149$ mm Hg.

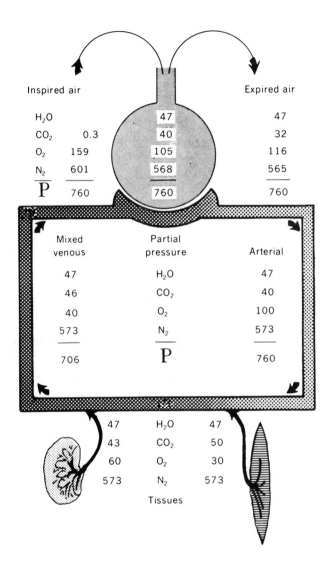

Figure 5–5. Typical values of gas tensions in inspired air, alveolar air (encircled), expired air, and blood, at rest. Barometric pressure, 760 mm Hg; for simplicity the inspired air is considered free from water (dry). Tension of oxygen and carbon dioxide varies markedly in venous blood from different organs. In this figure gas tensions in venous blood from the kidney and muscle are presented. (From *Textbook of Work Physiology*, 2nd Ed., by Astrand and Rodahl, page 239. Copyright © 1977 by McGraw-Hill Inc. Used with permission of McGraw-Hill Book Company.)

If you are in the mountain states, the total pressure may decrease to 630 mm Hg. In this case, the pressure of oxygen in the trachea would be approximately 132 mm Hg because of the reduced total pressure.

Theoretically, the partial pressure of oxygen (PO_2) in the lungs at 760 mm Hg should be about 149 mm Hg. This is not the case. The actual PO_2 in the alveoli is about 105 mm Hg. The reason for this is the fact that the gas in the lungs is a mixture of atmospheric air and used air (air already affected by the gaseous exchange). For that same reason, the PCO_2 is about 40 mm Hg because of the return of carbon dioxide from the cells to the alveolar surface. The water vapor pressure (PH_2O) is about 47 mm Hg, and the pressure of nitrogen (PN_2) is about 568 mm Hg (at an atmospheric pressure of 760 mm Hg). At rest, these partial pressures are surprisingly constant because of the dilution of incoming air with residual air, or air trapped in the lung spaces. During work, with the increased rate and depth of breathing, the variations become much larger. Figure 5–5 shows the partial pressure of gases in both inspired and expired air, as well as at different points throughout the body.

The partial pressures in the tissues vary widely with the particular need of the tissues. The PO_2 in muscle tissue may decrease to almost zero when muscles are at maximal work, and the PCO_2 may increase dramatically. Other tissues, which are not very active, may show almost no change in partial pressure. However, the partial pressures shown for mixed venous blood are fairly constant and represent an average of all the different tissues in the body.

Transport of Oxygen

Three percent of the total O_2 is carried in the dissolved state in the water of the plasma and the cells. About 97% of the oxygen is in combination with hemoglobin, the iron-protein molecule found in the red blood cells. Oxygen combines loosely and reversibly with the heme portion of hemoglobin with a ratio of one ferric atom (Fe^{+++}) to each molecule of oxygen.

The blood of the average man carries about 15 gm of hemoglobin/100 ml of blood (15 gm %). Each gram of hemoglobin can combine with about 1.3 ml of oxygen. Therefore, the average person carries about 20 ml of oxygen/100 ml of blood, or 20 volumes percent of oxygen.

During normal conditions, the venous blood returns to the lungs with about 15 volumes percent of oxygen. This means that about 5 ml of oxygen/100 ml of blood were released to the tissues of the body. During heavy exercise, this figure can be increased, so that about 15 ml of oxygen are released per 100 ml of blood. Physiologists often describe this relationship using the term a-v̄ O_2 difference (see p. 13). The a-v̄ O_2 diff. is 50 ml/liter (5 vol %) at rest or 150 ml/liter (15 vol %) during work.

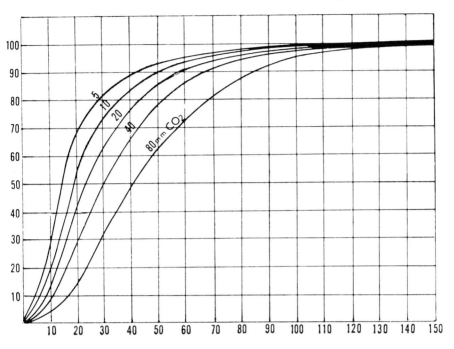

Figure 5–6.   Oxygen dissociation curve. The ordinate represents percentage of saturation of the blood with O_2; the abscissa represents partial pressure of O_2. (DeVries, H. A.: *Physiology of Exercise for Physical Education and Athletics.* Dubuque: Wm. C.Brown Co., 1967.)

Blood coming from the muscles being used maximally may be almost completely depleted of oxygen. The fraction of hemoglobin that gives up oxygen is referred to as the *utilization coefficient.* During rest this coefficient is about 25%; during work, it can rise to about 77%.

Figure 5–6 illustrates the oxygen dissociation curve. This curve is important to an understanding of the loading and unloading of hemoglobin with oxygen. Note that the blood at the alveoli (PO_2 104) is 97% saturated; because of the shape of the curve, the PO_2 must drop significantly to cause a serious change in saturation. However, at the tissue, where the PCO_2 is about 40 mm Hg, the blood is about 70% saturated, showing a drop of 30% of the oxygen under these conditions. Of course, when the PCO_2 increases (lower curve) because of a metabolic rate increase, the percentage of saturation is drastically decreased to release sufficient oxygen for the new metabolic level.

Transport of Carbon Dioxide

The processes involved in carbon dioxide transport are very complex as compared to those of the transport of oxygen. However, this does not present any particular problem, because carbon dioxide usually can be transported by the blood in far greater quantities than oxygen.

Carbon dioxide is transported in four different chemical forms; (1) as dissolved carbon dioxide, (2) as carbonic acid, (3) as bicarbonate ions, and (4) with hemoglobin as carbamino compounds.

About 7% of all carbon dioxide is carried by the blood in a dissolved state, and about 63% as bicarbonate ions (HCO_3^-). The initial reaction between carbon dioxide and water is accelerated by the action of carbonic anhydrase to form large quantities of carbonic acid (H_2CO_3) in the red blood cells. However, the carbonic acid formed in the cells immediately dissociates into hydrogen ions (H^+) and bicarbonate ions (HCO_3^-). This dissociation is so complete that little carbonic acid remains. Most of the hydrogen ions react with the hemoglobin which acts as an acid buffer, and many of the bicarbonate ions diffuse into the plasma.

The remaining 30% of carbon dioxide is carried in a loose, reversible chemical combination with hemoglobin called *carbaminohemoglobin*. It should be pointed out that the carbon dioxide does not bind with hemoglobin on the same site used by oxygen, but has its own specific site. Therefore, hemoglobin can combine with oxygen and carbon dioxide at the same time.

During intense exercise there is a hemoconcentration of the blood. This thickening is caused by a withdrawal of fluid to the active muscle cells and by the interstitial fluid. This raises the hematocrit and increases the oxygen capacity of the arterial blood by about 10%. However, there is not a 10% increase in oxygen saturation because of the decreased pH and an increase in heat, both of which shift the O_2 dissociation curve downward. The overall effect is a slight increase in oxygen delivery during maximal work.

ACID-BASE BALANCE

One of the most important functions of the body is the regulation of acid-base balance (pH), because only slight deviations in this balance can cause changes in cellular activity that are harmful to the organism. The by-products of cellular activity, such as carbon dioxide, lactic acid, phosphoric acid, and the like, tend to drive the pH down to a more acidic level, whereas certain illnesses tend to move the pH toward a more alkaline level.

The pH scale extends from 0 to 14.0, with a low number indicating an acidic condition, and a high number indicating an alkaline condition. A neutral solution would have a pH of 7.0. The pH of the body is normally about 7.4, or slightly toward the alkaline side of the scale.

To prevent acidosis or alkalosis, several systems are available: (1) the blood buffer systems, (2) the respiratory system, and (3) the kidneys.

The buffer systems of the blood act within a fraction of a second to prevent a drastic change in pH, and they are important to the maintenance of homeostasis. The respiratory system is stimulated by an increase in carbon dioxide to increase the rate of removal of carbon dioxide through the lungs. The kidneys can excrete either an acidic or alkaline urine to help readjust the hydrogen ion concentration (the pH).

A strong acid dissociates almost completely to form many hydrogen ions (H^+). When many hydrogen ions are released into a solution without a buffer, the pH drops drastically. The buffer systems of the body contain chemicals which absorb the excess hydrogen ions so that little change occurs in pH. A typical buffer system in the blood is the bicarbonate system. This system contains a mixture of carbonic acid (H_2CO_3) and sodium bicarbonate ($NaHCO_3$). If a strong acid such as hydrochloric acid (HCl) were added to this buffer system, the following reaction would take place:

$$HCl + NaHCO_3 \longrightarrow H_2CO_3 + NaCl$$

From this you can see that the strong HCl would be converted to a weak acid (H_2CO_3) which causes little change in the pH of the solution. In the blood there are other bicarbonate salts such as potassium bicarbonate, calcium bicarbonate, and magnesium bicarbonate which perform the same function as sodium bicarbonate.[4]

The most powerful buffer system in the blood is probably the protein buffer system. This method of buffering is the same as with the bicarbonate system. Because of the chemical makeup of proteins, there are free basic radicals of amino acids which can combine with hydrogen ions to buffer a solution. It is an extremely powerful system because of the great quantity of protein in the body.[6]

SELECTED REFERENCES

1. Astrand, P.-O., and Rodahl, K.: *Textbook of Work Physiology.* New York: McGraw-Hill Book Co., 1970.
2. Bloom, W., and Fawcett, D. W.: *A Textbook of Histology,* 9th ed. Philadelphia: W. B. Saunders Co., 1968.
3. Comroe, J. H.: *Physiology of Respiration.* Chicago: Year Book Medical Publishers, Inc. 1968.
4. DeVries, H. A. : *Physiology of Exercise,* 2nd ed. Dubuque: Wm. C. Brown Co., 1974.
5. Falls, H. B. (Ed.): *Exercise Physiology.* New York: Academic Press, 1968.
6. Guyton, A. C.: *Textbook of Medical Physiology,* 4th ed. Philadelphia: W. B. Saunders Co., 1971.
7. Kao, F. F.: *Introduction to Respiratory Physiology.* New York: American Elsevier Publishing Co. Inc., 1974.
8. Karpovich, P. V., and Sinning, N. E.: *Physiology of Muscular Activity,* 7th ed. Philadelphia: W. B. Saunders Co., 1971.

9. Morehouse, L. E., and Miller, A. T.: *Physiology of Exercise*, 7th ed. St. Louis: C. V. Mosby Co., 1976.
10. Ruch, T. C., and Patton, H. D.: *Physiology and Biophysics*, 19th ed. Philadelphia: W. B. Saunders Co., 1966.

Chapter 6
Physiological Response to Exercise

The purpose of this chapter is to summarize the responses of the body to exercise. Many of the responses have been mentioned in previous chapters, but they are sometimes hidden among the control factors and problems. Every student of exercise should be able to discuss both the acute and chronic responses of the body systems to exercise.

ACUTE RESPONSE TO EXERCISE

When exercise is begun, many changes occur in the body to support the increased need of the muscle cells for energy. These changes are controlled so fantastically that the correct volumes, beats, breaths, and forces are provided at the proper time.

HEART RATE.   Heart rate increases from about 60 beats/minute to a maximum of about 200 beats/minute during intense work. The resting heart rate is influenced by age, body position, fitness level, and environmental factors such as altitude, heat, and cold.

As exercise is begun, the heart rate increases. At moderate exercise, the heart rate will plateau, or level off, at some submaximal level and will stay at that level for some time if the work is not above the anaerobic threshold. As work is increased, so will the heart rate until a maximal heart rate is reached. The maximal heart rate can be predicted by subtracting a subject's age from 220. Thus, a 30-year-old would have a predicted maximal heart rate of 220 minus 30 or 190 beats/minute.

Since stroke volume increases to a heart rate of 110 to 120 (about 40% of the way between rest and maximal work), most heart rate tests of fitness measure the heart rate above this level because the relationship between heart rate and work is more linear.

STROKE VOLUME.   The stroke volume (SV) is the amount of blood ejected by the ventricle with each beat. There is a real difference in highly trained athletes and normal subjects in stroke volume. The SV of highly trained athletes may be twice as large as those of normal subjects. The average values are about 70 to 100 ml/beat for normal subjects and as high as 200 ml/beat in trained athletes.

The factors affecting stroke volume are related to the amount of blood returned to the heart (to distend, or stretch, the fibers), how hard the heart contracts, and how much pressure the heart works against.

The heart probably works at its largest size when a person lies down or exercises. It is smallest when the person is standing. When exercising, the venous return is large and the heart beats with more force. This yields the largest stroke volume that can be achieved.

Large venous return is associated with the training effect of the heart. Most exercise physiologists have guidelines for intensity which ensure large stroke volumes to overload the myocardium. These programs are more effective for cardiovascular training than programs of low intensity.

The idea that the heart gets much larger during exercise is false. The increase in stroke volume probably occurs as a result of more complete emptying of the ventricle during exercise, since the ventricle is only partially emptied at rest.

CARDIAC OUTPUT.   Cardiac output ($\dot{Q}$) is the total amount of blood ejected from one ventricle per minute and may be defined by the formula:

$$\dot{Q} = SV \times HR$$

where HR is the heart rate. Resting cardiac output is 4 to 6 l/minute. It increases with oxygen consumption (which makes sense, since the blood carries the oxygen used by the cells). Maximal cardiac outputs of nearly 40 l/minute have been measured in highly trained endurance athletes. Most people would have maximal $\dot{Q}$s of between 20 and 30 l/minute.

There is strong evidence that a large cardiac output capacity is inherited and is related to ventricular size. Although ventricular size can probably be increased through training, the large values mentioned previously may never be reached without some genetic help.

ARTERIOVENOUS OXYGEN DIFFERENCE. a–v̄ O_2 diff. is one of the factors that help explain the ability of the body to increase energy output so drastically from rest to maximal exercise. The difference between arterial blood and mixed venous blood at rest is about 50 ml of O_2/liter of blood. This difference increases as work is increased until the difference is 150 or 160 ml of O_2/liter of blood. In heavily worked muscles, the difference may even exceed these figures. Luckily, the body is able to increase the extraction of oxygen from the hemoglobin and does not have to depend entirely on increased flow for its supply.

It should be mentioned that the a–v̄ O_2 diff. in the heart is fairly large even at rest (150 ml/liter). During work, the increased oxygen demand is met almost entirely by increased flow. This is one reason why blockage of coronary arteries is such a troublesome matter.

OXYGEN CONSUMPTION. Oxygen consumption, or $\dot{V}O_2$, is the measurement of metabolic rate. As work is increased, so is $\dot{V}O_2$ (Fig. 6–1). $\dot{V}O_2$, expressed in liters/minute, is rather nondescript. Large persons may have large metabolic rates but not be in good condition.

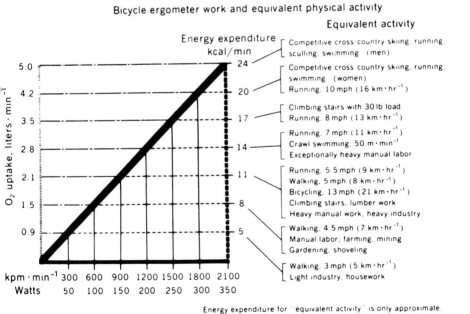

Figure 6–1. Relationship between $\dot{V}O_2$ and work. (From *Textbook of Work Physiology* by Astrand and Rodahl, page 454. Copyright © 1977 by McGraw-Hill, Inc. Used with permission of McGraw-Hill Book Company.)

That is why $\dot{V}_{O_2}$ is normally expressed in milliliters/kilograms/minute. Even this expression has limited interpretation. Saying that a person has a maximal $\dot{V}_{O_2}$ of 60 ml/kilogram/minute does not mean that he is well or poorly trained. It does mean, however, that he has a certain potential for aerobic work, and if he has increased to this level from 40 ml/kilogram/minute, it would indicate a marvelous training effect.

There is a large range of $\dot{V}_{O_2}$ maximum. Highly trained athletes may have values as high as 88 ml/kilograms/minute. Sedentary individuals may be as low as 20 ml/kilograms/minute. Females are 15% to 20% lower in comparable situations. Like many other functions of the body, $\dot{V}_{O_2}$ max decreases with age after about 30 years. However, there are many well-trained 60-year-olds whose $\dot{V}_{O_2}$ max is higher than that of sedentary 30-year-olds.

Oxygen consumption can be predicted fairly accurately by various tests. Performance tests, such as Cooper's 12-min or 1.5-mile run, and the 600-yard run-walk in the standard fitness test batteries, are based on the idea that the higher the $\dot{V}_{O_2}$, the faster the person can run a given distance. Tests such as the Astrand-Rhyming test and the various step tests which use heart rate during the test or during recovery estimate oxygen consumption potential based on the heart rate response to exercise. A lower heart rate for any given work load or a quicker recovery indicates a higher maximal oxygen uptake.

RESPIRATORY RESPONSE.   Since the exchange of respiratory gases occurs in the lungs, it is important that the amount of air ($\dot{V}_E$) moved by the lungs is sensitive to increased oxidative need. Resting $\dot{V}_E$ is about 5 to 7.5 l/minute. The V_T is about 0.5 l/breath and the frequency (f) of breathing, about 10 to 15 times/minute. $\dot{V}_E$ increases fairly linearly with increased activity, in the ratio of about 20 to 25 l of air/l of oxygen uptake in moderate work to about 30 to 35 l of air/minute/l of oxygen uptake at maximal work. Most people have a maximum V_E of between 100 and 200 l, depending on their VC, since normal tidal volume at work is about one-half VC with a breathing rate of 45 to 50 breaths/minute. Of course, since VC is related to size and age, a large young subject will have a larger maximum$\dot{V}_E$ than a smaller, older subject. $\dot{V}_E$ cannot be used as an indication of fitness.

The cost of breathing increases from about 1% to 3% of the total metabolic cost at rest to about 10% at maximal work. Normally, the lungs have much more capacity to move air than is needed, and most subjects hyperventilate at maximal work.

BLOOD PRESSURE.   Blood pressure is the pressure inside the vessels of the body caused by the pumping action of the heart. The systolic pressure at rest is about 120 mm Hg and the diastolic pressure, about 80 mm Hg. This indicates that the heart pushed blood into the vessels with a force of about 120 mm Hg and that the residual pressure

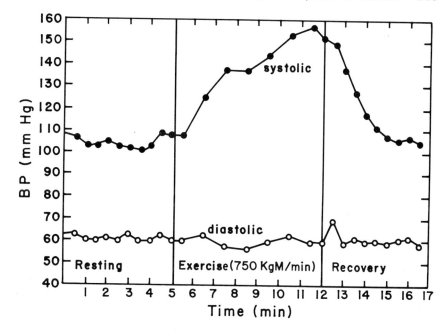

Figure 6–2.   Response of blood pressure to exercise.

in the vessels was about 80 mm Hg between beats. The systolic pressure rises with increased work to about 200 mm Hg, whereas the diastolic usually remains the same or decreases slightly (Fig. 6–2).

The pressures in the pulmonary system also increase during work, but it is difficult to monitor pulmonary pressure, and these pressures are not often mentioned. Resting pulmonary pressure may be about 20 mm Hg systolic and 3 or 4 mm Hg diastolic. The pulmonary systolic pressure may rise to 35 or 40 mm Hg, but the diastolic pressure will remain fairly constant.

Blood pressure measurements are extremely difficult to take while a subject is running. However, walking measurements are routinely taken, especially when testing high-risk or coronary heart disease patients on the treadmill.

Hydrostatic pressures in the lower body may increase the blood pressure in the ankle to 200 mm Hg or more. Any exercise of the legs decreases this pressure abruptly as the muscles of the legs pump blood through the one-way valves of the venous system. It is estimated that 30% of the total pumping action during exercise is supplied by the venous pump.

CIRCULATORY RESPONSE.   Since the vascular system is much too large for the amount of blood in it, the blood must be shunted to the system or systems which need it the most. The sympathetic nervous system sends vasoconstrictor and vasodilator fibers to the smooth muscles of the arterioles. As work is begun, the blood is shifted from the gut and other nonessential areas to the muscle beds. At the same time, the heart is stimulated by the accelerator nerve and the vagus nerve is inhibited to increase the total flow of blood. The precapillary sphincters are then dilated in the areas needing blood by the buildup of metabolites, and the blood flow serves the tissues which have the need. As heat builds up, some of the blood is shifted to the skin to help maintain internal temperatures within acceptable limits.

BLOOD RESPONSE.   During moderate to intense exercise, there is a hemoconcentration of the blood. This serves to increase the carrying capacity of the oxygen. However, there is also an increase in temperature and a decrease in pH. These two factors tend to decrease the oxygen-carrying capacity. The net effect is only a slight increase in the oxygen-carrying capacity.

Normal pH is about 7.4, which is slightly alkaline. Because of the rise in CO_2 and acidic by-products of metabolism, the pH may drop as low as 7.0. Lactic acid levels may increase from 10 mg/100 ml of blood to 200 mg/100 ml of blood during intense anaerobic work in highly trained athletes. Unconditioned subjects cannot attain these high values but may attain 80 to 90 mg/100 ml of blood.

The increased heat, lowered pH, high CO_2, and low O_2 tensions will increase the dissociation of O_2 at the cell, and the oxygen supplies of venous blood draining from the working muscles may be almost completely depleted.

FUEL FOR WORK.   The body prefers carbohydrate (CHO) to fats during high intensity work and can work three times as long at moderate work loads with a high-CHO diet as with a high-fat diet. This is not to say that fat is not an important energy source during work. Work of moderate intensity which lasts a long time will depend more and more on fat as a fuel as time goes by.

The respiratory quotient (R) reflects the fuel being used. In high-intensity activities, the R will rise and often will exceed 1.0 as the subject hyperventilates. In long duration, more moderate activities, the R will decrease slowly toward 0.7, indicating an increasing dependency upon fat.

Supersaturation of glycogen stores is an important preparatory step for athletes in activities lasting more than 1 hour. Although the initial speed will not be affected, the time that the speed can be maintained will be increased.

CHRONIC ADAPTATION TO EXERCISE

Many physiological changes associated with exercise and training are important to the performances of various activities. It must be remembered that the body responds specifically to the training stress placed upon it. If chronic adaptations are desired in the heart, the heart must be involved in the activity.

Holloszy classified the stimulus for change into three different categories:[11] (1) the learning of movement patterns for the development of skill; (2) strength exercise, which involves a few forceful contractions; and (3) endurance exercise, exemplified by activities such as long-distance running, swimming, or bicycling.

Since the primary adaptations to the first category take place in the central nervous system, the emphasis of this section will be on categories two and three.

Strength Training

Several important physiological changes consistently accompany increased strength.

INCREASED PROPORTION OF ACTIVE FIBERS.   Only a portion of muscle fibers is able to respond to impulses at a given time, but this portion can be altered by training. Many fibers are not able to contract; they are known as *inactive* (or *dormant* or *latent*) fibers. Fibers are dormant when the nerve pathways leading to them are not utilized or when the transmission of impulses over the end plates is poor. Extensive training improves the nerve pathways and the transmission of impulses, and this causes some dormant fibers to become active. It is believed that a poorly conditioned muscle may have as few as 60% active fibers, whereas a well-conditioned muscle may have over 90% active fibers. If this is true and if the individual fibers in the two different muscles are equally strong, the well-conditioned muscle could apply 30% more force. Dormant fibers, then, through increased demands on the muscle, become active and larger, and thereby contribute to strength.

INCREASED SIZE OF FIBERS AND CONNECTIVE TISSUE.   The individual muscle fibers increase in thickness as a result of strength training. This fact is supported by a number of research reports and much practical experience. The growth of the total muscle is due mainly to the increase in fiber size. Muscle fibers are not created through exercise, they are only enlarged. (Recent research indicates that perhaps some new fibers are created as a result of training, but this is not well substantiated.)

Numerous studies relative to muscle composition have shown that the amount of protein in muscles increases as a result of training. The amount of glycogen and various other substances also changes. Jokl cites evidence that there is a definite increase in actomyosin, the protein used most in muscle contraction.[14] The increased actomyosin would contribute to greater force of contraction, as well as an increase in size. Also, well-conditioned muscles possess a larger amount of water than other muscles. The increase is small, but even a small increase in fluid contributes proportionately to muscle growth.

Regular and heavy work places additional stress on connective tissue of the muscles and causes the tissue to thicken and toughen. The sarcolemma, which surrounds each muscle fiber, grows thicker. Strain, such as that caused by strength building, causes primary cellular multiplication in ligaments and tendons, and this results in growth and toughening of these tissues.

INCREASE IN CAPILLARIES.   An increased supply of capillaries within the muscles is another result of muscle training. However, this result relates even more to endurance training than to strength. The increase in capillaries is necessary to supply adequate oxygen and nutrients to the enlarged muscle fibers and the fibers that have been reactivated. Training usually produces more than the number of capillaries needed to supply the increased amount of muscle tissue, and the final result is improved muscular function.

DECREASED FAT WITHIN THE MUSCLE TISSUES.   Fatty tissue of the body accumulates around visceral organs, on the surface of skeletal muscles (between muscles and skin), and within muscles. Fat within the muscles creates friction and reduces the efficiency of contraction. Fat tends to accumulate in muscles that receive inadequate use and are poorly conditioned. Muscle training reduces the amount of fat within the muscles, thus causing the muscles to contract more efficiently and effectively. Loss of fat tends to reduce the size of the cross section of the muscle, but if heavy work is done, this reduction is often more than offset by increased muscle tissue.

CHANGES IN MUSCLE CHEMISTRY.   In addition to increases in protein and water, several other changes occur in the chemical composition of muscles as a result of training. Increases definitely occur in glycogen, ATP, phosphocreatine, and hemoglobin. There is an increase in the effectiveness of enzymes and coenzymes in the decomposition of the reserve nutrients in the muscle, and this frees more energy for work. Further, well-conditioned muscles produce less lactic acid per amount of work than poorly conditioned muscles.

DECREASED INHIBITORY CONTROL OF MUSCLES.   Strength training may reduce the effect of the inhibitory mechanism of muscle contraction. Since the end point of a brief maximal strength effort may be set by inhibitory functions, training should be directed toward reducing the inhibitory controls. This lessening of inhibitory sensitivity would permit a higher degree of tension to occur, thus increasing the strength of the movement. Two methods of modifying inhibitory mechanisms have been suggested, behavioral and morphological. The behavioral method is based on psychological conditioning which results in the ability to "relax" (release tenseness in antagonistic muscles) while performing. A morphological result of muscular exercise of the repeated overload variety is a thickening and toughening of the muscles' fibrous connective tissue. Embedded in the connective tissue throughout the muscle are the Golgi sensory organs of inhibition. The Golgi organs are believed to discharge inhibitory impulses whenever muscle tension rises above their threshold level of stimulus. The resulting Golgi inhibitory impulses act as an emergency brake to bring further increases in muscle tension to a halt. The thickening and toughening of the fibrous connective tissue may shield the Golgi sense organs somewhat from the tension of maximal muscular contraction. This shielding may permit innervation of the muscles to proceed farther without inhibition, and thus permit higher muscle tension to be developed before the Golgi braking device is activated.

Endurance Training

The adaptations brought about by endurance-type activities affect both the oxygen transport system and biochemical changes in the muscles. The following discussion involves the changes that occur in the cardiovascular system and in the muscles as a result of endurance exercise.

OXYGEN TRANSPORT SYSTEM.   Endurance training seems to increase total heart volume. Well-trained endurance athletes, both young and old, have larger volumes than their untrained peers. The muscle mass of the heart also is increased. Apparently, the heart hypertrophies as a result of a volume or pressure overload. Studies by investigators using echocardiography have shown that athletes who work against a pressure overload (weight lifters, football players, and so forth) tend to have a thicker ventricular wall and smaller ventricular volume than the endurance athlete.[18,19] The endurance athlete (long-distance runner, swimmer, and the like) is characterized by a large ventricular volume and normal wall thickness. The large heart of the endurance athlete is probably associated with long periods of intense training and could be partly genetic in nature.

The large ventricular volume of the endurance athlete yields increases in stroke volume both at rest and at any exercise level. Larger end diastolic volume and increased myocardial performance also increase the amount of blood pumped each beat. It is clear that trained hearts exhibit increased contractility, which probably results in smaller end systolic volumes during work. The large cardiac output of trained subjects is due almost entirely to the increased stroke volume.

Resting heart rate decreases, as does the heart rate at any given submaximal work load with training. Maximal heart rate may be slightly decreased or show no change.

It appears that young persons undergoing a training program increase their ability to extract oxygen from the blood (increased $a-\bar{v}\ O_2$ difference) but that older subjects do not. The mechanisms for increasing the $a-\bar{v}\ O_2$ difference are probably related to increased capillary density and increased number and activity of mitochondria within the active tissues.

The hearts of trained rodents have shown an increase in the amount of glycogen stored. There was also an increased turnover of fatty acids associated with an increased capacity to utilize lipid for fuel.[9]

Active men have been shown to have lower resting blood pressure than inactive men. Significant reductions also have been reported in hypertensive individuals who have completed an exercise program. Maximal blood pressures are not significantly different among groups of trained, slightly trained, and untrained individuals. However, trained individuals have lower blood pressure at any given submaximal work load.

Despite much research, it is unclear whether training will result in an increased blood volume. Hematocrit and hemoglobin concentrations also are similar in athletic and nonathletic populations.

There are significant increases in maximal oxygen consumption in trained individuals. The amount of increase in max $\dot{V}O_2$ is still unclear. However, increases of 20% to 30% seem reasonable.[5] Well-trained athletes often have $\dot{V}O_2$ maximums over 70 ml/kilograms/minute, whereas those of untrained subjects may be as low as 20 ml/kilograms/minute. Some of this difference seems to be the result of hereditary factors. Oxygen consumption at submaximal work loads is similar in subjects of the same body mass. However, slight differences may exist because of differences of movement.

At a given submaximal $\dot{V}O_2$ the content of lactic acid will be lower in a trained subject than in an untrained one. Trained subjects also can work at a higher percentage of their maximum than can untrained subjects. Higher concentrations of lactate can be tolerated by trained subjects.

The V_E required per liter of oxygen consumed does not change materially, but the total maximum V_E increases with training. V_E at rest is not significantly changed. However, at a submaximal work load, there is a slight increase in V_E. Frequency of breathing is usually decreased slightly at rest and during submaximal work.

See Table 6–1 for typical physiological changes associated with endurance training. These values are compared to those of a world-class endurance runner on the right.

BIOCHEMICAL CHANGES.   Total *myoglobin* increases significantly following endurance training. Myoglobin content generally parallels respiratory capacity in skeletal muscles and is found in all muscles with high respiratory capacity. Although oxymyoglobin is a

TABLE 6–1
Hypothetical Physiological and Body Composition Changes in a Sedentary Normal Individual Resulting from an Endurance Training Program*, Compared to the Values of a World-class Endurance Runner of the Same Age

Variables	Sedentary Normal Pre-Training	Post-Training	World-Class Endurance Runner
Cardiovascular			
HRrest, beats/min	71	59	36
HRmax, beats/min	185	183	174
SVrest, ml†	65	80	125
SVmax, ml†	120	140	200
Qrest, liters/min	4.6	4.7	4.5
Qmax, liters/min	22.2	25.6	34.8
Heart volume, ml	750	820	1,200
Blood volume, liters	4.7	5.1	6.0
Systolic BPrest, mmHg	135	130	12.0
Systolic BPmax, mmHg	210	205	210
Diastolic BPrest, mmHg	78	76	65
Diastolic BPmax, mmHg	82	80	65
Respiratory			
$\dot{V}$Erest, liters/min (BTPS)	7	6	6
$\dot{V}$Emax, liters/min (BTPS)	110	135	195
f rest, breaths/min	14	12	12
f max, breaths/min	40	45	55
TVrest, liters	0.5	0.5	0.5
TVmax, liters	2.75	3.0	3.5
VC, liters	5.8	6.0	6.2
RV, liters	1.4	1.2	1.2
Metabolic			
a-$\bar{v}$ O_2 diff rest, ml/100 ml	6.0	6.0	6.0
a-$\bar{v}$ O_2 diff max, ml/100 ml	14.5	15.0	16.0
$\dot{V}O_2$ rest, ml/kg·min	3.5	3.7	4.0
$\dot{V}O_2$ max, ml/kg·min	40.5	49.8	76.7
Blood lactate rest, mg/100 ml	10	10	10
Blood lactate max, mg/100 ml	110	125	185
Body Composition			
Weight, lb	175	170	150
Fat Weight, lb	28	21.3	11.3
Lean Weight, lb	147	148.7	138.7
Relative Fat, %	16.0	12.5	7.5

*6-month training program, jogging 3–4 times/week, 30 min/day, at 75% of his $\dot{V}O_2$ max.
†Upright position.
Wilmore and Norton: *The Heart and Lungs at Work.* Schiller Park, Ill.: Beckman Instruments, Inc., 1974, page 364.

storage form of oxygen in the muscle, the main function of myoglobin is to facilitate oxygen utilization in muscle by increasing the rate of its diffusion through the cytoplasm to the mitochondria.[22]

Training increases the capacity of skeletal muscle to oxidize glucose and fat for energy during work. Not only is there an increase in the number and size of the mitochondria, but the enzymes in the Krebs cycle and the hydrogen-electron transport system are increased in activity and in number. For example, there is a twofold increase in the levels of the mitochondrial respiratory chain enzymes involved in the oxidation of reduced nicotinamide adenine dinucleotide (NADH) and succinate,[12] as well as various citric acid cycle enzymes such as citrate synthase, aconitase, and succinate dehydrogenase.[1] Twofold increases in the enzymes involved in fatty acid metabolism (carnitine palmityl transferase, palmityl CoA dehydrogenase) have also been reported.[17]

Training also increases the amount of glycogen in the muscle.[8] This provides a ready store of energy for the increased metabolic capacity of the mitochondria. This change is probably brought about by an increase in the activity of an enzyme called glycogen synthetase.[23]

The importance of the biochemical changes can best be appreciated in terms of how they affect the ability to do work. Not only do these changes result in an increased maximum $\dot{V}O_2$, but work at submaximal levels becomes accomplished more easily. For instance, trained individuals deplete their glycogen stores more slowly than do untrained ones.[9] This glycogen sparing effect comes about by virtue of the increased oxidative capacity for fatty acids. Because of this, trained men have lower Rs at any given submaximal work level than do the untrained, even at the same percent of maximal capacity.

Of course, a decrease in a dependence upon glycogen yields a lowered lactate production in trained individuals. This relationship is true whether at a given percent of maximal work, or at any related work load. This phenomenon is probably not related to greater tissue hypoxia in the untrained, for the VO_2 is nearly the same at any given submaximal work load. The cause is probably related to the balance between the rate of glycolysis and the rate at which the smaller oxidative system of the untrained can handle pyruvate.

It is interesting to note that cardiac muscle does not undergo the same kind of enzymatic changes following training that skeletal muscle does. This lack of change can probably be explained by the fact that the cardiac muscle is a highly oxidative muscle in the first place and responds by increasing its size and force of contraction. The increased force of contraction is related to an increase in myosin ATPase activity in trained hearts.[24]

It should be pointed out that biochemical changes also occur in the anaerobic system owing to training. Stores of ATP are known to increase by 25% as a result of training.[15] Muscle levels of creatine phosphate (CP) are also increased,[6] as well as the enzymes associated with the use of these high-energy molecules.

Training also increases glycolytic capacity, as shown by the greater levels of lactic acid developed in trained subjects versus untrained persons. Activity levels of various glycolytic enzymes (phosphofructokinase, hexokinase, glyceraldehyde-3-phosphate dehydrogenase) also have shown an increase as a result of training (see reference 11 for a more detailed discussion concerning biochemical changes).

SELECTED REFERENCES

1. Baldwin, K. M., Klinkerfuss, G. H., Terjung, R. L., et al.: Respiratory capacity of white, red and intermediate muscle: Adaptive response to exercise. Am. J. Physiol., 222:373–378, 1972.
2. Berger, R. A.: Comparison of static and dynamic strength increases. Res. Q., 33:329, 1962a.
3. Berger, R. A.: Effect of varied weight training programs on strength. Res. Q., 33:168, 1962b.
4. Berger, R. A.: Leg extension at three different angles. Res. Q., 37:560, 1966.
5. Ekblom, B., Astrand, P., Saltin, B., Stenberg, J., and Wallstrom, B.: Effect of training on circulatory response to exercise. J. Appl. Physiol., 24:518–528, 1968.
6. Eriksson, B., Gollnick, P. , and Saltin, B.: Muscle metabolism and enzyme activities after training in boys 11–13 years old. Acta Physiol. Scand., 87:485–497, 1973.
7. Fox, E., Bartels, R., Billings, C., Mathews, D., Bason, R., and Webb, W.: Intensity and distance of interval training programs and changes in aerobic power. Med. Sci. Sports, 5:18–22, 1973.
8. Gollnick, P., Armstrong, R., Saltin, B., Saubert, C., Sembrowich, W., and Shepherd, R.: Effect of training on enzyme activity and fiber composition of human skeletal muscle. J. Appl. Physiol., 34:107–111, 1973.
9. Hermansen, L., Hultman, E., and Saltin, B.: Muscle glycogen during prolonged severe exercise. Acta Physiol. Scand., 71:129–139, 1967.
10. Hettinger, T.: Physiology of Strength. Springfield, Ill., Charles C Thomas, 1961.
11. Holloszy, J. O.: Adaptations of muscular tissue to training. Prog. Cardiovasc. Dis., 18:445–458, 1976.
12. Holloszy, J. O.: Biochemical adaptations in muscle. Effects of exercise on mitochondrial oxygen uptake and respiratory enzyme activity in skeletal muscle. J. Biol. Chem., 242:2278–2282, 1967.
13. Johnson, B. L., et al.: A comparison of concentric and eccentric muscle training. Med. Sci. Sports, 8:35–38, 1976.
14. Jokl, E.: Physiology of Exercise. Springfield, Ill., Charles C Thomas, 1964.
15. Karlsson, J., Nordesjo, L., Jorfeldt, L., and Saltin, B.: Muscle lactate, ATP, and CP levels during exercise after physical training in man. J. Appl. Physiol., 33:199–203, 1972.
16. Mathews, K. D., and Fox, E. L.: The Physiological Basis of Physical Education and Athletics. Philadelphia: W. B. Saunders Co., 1976.
17. Mole, P. A., Oscai, L. B., and Holloszy, J. O.: Adaptation of muscle to exercise. Increase in levels of palmityl CoA synthetase, carnitine palmityl-transferase, and palmityl CoA dehydrogenase and in the capacity to oxidize fatty acids. J. Clin. Invest., 50:2323–2330, 1971.

18. Morganroth, J., Maron, B., Henry, W., and Epstein, S.: Comparative left ventricular dimensions in trained athletes. *Ann. Intern. Med., 82*:521–524, 1975.
19. Nutter, D., Gilbert, C., Heymsfield, S., Perkins, J., and Schlant, R.: Cardiac hypertrophy in the endurance athlete. *Physiologist, 18*:336, 1975.
20. Saltin, , B., and Astrand, P.-O.: Maximal oxygen uptake in athletes. *J. Appl. Physiol., 23*:353, 1967.
21. Scheuer, J., and Tipton, C. M.: Cardiovascular adaptation to physical training. *Am. Rev. Physiol., 39*:221–251, 1977.
22. Scholander, P. F.: Oxygen transport through hemoglobin solutions. *Science, 131*:585–590, 1960.
23. Taylor, A., Thayer, R., and Rao, S.: Human skeletal muscle glycogen synthetase activities with exercise and training. *Can. J. Physiol. Pharmacol., 50*:411–412, 1972.
24. Wilkerson, J. E., and Evonuk, E.: Changes in cardiac and skeletal muscle myosin ATPase activities after exercise. *J. Appl. Physiol., 30*:328–330, 1971.

PART II
CONDITIONING
GUIDELINES

Certain human traits are basic to excellence in performance, and the lack of an adequate amount of these traits will restrict performance ability. Among these traits are strength, endurance, power, agility, speed, fast reaction time, flexibility, and coordination. Each of the traits can be improved considerably by correct training methods. In Part II are described the importance of the various traits, the best methods for developing them, and factors that influence the traits. Each of the chapters in Part II deals with one or more of the selected traits. Also included is a chapter on special training considerations for women, and one for adults of various ages.

Chapter 7

Strength and Muscular Endurance

The prize does not always go to the strongest and the most durable person, but it often does. It has been learned through experience and research that a high level of strength and endurance is essential to good performance in almost all athletic events, and in some events strength is of utmost importance. The relative significance of these qualities varies, depending on the nature of the particular activity.

STRENGTH

Strength is the ability of the body or its segments to apply force. Some persons have the impression that strength is only the contractile force of muscles. But strength involves a combination of three factors: (1) the combined contractile forces of the muscles causing the movement (agonists); (2) the ability to coordinate the agonistic muscles with the antagonistic muscles, and the neutralizer and stabilizer muscles; and (3) the mechanical ratios of the lever (bone) arrangements involved. The *first* factor depends on the maximal contractile force of each muscle agonistic to the movement. This force can be increased significantly through progressive resistance training. The *second* factor depends on the ability to coordinate the contractions of the individual muscles. This can be improved a limited amount by practicing the particular movements (developing skill). The *third* factor depends on the angle of pull of the muscles and the relative length of the resistance arm and effort arm of each lever. Sometimes this ratio can be altered advantageously by changing the positions of certain body parts.

There are two basic kinds of strength: *static* (isometric) and *dynamic* (isotonic). Dynamic strength can be classified further as *concentric* (muscle shortens) or *eccentric* (muscle lengthens).

Static strength and dynamic strength are somewhat related, but they are not synonymous, and it is possible to develop either kind of strength without developing the other kind to the same degree. Static strength can be measured more accurately than can dynamic strength, and most of the strength-testing instruments are designed to measure static strength. But dynamic strength is utilized far more frequently in performance.

Significance of Strength

The definition of strength—"to apply force"—implies its importance in performance. Even though nearly all movements are performed

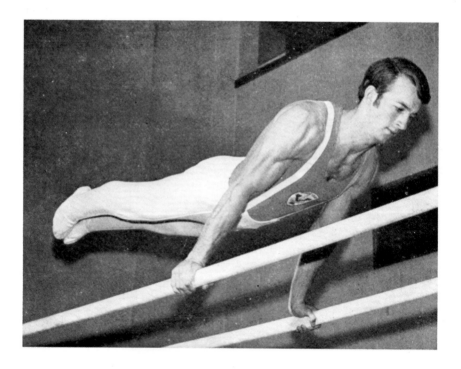

Figure 7–1. Gymnastic performances require great strength. This pose on the parallel bars demonstrates superior strength of the total body.

against some resistance, athletes perform movements against much greater resistance than usual. For example, in the shot put, discus throw, pole vault, various gymnastic movements, jumping, running, swimming, and leaping, the body segments must exert maximal force. If all else remains equal, greater strength often results in better performance than normal. In some athletic events, strength is the primary contributor and is therefore fundamental to excellence in these events.

In addition to being an important trait by itself, strength is an element in several other performance traits. It is a contributor to power, because power = force × velocity. Increased strength results in the ability to apply more force, and thereby it contributes to power.

Strength is also a factor in *muscular endurance*, which is the ability of the muscles to resist fatigue while doing work. Suppose a person moves a given resistance through a range of motion 100 times. If his strength increased 50%, he would then be able to move the same resistance with greater ease; thus, he could repeat the movement considerably more than 100 times. This illustrates how strength contributes to muscular endurance.

Strength contributes to *agility* because adequate strength is required to control the weight of the body against the force of inertia and to maneuver the body and its parts rapidly. Also, strength is a factor in *running speed*, because great force is required to accelerate the body and to keep it in motion at top speed. There is no doubt that lack of sufficient strength is a serious handicap to many would-be good athletes.

In addition to its importance in athletic performance, muscular strength also plays an important role in protecting athletes from injury. Strong muscles enable an athlete to move quickly and avoid accidents, and they also increase joint stability. The knee joint is the one that deserves the most attention relative to injury. In addition to overall strength of the muscles whose tendons cross over the joint, one also must be concerned about the relative strength of opposing muscle groups (antagonists). There is substantial evidence to support the idea that a knee joint is more prone to injury when there is an imbalance of strength in either group.

A prolonged study done at West Point Military Academy showed that a high percentage of athletes sustaining knee injuries had strength imbalance of 10% or more. Klein did a 5-year study of 515 college football players and found that those who were not injured had approximately a 4% strength imbalance, whereas of those who were injured, 79.5% had a strength imbalance of approximately 10% or more, and all were injured on the weak side.[24]

Klein recommends that every training program for vigorous sports,

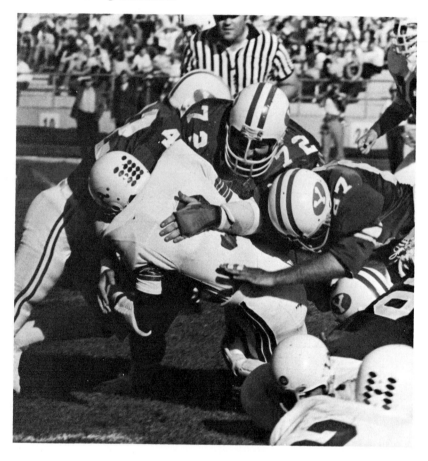

Figure 7–2.   Strength is of fundamental importance in contact sports
such as football.

especially contact sports, include strength testing and strength-
building programs.[24] The strength building should concentrate on the
development of overall strength to add stability to joints, and emphasis
should be placed on development of the muscles on the weak side
where excessive strength imbalances exist.

How to Increase Strength

To increase rapidly in strength, muscles must be contracted against
heavy resistance, and the resistance must be increased as the muscles
become stronger. In other words, the muscles are *overloaded*, meaning
they are loaded beyond their normal requirements, and *progressive*

resistance is applied, meaning that as the muscles become stronger they are worked against correspondingly greater resistance.

There are several approaches to developing strength. In fact, any form of exercise that applies heavier than usual resistance will stimulate an increase in strength. Strength-building stimuli may be provided by:

1. Hard manual labor or vigorous athletic performance. (It is not possible to approach maximal strength by this method because of the absence of progressive resistance.)
2. Specific exercises against body weight, as in pull-ups or dips. (Additional weight must be added to body weight in order to get sustained gains in strength.)
3. Heavy resistance exercises against external movable resistance, such as weight-training equipment. (This method provides the greatest potential for gaining strength, because the resistance can be increased progressively.)
4. Application of muscle tension (isometric contractions) against a fixed object or another body part. (This method has proven to be effective, but it has some pronounced limitations.)

The first three methods result in isotonic (dynamic) contractions, meaning the muscles change in length, and movement of body segments occurs. The fourth method results in isometric (static) contractions, in which the muscles apply tension but do not shorten, and do not move the body segments.

UNDERLYING CONCEPTS. The objective of most athletes who engage in strength programs is to gain usable strength in the most efficient manner. To accomplish this, a few basic concepts should be understood.

1. Although the contractile force of a muscle is maximal when the muscle is fully extended, the mechanical advantage is less than optimal in that position, thus strength is less than maximal when the muscles are extended. As the muscles go through their range of contraction, the mechanical ratio changes, and this results in a strength curve. To experience maximal strength gains, a variable resistance to match the strength curve would seem to be an advantage.
2. The resistance should directly oppose the direction of the body movement (omnidirectional resistance) and be carried through the full range of motion.
3. In order for a muscle group to apply maximal force, it cannot depend on weaker muscles to transmit the resistance. In other words, to get maximal results some body parts need to be isolated so that sufficiently heavy resistance can be applied.
4. Regardless of the strength-training method used, the two fun-

damental concepts, *overload* and *progressive resistance,* must be applied.

5. Usually, strength develops more rapidly in muscles that are a long way from their strength potential (end strength), and the rate of strength development decreases as the muscles approach end strength.

6. Each strength-training method has certain advantages. The final selection of the method to use should be based on purpose, administrative feasibility, and personal preference.

Programs for Developing Strength

Many programs for developing strength are used by athletes and coaches. The following are the most common of the structured programs:

ISOTONIC (DYNAMIC) STRENGTH TRAINING (WEIGHT TRAINING). Prior to World War II, strength-building exercises were used little in athletic training. In fact, it was believed that "muscle-boundness" resulted from such programs, and they were taboo to those seeking to improve athletic performance. During World War II, Thomas DeLorme and his co-workers experienced great success with heavy resistance exercises in the rehabilitation of hospital patients. Following his work, much research was done to determine the effects of this kind of training on athletic performance. It was learned that increased strength was highly beneficial to athletic performance, and that heavy resistance exercise was the most expedient method of increasing strength. Thus, weight training gained popularity among athletes and coaches.

It is an established fact that strength can be increased rapidly by exercising against heavy resistance for a few repetitions. After much study and experimentation, DeLorme and Wilkins recommended the following program be done every second day:[10]

One set of 10 repetitions with 1/2 RMs*
One set of 10 repetitions with 3/4 10 RMs
One set of 10 repetitions with 10 RMs

Even though DeLorme and Wilkins' method is still considered effective, more recent evidence supports the idea that a program of fewer repetitions with heavier weight is better. Berger found that strength increases more rapidly when 6 to 8 RMs are used with 3 sets.[5] Several other studies done since have added support to Berger's findings, although there is still some lack of agreement among experts

---

* *Repetition* (rep) means one execution of an exercise.
Set means a group of reps done in succession.
RM means repetition maximum. Ten RMs = 10 repetitions of an exercise using the maximal weight that can be lifted successively 10 times.

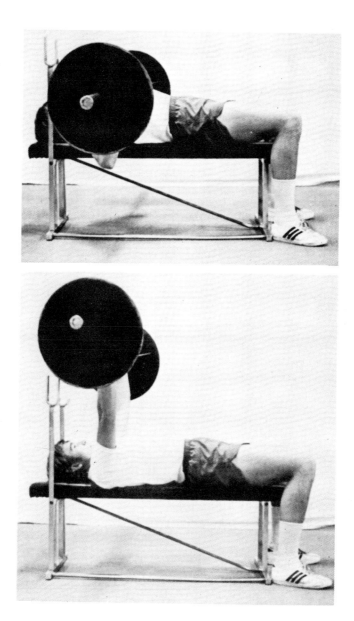

Figure 7–3. Bench press exercise using free lift equipment. (Robinson, C. F., Jensen, C. R., James, S. W., and Hirschi, W. M.: *Modern Techniques of Track and Field*. Philadelphia: Lea & Febiger, 1974, page 306.)

about the exact program that is best for building strength. However, the following guides are generally agreed upon, and they are supported by research and practical experience.

1. Exercises must be selected to work the particular muscles in which strength is to be developed, because significant strength gains result only in the exercised muscles.
2. Muscles should be contracted regularly (at least every second day, i.e., Monday, Wednesday, Friday) against *heavy* resistance.
3. Near-maximal weight for few repetitions (6 to 8) should be used.

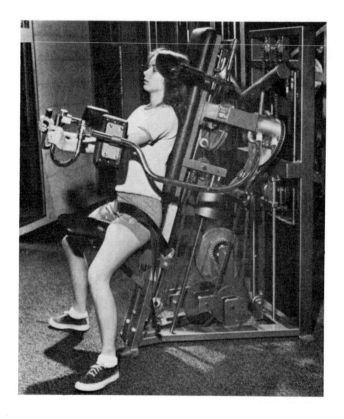

Figure 7–4. Nautilus equipment being used in muscle training. This sophisticated machinery is highly useful for the development of muscular strength, endurance, and power. Several different machines have been designed for developing different muscle groups. (From *Applied Kinesiology: The Scientific Study of Human Performance* by Jensen and Schultz, page 171. Copyright © 1977 by McGraw-Hill, Inc. Used with permission of McGraw-Hill Book Company.)

4. As strength increases, the weight must be increased progressively to provide continual overloading (progressive resistance).

Suppose you want to design a strength-building program for a discus thrower, an athlete who requires great strength and speed. A typical procedure would be as follows:

1. Analyze the throw, and determine the contributing movements.
2. Select exercises that work the muscles that cause these movements.
3. Determine the maximal amount of weight that can be lifted for one rep with each exercise, and use 70% to 80% of maximal weight.
4. Have the athlete perform at least three sets of each exercise, doing as many reps as possible in each set. (If more than 8 reps can be done, the weight is too light.) Some mature athletes prefer to do more sets (5 to 15) with fewer reps (2 or 3) and very heavy weight (80% to 90% of 1 RM).
5. Have him rest 2 to 3 min between sets.
6. Have him perform the workout on alternate days (Monday, Wednesday, Friday).
7. Increase the resistance each week (progressive resistance), as increases in strength permit.

Specific exercises for strengthening certain muscles can be found on weight-training charts and in books on weight training. However, by analyzing the actions involved in a particular performance, a person should be able to design an exercise program to suit his specific purpose. If in doubt, the exercise movements that most closely resemble the particular skill will probably be the correct choices.

ISOMETRIC (STATIC) STRENGTH TRAINING. Studies that support strength-building programs composed of static muscular contractions were conducted by Hettinger and Muller of Germany.[15] Soon afterwards, coaches and athletes were almost too enthusiastic about adopting isometric programs. Implementation was more rapid than the development of knowledge about the effectiveness of this approach. The original study by Hettinger and Muller indicated that static contractions of two-thirds maximum held for 6 sec were effective; they claimed an increase of 5% a week. Subsequent studies generally support the belief that strength can be increased with isometric exercises; however, the later studies have not shown increases of the magnitude of 5% a week, as claimed in earlier studies. It is difficult to use the percentage of improvement as an objective comparison. This is due to the widely accepted belief that the closer one is to theoretical maximal strength, the more difficult it is to show a high percentage of

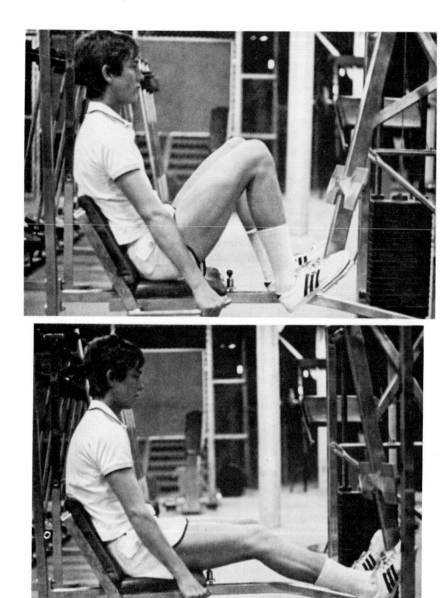

Figure 7–5. Leg press exercise being performed on Universal Gym. (Robinson, C. F., Jensen, C. R., James, S. W., and Hirschi, W. M.: *Modern Techniques of Track and Field*. Philadelphia: Lea & Febiger, 1974, page 317.)

improvement. Thus, the same procedure may result in a 2% increase in a highly trained athlete and a 5% increase in a sedentary individual.

Research by Muller and Rohmert of Germany, reported by Royce,[32] showed that strength increases more rapidly when the muscles contract at near maximum, and 5 to 10 reps are used. They also established the idea that strength increases more evenly throughout the range of motion if the contractions are done at various positions. Subsequent studies were performed in the United States by Ball and associates,[3] Rasch and Morehouse,[30] and Rich[31] who employed varying amounts of tension and varying lengths and numbers of contractions, and the procedures all produced significant strength gains.

McGlynn reviewed the research that had been done prior to that time on isometric training.[26] He claims that the available research does not

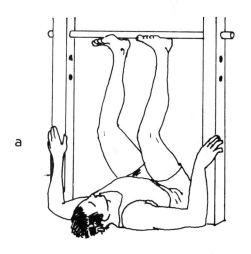

a

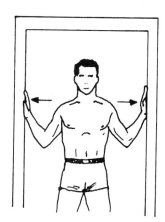

b

Figure 7–6. Isometric exercises to condition certain muscle groups: A, leg press; B, lateral arm press.

warrant the indiscriminate use of isometric training for strength development in athletes. Further, he points out that the research has not resulted in agreement upon the optimal percentage of maximum of each contraction, or the number of repetitions a day, or whether the training should be done every day or alternate days. We agree that additional research needs to be done to determine the value of isometrics more clearly. However, it is clear that isometric training can be highly useful when isotonic or isokinetic equipment is not available. We do not recommend that athletes substitute isometric exercises for isotonic or isokinetic training when equipment is available.

In spite of the fact that there is some uncertainty about the best approach to isometrics, the available evidence supports the following guidelines:

1. The best isometric method for increasing strength at a particular body position is 6 to 8 reps of near maximal contraction *daily*. Even though good results have been obtained with contractions of two-thirds maximum, it has been found that individuals are poor judges of how much tension they apply, so the safe thing to do is use near maximal tension.

2. If increased strength is desired throughout the full range, then the contractions should be done at various positions. When strength is needed only at the beginning of the motion, as in ballistic movements, the exercises should be designed accordingly.

3. If *rapid* development of strength is the primary concern, then training should be done daily. However, if the objective is more long range, training may be done on alternate days. Strength gained slowly tends to be more permanent.

4. One workout a day, as described in item 1, will produce as much strength as will multiple workouts.

5. The best breathing technique is to take a deep breath at the beginning of the contraction, hold it for a few seconds, then exhale slowly during the latter part of the contraction.

ISOKINETIC STRENGTH TRAINING. A distinct disadvantage of conventional isotonic strength training is that the muscle being trained is not stressed effectively through the whole range of motion. This is due to changes in leverage combined with changes in the direction of movement of the resistance in relation to the line of gravity. At certain points in the range of motion a muscle might contract at maximum, but at other points the contraction is only a percentage of maximum. Thus, the training effect is not consistent throughout the range of motion.

Isokinetic exercise is a form of isotonics performed with equipment that automatically adjusts the resistance to the force exerted against it, so that at every angle through the range of motion the resistance is

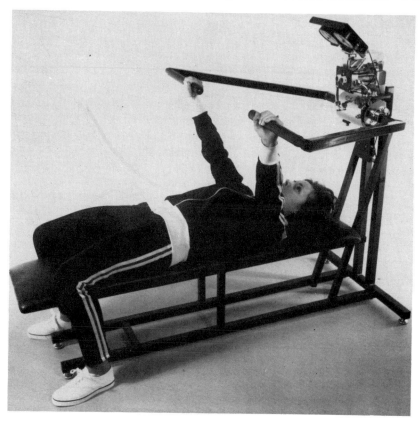

Figure 7–7. Isokinetic strength exercise being performed on a Cybex machine. (Courtesy of Lumex Corporation.)

equal to the muscular force. There is no ballistic effect, as there is when exercising with barbells. The use of the isokinetic method results in a varying amount of resistance through the range of motion which corresponds to the strength curve of the movement. The resistance accommodates the force. In other words, it applies the principle of work against resistance equally, all the way through the range of motion. Isokinetic exercise devices have variable speed adjustments so that exercises can be done at slow, intermediate, or fast speeds.

Thistle and associates compared isokinetic training with isotonic and isometric procedures and found that, after 8 weeks of training, the isokinetic group had gained approximately 35% in quadriceps strength as compared with 27.5% for the isotonic group and 9.2% for the isometric group.[35] A control group decreased 9.4% over the time interval. Moffroid found that isokinetic training over a 4-week period was approximately equal in effectiveness to isotonic and isometric training.[27] DeLateur and co-workers compared an isokinetic strength program with an isotonic program involving the quadriceps muscles, and the results showed that the two programs were equally effective for developing strength.[9]

Van Oteghen[34] measured the effectiveness of two speeds of isokinetic exercises on vertical jump performance and, after the athletes trained for 8 weeks, found that both slow-speed and fast-speed isokinetics caused significant increases in the vertical jump.[36] Shepherd compared the effects of isotonic, isokinetic, and negative (eccentric) resistance strength-training programs.[33] He found that all three programs produced significant improvements in both isotonic and isometric strength with no significant difference in their relative effectiveness.

Pipes and Wilmore studied the changes in strength, body composition, anthropometric measurements, and selected motor performance tasks between groups trained isotonically and isokinetically.[28] The results demonstrated a clear superiority of isokinetic training over isotonic training. The *isokinetic high-speed* group demonstrated the greatest gains.

Even though the optimal isokinetic strength program is not known, it is generally agreed that each exercise should be performed with 6 to 8 reps and 3 sets on alternate days. Other combinations of reps and sets close to this will cause similar results. *Fast-speed* contractions are more effective than slow or intermediate speeds.

There seems to be little doubt that isokinetic exercise is just as effective as conventional isotonic exercise or isometric exercise for building strength. Further, it is quite possible that additional research will support isokinetic strength training as the superior method.

NEGATIVE (ECCENTRIC) RESISTANCE EXERCISE.   Negative resistance exercises have been used by some athletes because of the great overload involved. A load greater than the maximal 1 RM is used, and the athlete is helped into an extended position by his spotters. He then resists the load as he is forced back to his starting position. These techniques work best when a Universal Gym or Nautilas machine is used because it decreases the danger of injury.

Although eccentric exercises for strength and endurance have not been of prime interest to exercise physiologists, coaches, or athletes, a few investigators have given attention to this topic. Johnson and associates compared concentric and eccentric strength training, using concentric exercises that were 80% of one repetition maximum for 10 reps and 2 sets, and eccentric exercises that were 120% of one concentric repetition maximum for 6 reps and 2 sets.[22] Both routines produced significant gains in strength in all subjects, but neither

training procedure produced dynamic or static strength gains significantly greater than the other.

Rasch did a thorough review of the literature on this topic, and he
stated these interesting observations:[29]

1. The energy costs of performing against a constant amount of
    resistance are much less using eccentric contractions than using
    concentric contractions. This means that in order to apply the
    same amount of overload, eccentric contractions must be per-
    formed against considerably greater resistance than that for
    concentric contractions.

2. At practically all angles of pull, measured muscle tension that
    can be applied is consistently greater for eccentric movements
    than for concentric movements or isometric contractions. This
    means that eccentric strength measures cannot logically be
    compared to concentric or isometric measures.

3. From the limited studies reported, it would appear that the
    amount of strength that can be developed through eccentric
    exercise is not statistically different from the amount that can be
    developed with concentric exercise.

4. Some experts believe that, all else being equal, concentric

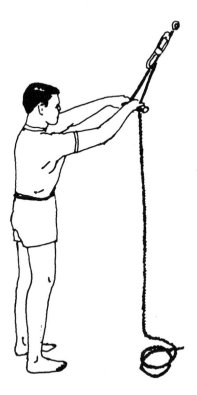

Figure 7–8. Use of Exer-Genie to
combine isometric and isotonic exercises.

exercises are preferred because they relate more closely to the movement patterns involved in performance. Strength is almost always employed in the performance of positive work, and only rarely are muscles called upon to do heavy resistive negative work during performance.

OTHER STRENGTH-BUILDING METHODS.   A limited amount of research supports the claim that strength can be gained at a rapid rate by combining isometrics and isotonics. This is done by contracting the muscles isometrically against a rope or cable arrangement for about 10 sec, then reducing the resistance to allow a slow-motion isotonic contraction to occur. Several mechanical devices for use with this approach have been developed and sold commercially. With this method it is recommended that each exercise be repeated 8 to 10 times daily.

A less effective and seldom-used method is functional overload. The activity itself is performed under resistive conditions. Weighted vests, ankle weights, and other weighted objects and implements have been used in the past. Throwing weighted baseballs and swinging weighted bats are still used by some. These methods have the advantage of closely coordinating the strength gains into the movement patterns, but some experts think it reduces coordination and timing. Only mild strength gains result from this method, because typically the resistance is too little to provide a strong stimulus for strength.

Factors That Influence Strength

Numerous factors relate to and influence strength. It is important to know what has been learned through research and observation about these factors.

MUSCLE SIZE.   The contractile force of a muscle is related to the muscle's cross-sectional measurement (diameter). As strength increases, the cross sections of the individual muscle fibers increase, resulting in a greater cross-sectional area of the muscle. The increase in size is in approximate proportion to the increase in strength. However, there are other influencing factors. For instance: (1) two muscles having equal cross sections may differ in their ability to apply tension owing to varying amounts of fatty tissue. Fat lacks ability to contract, causes friction, and interferes with the shortening of muscle fibers. (2) The proportion of active fibers in different muscles influences contractile force. (3) The efficiency of contraction has an important influence on strength. Nevertheless, muscle size and strength are closely related. Typically, significant strength gains will cause approximately corresponding increases in muscle size.

It has been noted that growth in muscle girth is related to body type. Those with a high degree of ectomorphy (leanness) appear to respond less to strenuous strength exercises than the athletic type or those with a high degree of mesomorphy (muscular with heavy skeletal systems) who appear to respond the most. Further, muscular training has a positive effect on the development of various connective tissues. Of particular interest has been the strength of ligaments supporting various vulnerable joints. It has been found that exercise increases the thickness of ligaments, tendons, and other connective tissues. In fact, the hypertrophy of the tendons may be as great as that of the muscles. Also, the hyaline cartilage which covers the articulating surfaces of bones in joints shows similar changes. In addition, there is indication that long periods of vigorous training contribute to larger and stronger bones.

MECHANICS OF STRENGTH.   Strength has a mechanical element because the body functions as a system of levers. A force applied at a right angle to a lever gives the maximal mechanical efficiency. The greater the deviation from the right angle, the less efficient is the force. In flexing a fully extended arm, most of the initial force is wasted by

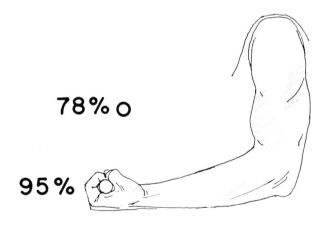

Figure 7–9.   Approximate percentage of maximal strength at different angles of pull through the elbow flexion movement.

pulling the radius and ulna against the humerus. The greatest strength occurs at the position offering the best combination of contractile force and angle of pull. Since the tension applied by muscles lessens as the muscles shorten, and because the muscles pull at varying angles as the lever moves through its range of motion, it is apparent that strength varies at different positions. In other words, there is a strength curve for each movement. When maximal force is needed, it is important to have the body segments positioned where they can apply their greatest force. Linford and Rarick[24] found that leg strength remains about the same when the knee is bent at an angle between 164° and 130°, but as the angle decreases beyond 130°, strength diminishes.[25] Berger's studies produced evidence that supports Linford's findings.[6]

Another aspect of strength with some relationship to mechanics is the direction of pull of muscle fibers. The structural arrangement of fibers bears an important relationship to the force and distance of contraction. There are two main kinds of fiber arrangements, the *fusiform* (longitudinal) and the *penniform* (diagonal), but there are several variations from these two basic forms. Even though there is lack

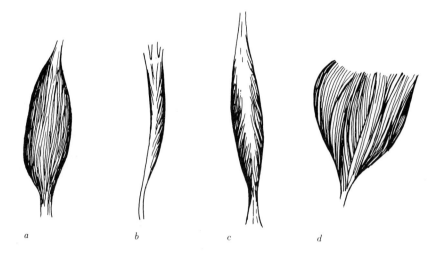

a   *b*   *c*   *d*

Figure 7–10.   Variations in the arrangement of muscle fiber. a, Fusiform—examples are brachialis and brachioradialis of the arm, and the sartorius muscle of the leg. b, Unipenniform—examples are the extensor digitorum longus and the tibialis posterior muscles of the leg. c, Bipenniform—the best example is the rectus femoris. d, Multipenniform—examples are the deltoid and pectoralis major. In these muscles the tendon runs into the center of the muscle, and diagonal fibers attach to it from all directions. (From *Applied Kinesiology: The Scientific Study of Human Performance* by Jensen and Schultz, page 13. Copyright © 1977 by McGraw-Hill, Inc. Used with permission of McGraw-Hill Book Company.)

of agreement among experts about the variations, the forms illustrated in Figure 7–10 are representative.

The fusiform muscle is the simplest structurally. Because the fibers of a fusiform muscle run longitudinally along the muscle, there is a one-to-one relationship between shortening of the muscle and the amount of movement it causes. This is an advantage in speed of movement, but it is a disadvantage in the application of force. Conversely, the fibers of penniform muscles are arranged like the structure of a feather, with the tendon in the place of the shaft and the muscle fibers in the place of the barbs. With the muscle fibers arranged diagonally to the direction of pull, more fibers can be brought into play, but the range of motion is reduced. Therefore, penniform muscles are designed primarily for the application of force through short ranges of motion, and fusiform muscles are designed for less force through greater ranges of motion.

LENGTH OF MUSCLE.   The tension a muscle can apply (contractile force) increases with the extension of the muscle. This means that the contractile force is greatest when the muscle is fully extended. Force steadily diminishes as the muscle shortens, and the muscle is unable to apply any force beyond its fully contracted position. Muscle contraction may be paralleled to a rubber band, which applies its greatest tension when stretched. Contractile force is not reduced in the same proportion as is the length of the muscle; during the early phase of contraction the force reduces slowly, whereas during the late phase force reduces proportionately faster.

It is interesting to know that the initial contractile force can be increased by placing the muscle on *sudden stretch*. This activates the *stretch reflex* mechanism and causes an additional volley of impulses to supplement those that originate in the central nervous system. The stretch reflex is primarily a postural reflex, but it is used effectively to aid contractions in voluntary movements. For example, when a pitcher throws a baseball, the muscles used to drive the ball forward are placed on sudden stretch at the completion of the windup, and the contractions are stronger than they would have been otherwise.

The stretch reflex also is well illustrated in vertical jumping. Just prior to the jump the performer dips, placing the jumping muscles on sudden stretch and activating the stretch reflex. If the dip is purposely eliminated, or if there is a pause at the bottom of the dip, the height of the jump will be less than expected.

STRENGTH TRAINABILITY OF MUSCLES.   There is much variation in the strength increases reported by different researchers under varying conditions. For example, Hettinger and Muller reported phenomenal gains of as much as 160% during the first week of training.[15] A few other researchers have reported less but still unusually large gains. Such fantastic results should not be expected, because large strength gains do not come easily or rapidly. A 5% gain a week over a period of a few weeks should be considered excellent or extraordinary. After a few weeks of training, the gains will decline to a leveling-off point, beyond which additional strength is gained very slowly.

There are several interesting points about strength trainability:

1. Some persons are more responsive to training than others simply because of their physiological makeup, which influences their capacity for strength development.

2. The same person responds differently to training as his state of conditioning changes. Generally, muscles in poor condition respond rapidly, whereas already well-conditioned muscles respond more slowly. Gains in strength become increasingly more difficult as the strength level gets closer to strength potential (end strength).

3. The same person responds differently to training at different ages. Men are the most trainable during the formative years, up to about age 25, after which they become less responsive year by year. However, as long as the organism is healthy and normal, it will respond to strength stimuli by some amount. Women are the most responsive to training during the formative years, up to about age 21, after which they become progressively less responsive.

4. Not all muscles respond at the same rate even when optimal strength stimuli are provided. Some muscle groups might increase 5% a week but others only 1% or 2%. This is apparently due to two factors: (1) in the same individual some muscle groups are naturally more trainable than others; and (2) muscle groups vary in their level of conditioning because of the amount of use they receive during daily living. This difference causes them to respond at different rates.

RED AND WHITE MUSCLE FIBERS.   There is little doubt that red and white muscle fibers are recruited selectively, depending upon the intensity and type of activity (see Chapter 2 for a discussion of red and white fibers). It is possible that training programs for strength need to emphasize speed if the goal is to develop the white fast-twitch fibers, and that the traditional strength-training programs may develop the red slow-twitch fibers preferentially.

The changes in aerobic potential associated with training apparently come about by increases in both red and white fibers. However, changes in glycolytic capacity appear to be much more specific.[2]

There is also evidence to suggest selective hypertrophy of red and white fibers. Red fibers occupy a greater area of the muscle in an endurance athlete than do white fibers. Conversely, white fibers occupy a greater area in weight lifters and sprinters than do red. Much research remains to be done in this area.

Experiments conducted at Indiana University showed that both expert swimmers and expert basketball players increased their vertical jump ability between 3 and 5 inches as a result of muscle training that emphasized the development of white fibers.[8] Athletes on training programs that emphasized the development of red fibers did not increase in vertical jump ability. (However, it should be assumed that those who emphasized red fiber development better prepared their muscles for endurance-type performance.)

WHEN TRAINING IS STOPPED. If a strength-training program is terminated, much of the strength that was gained will be lost at approximately one third of the rate it was gained. This means that strength gained rapidly is lost rapidly when training is stopped, whereas strength gained more gradually lasts longer after training is ended. Even though much of the increased strength is lost in the absence of training, a portion of it is retained for a long period, and a small amount is retained indefinitely.

Hettinger claims that the rate of strength loss can be retarded considerably with only one training session every 6 weeks, and that all of the strength gained can be retained with one training session every 2 weeks.[14] However, the truthfulness of this claim would depend on how close one is to strength potential. A person who is near end strength has to work hard and regularly in order to maintain that level. Whereas one who is far from his strength potential can maintain the level much more easily, perhaps by training only once every 2 weeks.

It is an interesting fact that the conditions under which strength is developed do not seem to influence its retention. For example, the rate at which strength is lost is unrelated to the number of workouts per day during the period the strength was gained or the amount of fatigue incurred in each workout, or other such specifics. But it is related to the rate at which the strength was gained.

RELATIONSHIP OF STRENGTH TO AGE. Research, combined with practical experience, indicates that under normal conditions boys increase in strength rather consistently until they reach age 20 years. After this age, strength increases at a slower rate until about the age of 25, when maximal strength is attained. Soon after the maximal level is attained, strength begins to diminish. Strength normally varies less between 20 and 30 years than at any other comparable age range.

It has been observed that after the age of 25 years, a person loses nearly 1% of his remaining strength each year, and at age 65 most persons are 65% to 70% as strong as they were at age 20 to 30. However, the rate of loss is influenced considerably by one's activity level.

As a child grows from infancy to adulthood, strength increases in approximate proportion to the increase in muscle size. Apparently there is no significant change in muscle quality, because practically all the increased strength can be accounted for by muscle growth. However, it seems likely that part of the loss of strength in later life can be attributed to decreased quality of muscle tissue, along with some decrease in quantity.

It is important to recognize that the strength curve in Figure 7–11 is what can be expected under normal living conditions. The curve can be altered at any point in life by using effective strength-building methods. As a result of training, a person can be significantly stronger at any particular age than he would otherwise have been, and he can retard the decline of strength that normally occurs. Some "strength builders" (those dedicated to maximal strength) continue to increase in strength until they reach the mid 30s.

Girls increase in strength at about the same rate as do boys to approximately the age of 12, after which the rate of increase in girls begins to level off. After puberty girls still gain strength, but at a slow rate. They typically reach maximal strength at about the age of 21, and soon after that strength begins to decline at about the same rate as that in men.

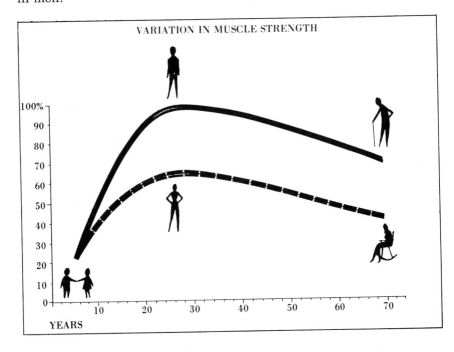

Figure 7–11.   Muscle strength in relation to age and sex.

STRENGTH DIFFERENCES OF THE TWO SEXES.   Research supports the claim that on the average, women are about two thirds as
strong as men, and they have about two thirds as much muscle tissue as
men. However, this percentage is not consistent among all muscle
groups. For example, it has been found through research that on the
average women are 80% as strong as men in the hip flexors and hip
extensors, and they are about 55% as strong in the forearm flexors and
extensors.

Probably there are two reasons why the proportionate strength of
women as compared to men varies with different muscle groups. (1)
The natural differences in body proportions of the two sexes cause
some muscle groups in women to be nearly as large as those in men,
whereas other muscle groups are much smaller in women. (2) Daily
activity patterns influence the amount of use that different muscle
groups receive and thereby influence their strength levels. Typically,
daily activity patterns of women are different from those for men,
although this difference has diminished during recent decades. The
strength differences between the two sexes can be accounted for mostly
by the differences in muscle mass. There is probably no substantial
difference in the quality of muscle tissue of women and men.

EFFECTS OF TEMPERATURE.   Muscular contraction is both
greater and faster when the temperature of muscle fibers is slightly
higher than normal body temperature. In this slightly warmed condition, the muscle viscosity is lower, the chemical reactions of contraction and recovery are more rapid, and circulation is improved. The heat
produced by muscular contraction seems to improve the condition of
the muscle for further work. Conversely, muscle temperature below
normal elevates the irritability threshold and increases viscosity, thus
contributing to more sluggish and slightly weakened contractions.

A. V. Hill found that a 2° increase in body temperature increased
strength a measurable amount.[20] Grose found that when the arm was
immersed in hot water (120° F) for 8 min, small gains in strength
resulted.[13] Immersion in cold water (50° F) resulted in a mean decrease
of 11% in strength.

RESERVE STRENGTH.   The reserve-strength theory is supported by
observations of persons who have performed great feats of strength
while under emotional stress or excitement, and who were unable to
perform voluntarily the same feats after the emotional state had passed.
This idea has little support from research, probably because conditions
are difficult to reproduce experimentally. Physiologists have explained
reserve strength as a condition resulting from (1) increased secretion of
epinephrine (Adrenalin), causing the muscles to become more irritable,
or (2) a stronger stimulus from the central nervous system and a
reduction of inhibition, causing more muscle fibers to respond.

If the reserve-strength theory is true, coaches and athletes ought to capitalize on it when maximal strength is needed. We believe that the theory is true, and that it partly accounts for the fact that athletes usually perform feats of greater strength (and endurance) under the stress of competition than in practice.

CROSS-TRAINING EFFECTS.   Several studies have indicated that by training certain muscles on one side of the body a lesser but measurable gain in strength (and endurance) results in the corresponding muscles on the opposite side. Hellebrandt and her co-workers did considerable research in this area.[17-19] Hettinger and Muller concluded that cross training in strength occurs only when isotonic methods are used.[16] They found no cross effects whatsoever from isometric training. Conversely, Coleman found that cross effects resulted from both isotonic and isometric training.[7] Gardner, who experimented with five different strength programs, obtained no significant cross effects.[12]

The following facts should be pointed out: (1) Cross-training effects on strength have been observed only from exercises that cause overloading of the muscles. A light load does not produce strength, and neither does it cause cross-training effects. (2) It has been observed that during heavy resistance exercise the muscles of the untrained side experience slight isometric contractions during the contractions of the muscles on the side being trained. (3) In some experiments on this topic, strength tests were given at various intervals throughout the experimental period, and the tests themselves might have resulted in strength stimuli, accounting for at least part of the cross-training results.

The rationale for cross training is not clear, but it is known that isotonics involve more complex patterns of innervation than isometrics. Because of this, some motor learning might result in the muscle groups opposite those being trained. DeVries states: "it seems likely that the cross-education is brought about by an overflow of nervous energy from neurons in the motor cortex which innervate the crossed pyramidal fibers, to a smaller number of neurons that supply the uncrossed fibers."[11] This statement indicates that cross training is centered in the nervous system and not in the muscle tissue.

SEASONS AND ULTRAVIOLET RADIATION.   It has been found that persons display greater fitness during the summer than during other seasons. A practical question then is whether they are more responsive to training during the hot months. To answer the question, Hettinger compiled data showing that individuals training under experimental conditions gained strength faster during July, August, and September than during other months.[14] He theorized that the main reasons were that (1) the subjects got more ultraviolet radiation from the sun during the hot summer months, and (2) they ate considerably more fresh fruit and vegetables during the summer, thus increasing their intake of vitamins.

Ultraviolet radiation has been administered artificially to athletes in training for vigorous sports on several occasions, and in each case positive effects have been reported. Even though there is evidence that an abundance of radiation is beneficial to strength development, the evidence is not really conclusive, and the topic deserves additional experimentation. (When sunlamps are used for ultraviolet radiation, caution against overexposure should be exercised.)

DIET AND FOOD SUPPLEMENTS. It is well established that the ability to maintain a high level of conditioning and to improve conditioning is greatly hindered by inadequate diet. Some researchers claim that certain food supplements make significant contributions to conditioning. However, when all information on this topic is put together, it indicates that if a person has a sound diet to begin with, food supplements contribute little, if any, to trainability. Specifically, there is no evidence that supplements increase the rate of strength gains, provided the person eats a well-rounded diet, including ample amounts of animal products, fresh fruits, and vegetables (see Chapter 14 for a more complete discussion on this topic).

During the past few years more and more athletes have turned to the use of a group of drugs called *anabolic steroids*, which supposedly contribute to greater strength and weight gains. Even though some research indicates that steroids might enhance strength training, the use of such drugs by athletes is highly questionable.

Steroids are drugs that chemically resemble male sex hormones. We do not know precisely how hormones work; thus, all possible side effects are not known. Some recent studies have shown that if the dosage is kept small and the duration of use short, no immediate undesirable effects are *apparent*. But the long-range effects still remain in question (see Chapter 14).

MUSCLE ENDURANCE

Endurance is defined as resistance to fatigue and quick recovery after fatigue. A high level of endurance implies that a given level of performance can be continued for a relatively long time. Increased endurance postpones the onset of fatigue. Endurance contributes to improved performance in instances in which fatigue is a limiting factor. The definition of endurance may apply to the body as a whole, to a particular body system, or to a local area of the muscle system.

Cardiovascular endurance is of vital concern in athletics and the following chapter is devoted to this important topic. This section covers muscular endurance, which is closely related to strength.

Muscular endurance is dependent upon (1) the quality of the mus-

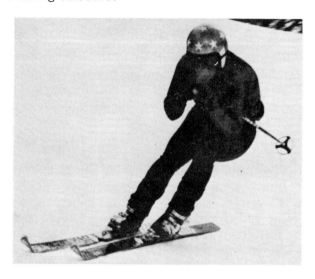

Figure 7–12. Downhill racer in action. (Tucker, K., and Jensen, C. R.: *Skiing,* 3rd ed. Dubuque: Wm. C. Brown Co., 1976, page 53.)

cles, (2) the extensiveness of their capillary beds, and (3) the nerve mechanisms supplying them. There are three potential sites of muscular fatigue (more correctly, of neuromuscular fatigue): (1) the synapses in the central nervous system, (2) the myoneural junction, and (3) the muscle tissue. The best available evidence points to the muscle tissue itself as the site of potential fatigue. It is doubtful that fatigue ever occurs at the myoneural junction. Asmussen stresses that muscular fatigue involves the chemical reactions, both aerobic and anaerobic, that are responsible for delivering energy to the contractile mechanism of the myofibrils of the muscle tissue.[1]

It has been well established that strength contributes to muscle endurance. In fact, there is a high correlation (.75 to .97) between strength and *absolute muscle endurance,* which is the amount of time that a subject can work against a constant resistance without relating the resistance to the subject's strength.

Conversely, there appears to be a low negative relationship between strength and *relative* muscle endurance. In other words, when the resistance is adjusted to correspond with each person's strength, then a weaker person tends to demonstrate more endurance than a stronger one. The research supports the following important conclusions about the relationship of strength and endurance:

1. There is a strong positive relationship between isotonic strength and *absolute* isotonic endurance (the same kind of

relationship exists between isometric strength and *absolute* isometric endurance).

2. There is a low negative relationship between isotonic strength and *relative* isotonic endurance (the same kind of relationship exists between isometric strength and relative isometric endurance).

Since increasing strength is an effective method of increasing absolute muscle endurance, the strength-building methods described previously may be used for this purpose (heavy resistance with few reps). The long accepted method of increased repetitions with decreased weight also may be used as long as the resistance is not decreased too much. Surprisingly, comparisons of strength and endurance programs have shown that both strength *and* endurance can be developed from either approach.[34]

Even though weight training has been used for illustration, it should be recognized that muscle endurance can be increased by any form of exercise that results in *overloading* the muscles either in *weight* or in *repetitions*. For example, calisthenic exercises, regular vigorous sports participation, and hard manual labor are all effective for developing endurance in the muscles. But it should be stressed that muscle endurance is highly specific, and significant increases will be limited to the muscles that experience regular overloading.

SELECTED REFERENCES

1. Asmussen, E.: The neuromuscular system and exercise. In *Exercise Physiology.* N. H. Balls (Ed.). New York: Academic Press, 1968, p. 39.
2. Baldwin, K. M., Winder, W. W., Terjung, R. L., et al.: Glycolytic enzymes in different types of skeletal muscle: Adaptation to exercise. *Am. J. Physiol.,* 225:962–966, 1973.
3. Ball, J. R., Rich, G. Q., and Wallis, E. L.: Effects of isometric training on vertical jumping. *Res. Q.,* 35:231, 1964.
4. Berger, R. A.: Comparison of static and dynamic strength increases. *Res. Q.,* 33:329, 1962a.
5. Berger, R. A.: Effect of varied weight training programs on strength. *Res. Q.,* 33:168, 1962b.
6. Berger, R. A.: Leg extension at three different angles. *Res. Q.,* 37:560, 1966.
7. Coleman, A. E.: Effect of unilateral isometric and isotonic contractions on the strength of the contralateral limb. *Res. Q.,* 40:490, 1969.
8. Councilman, J. E.: The importance of speed in exercise. *Athletic Journal,* May 1976, pp. 72–75.
9. DeLateur, B., et al.: Comparison of effectiveness of isokinetic and isotonic exercise in quadriceps strengthening. *Arch. Phys. Med. Rehabil.,* Feb. 1972, pp. 60–64.
10. DeLorme, T., and Wilkins, A. L.: *Progressive Resistance Exercise.* New York: Appleton-Century-Crofts, 1951.
11. DeVries, H. A.: *Physiology of Exercise for Physical Education and Athletics,* 2nd ed. Dubuque: Wm. C. Brown Co., 1974.

12. Gardner, H. W.: Specificity of strength changes of the exercised and non-exercised limb following isometric training. *Res. Q.*, 34:98, 1963.
13. Grose, J. E.: Depression of muscle fatigue curves by heat and cold. *Res. Q.*, 29:19, 1958.
14. Hettinger, T.: *Physiology of Strength.* Springfield, Ill.: Charles C Thomas, 1961.
15. Hettinger, T., and Muller, E. A.: Muskelleistung and Muskeltraining. *Arbeitsphysiologie*, 15:111, 1953.
16. Hettinger, T., and Muller, E. A.: Die Trainierbarkeit der Muskulatur. *Arbeitsphysiologie*, 16:90, 1955.
17. Hellebrandt, F. A.: Cross education: Ipsilateral and contralateral effects of unimanual training. *J. Appl. Physiol.*, 4:136, 1951.
18. Hellebrandt, F. A., Houtz, S. J., and Kirkorian, A. M.: Influence of bimanual exercise on unilateral work capacity. *J. Appl. Physiol.*, 2:446, 1950.
19. Hellebrandt, F. A., Parrish, A. M., and Houtz, S. J.: Cross education: The influence of unilateral exercise on the contralateral limb. *Arch. Phys. Med.*, 78:76, 1947.
20. Hill, A. V.: The mechanics of voluntary muscle. *Lancet*, 261:947, 1951.
21. Jensen, C. R.: The significance of strength in athletic performance. *Coach and Athlete*, December 1965, p. 22.
22. Johnson, B. L., et al.: A comparison of concentric and eccentric muscle training. *Med. Sci. Sports*, 8:35–38, 1976.
23. Jokl, E.: *Physiology of Exercise.* Springfield, Ill.: Charles C Thomas, 1964.
24. Klein, K. K.: Muscular strength in the knee. *The Physician and Sports Medicine*, December 1974, p. 29.
25. Linford, A. G., and Rarick, L.: The effect of knee angle on the measurement of leg strength of college males. *Res. Q.*, 39:582, 1968.
26. McGlynn, G. H.: A re-evaluation of isometric strength training. *Journal Sports Med.*, December 1972, pp. 258, 260.
27. Moffroid, M., et al.: A study of isokinetic exercise. *Phys. Ther.*, 49:735, 1966.
28. Pipes, T. B., and Wilmore, J.: Isokinetic versus isotonic strength training in adult men. *Athletic Journal*, June 1976, pp. 26–29.
29. Rasch, P. J.: The present status of negative (eccentric) exercise. *Am. Correct. Ther. J.*, May-June 1974, p. 77.
30. Rasch, P. J., and Morehouse, L. E.: Effect of static and dynamic exercises on muscular strength and hypertrophy. *J. Appl. Physiol.*, 11:29, 1957.
31. Rich, G. Q., Ball, J. R., and Wallis, E. L.: Effects of isometric training on strength and transfer of effect to untrained antagonists. *J. Sports Med. Phys. Fitness*, 4:217, 1964.
32. Royce, J.: Isometric fatigue curves in human muscle with normal and occluded circulation. *Res. Q.*, 29:204, 1958.
33. Shepherd, G. R.: A comparison of the effects of isotonic, isokinetic and negative resistance strength training programs. Doctoral dissertation. Provo: Brigham Young University, 1975.
34. Sorenson, M. B.: The Effects of Conventional and High-repetition Weight-training Programs on Strength and Cardiovascular Endurance. Unpublished doctoral dissertation. Provo: Brigham Young University, 1974.
35. Thistle, H. G., et al.: Isokinetic contraction: A new concept of resistive exercise. *Arch. Phys. Med. Rehabil.*, 48:279, 1966.
36. Van Oteghen, S. L.: Two speeds of isokinetic exercise as related to the vertical jump performance of women. *Res. Q.*, 46:78–84, 1975.

Chapter 8
Endurance and the Energy Systems

Three sources of energy for muscular activity have been mentioned and discussed in previous chapters. The first of these is the ATP and CP found in the cell. This is called the alactacid system and can support intense work only for 10 to 15 sec before it is used up. The second major source of energy is that produced by the glycolytic pathway. This is often referred to as the lactacid system, because lactic acid is produced as a by-product when it is used for energy production. Energy from this source can support intense work only for 45 to 60 sec. The third source of energy comes from the oxidative pathways in the cell and yields water and carbon dioxide as normal by-products. Of course, this system can support low levels of work almost indefinitely, and moderate levels for long periods. This is the most efficient of the energy systems, and is able to produce ATP from food products at an efficiency of about 50%.

Each of these systems can be trained to become more effective in the production of energy, and should be trained either alone or together for all athletic events. The purpose of this chapter is to discuss the techniques of training these energy systems and the principles involved in using these techniques.

SPECIFIC TRAINING GUIDELINES

Although few athletic events use a single system, it might be helpful to discuss first how each system can be trained with minimal involvement of other systems.

159

Alactacid System (ATP-CP)

The alactacid system can be improved best by short (10 sec or so) bouts of high-intensity work, followed by rest periods of at least the same duration and preferably longer. High-intensity work bouts of 10 sec, followed by 10-sec rest periods raised blood lactate only from 10 mg/100 ml of blood to 20 mg/100 ml of blood after 30 min of work. Fifteen-sec work bouts followed by 30 sec of rest only yielded an increase in lactate of 16 mg/100 ml of blood.[11] Athletes trained with short, high-intensity sprint training increase their power potential dramatically as measured by a test such as the Margaria-Kalamen power test. This would indicate that specific training of this system is accomplished easily. This increase in power is a result of increased levels of ATP-CP in the muscle. This increase has been reported at 25% to 40%.[24]

Lactacid System

The best way to train the lactacid system is to use longer bouts (45 to 60 sec) of high-intensity work, followed by recovery periods at least as long as the work period or longer. Four or five such work bouts increase the lactic acid levels to maximal values (20 mmoles/liter) and are strenuous for the subject. There is no doubt that training of this type increases the athlete's ability to develop high blood lactate levels. The enzymes of glycolysis also are increased significantly.[19]

Oxidative or Aerobic System

The best way to train the oxidative system *only* would be to work at moderate levels for long periods of time.

The following "rules" have been proven through research to yield changes in aerobic conditioning:

1. *Type.* Choose activities involving large muscle groups of the body in a rhythmic, continuous way. Jogging, walking, rope jumping, swimming, and bicycling are excellent activities which meet these criteria.

2. *Intensity.* The minimal level of intensity should be hard enough to cause a heart rate (HR) of 120 beats/minute. This is the point at which stroke volume is maximal and yields a volume overload on the myocardium. Karvonen found the minimal level of intensity to be 60% of the difference between resting HR and maximal HR, added to the resting HR.[22] Others have found that about 70% of the maximal heart rate yields good results.[1] Within limits, the higher the intensity, the better is the effect. Of course, as stress levels increase, the involvement of the anaerobic systems will also increase.

3. *Duration.* The workout must be at least 15-min duration at the

proper intensity. Longer durations are more effective yet.[30] Most errors in aerobic conditioning involve the violation of the duration principle. Short exercise bouts (4 or 5 min) followed by rest periods long enough to allow the heart rate to decrease below the minimal training intensity are not as effective for training the aerobic system as is continuous exercise at the proper duration.

4. *Frequency.* Workouts should be scheduled on a daily basis, if possible, for maximal effect. However, a frequency of three times a week or every other day will be effective if the duration is increased by 5 or 10 min.

It should be emphasized that aerobic conditioning can be accomplished using interval training techniques. Astrand and Rodahl suggested working from 3 to 5 min with equal periods of light work.[7] The tempo does not have to be maximal during these periods, nor does one need to be exhausted at the end of the workout. Astrand and Rodahl recommended that the work bout elicit heart rates that are within 10 beats of maximum. The rest period heart rates should not decrease below 120 beats/minute. These intensities and rest durations can be computed using heart rate or by timing the work interval at some percentage of the athlete's maximal time (see section on interval training in this chapter for more information).

These aforementioned increase the $\dot{V}O_2$ max, cardiac output, and stroke volume of the heart, and are associated with increased running speed, decreased submaximal and resting heart rates, and the number of mitochondria and the concentration of oxidative enzymes in the mitochondria of the muscle involved in the exercise.

SELECTION OF THE ENERGY SYSTEM

Most athletic events involve two, and sometimes all, energy systems. However, there is always a predominant system which must receive the most emphasis. How can you tell which system requires the most emphasis? Table 8–1 illustrates the relationship between different track events and the primary energy systems involved. From these data, it is apparent that an athlete who is training to run the mile should devote 20% of his program to speed (alactacid), 55% to lactacid programs, and 25% to aerobic work. Notice that the time of each performance also is included. This allows the coach or athlete to use this information for other events. For example, a swimming event lasting 4 to 5 min would require approximately the same training emphasis as the mile run, which also lasts 4 to 5 min. Of course, the training stimulus would vary depending on the activity involved. *The point is that the energy source to be emphasized is time-dependent.*

TABLE 8–1
Percentage of Training Time Spent in Developing the Energy Sources for Various Track Events

Event	Performance Time	Speed %	Aerobic Capacity %	Anaerobic Capacity %
Marathon	135:00 to 180:00	5	90	5
6 mile	30:00 to 50:00	5	80	15
3 mile	15:00 to 25:00	10	70	20
2 mile	10:00 to 16:00	20	40	40
1 mile	4:00 to 6:00	20	25	55
880 yards	2:00 to 3:00	30	5	65
440 yards	1:00 to 1:30	80	3	15
220 yards	0:22 to 0:35	95	3	2
110 yards	0:10 to 0:15	95	2	3

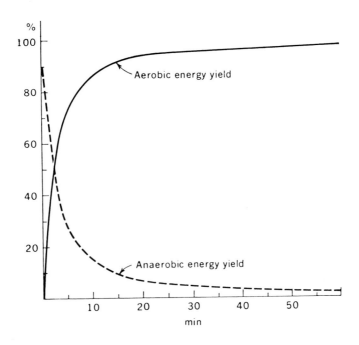

Figure 8–1. Relative contribution in percentage of total energy yield from aerobic and anaerobic processes, respectively, during maximal efforts of up to 60 min duration for an individual with high maximal power for both processes. Note that a 2-min maximal effort hits the 50 percent mark, meaning that both processes are equally important for success. (From *Textbook of Work Physiology* by Astrand and Rodahl, page 304. Copyright © 1970 by McGraw-Hill, Inc. Used with permission of McGraw-Hill Book Company.)

TABLE 8-2
Various Sports and Their Predominant Energy System (S)

Sports or Sport Activity	% Emphasis According to Energy Systems		
	ATP-PC and LA	LA-O_2	O_2
1. Baseball	80	20	—
2. Basketball	85	15	—
3. Fencing	90	10	—
4. Field Hockey	60	20	20
5. Football	90	10	—
6. Golf	95	5	—
7. Gymnastics	90	10	—
8. Ice Hockey			
a. forwards, defense	80	20	—
b. goalie	95	5	—
9. Lacrosse			
a. goalie, defense, attack men	80	20	—
b. midfielders, man-down	60	20	20
10. Rowing	20	30	50
11. Skiing			
a. slalom, jumping, downhill	80	20	—
b. cross-country	—	5	95
c. pleasure skiing	34	33	33
12. Soccer			
a. goalie, wings, strikers	80	20	—
b. halfbacks, or link men	60	20	20
13. Swimming and diving			
a. 50 yds., diving	98	2	—
b. 100 yds.	80	15	5
c. 200 yds.	30	65	5
d. 400, 500 yds.	20	40	40
e. 1500, 1650 yds.	10	20	70
14. Tennis	70	20	10
15. Track and field			
a. 100, 220 yds.	98	2	—
b. field events	90	10	—
c. 440 yds.	80	15	5
d. 880 yds.	30	65	5
e. 1 mile	20	55	25
f. 2 miles	20	40	40
g. 3 miles	10	20	70
h. 6 miles (cross-country)	5	15	80
i. marathon	—	5	95
16. Volleyball	90	10	—
17. Wrestling	90	10	—

Modified from Mathews, K. D., and Fox, E. L.: *The Physiological Basis of Physical Education and Athletics.* Philadelphia: W. B. Saunders Co., 1976.

This relationship is more graphically shown in Figure 8–1, which shows the total contribution of anaerobic energy (both alactacid and lactacid) and aerobic energy as related to time of the activity.

Using the information in Table 8–1, Mathews and Fox have developed a table showing their idea of the energy requirements of various activities (Table 8–2).[28] It is difficult to assess the contribution of the various energy systems in a sport such as football, however, because of several complicating factors. For instance, the energy needs for a lineman may differ significantly from those of a split end. It also is difficult to assess the contribution of the aerobic system in games that last for several hours. An increased emphasis on aerobic conditioning may be extremely valuable during the last quarter of a contest, during which the high aerobic capacity would result in a more rapid payoff of oxygen debt and allow the player to perform at his early game level of skill.

TRAINING PROGRAMS

It is easy to use time-energy relationships to train runners. Table 8–3 lists various types of training programs involving speed training, aerobic training, and anaerobic training. A coach or an athlete can refer to Table 8–1 for the type of program needed in training for his event, then to Table 8–3 for a description of the training program to be used. For example, a 2-miler should use a training program with 20% of the emphasis on speed, 40% on aerobic capacity, and 40% on the lactacid system. He would then attempt to match these percentages to a training program listed in Table 8–3. Speed play, or fartlek training, is the type of training most nearly matched to the training requirements of a 2-miler, but repetition running could be used with good results.

TABLE 8–3
Endurance Development Programs Specifying Type of Training

Types of Training	Speed %	Aerobic Endurance %	Anaerobic Endurance %
Repetitions of sprints	90	4	6
Continuous slow running	2	93	5
Continuous fast running	2	90	8
Slow interval	10	60	30
Fast interval	30	20	50
Repetition running	10	40	50
Speed play	20	40	40
Interval sprinting	20	70	10
Acceleration sprinting	90	5	5
Hollow sprints	85	5	10

The different types of training listed in Table 8–3 are described below:

Repetitions of sprints involve the repetition of short sprints as a means of preparation for competitive running. Since sprinting means running at absolute maximal speed, there is not an "easy sprint." The effect of sprinting as a means of training is the development of speed and muscular strength.

Continuous slow running refers to running long distances at relatively slow speeds. The distances covered in this type of training should be related to the racing event. For example, a miler might run five times his racing distance or more. The heart rate should be between 80% and 90% maximum during this type of training, and the speed depends upon the ability of the athlete.

Continuous fast running differs from continuous slow running in terms of speed. Because the pace is faster, fatigue is encountered sooner. This training develops aerobic endurance. It represents a form of effort that seeks gradually to condition the organism to tolerate the stress encountered in running at faster and faster speeds.

Slow interval develops aerobic endurance. The speed is faster than in continuous fast-running training, thus adapting the athlete to running at a more intense effort. In this type of formal fast-slow running, the heart beats at the rate of approximately 180 beats per min or more during the heavy work phase.

Fast interval develops anaerobic endurance or speed endurance. It is used after a background of aerobic or general endurance has been established. The heart should beat at maximal or near-maximal rate during the work phase. It develops the ability of the runner to withstand fatigue in the absence of an adequate oxygen supply.

Repetition running differs from internal training in terms of the length of the fast run and the degree of recovery following each fast effort. It involves repetitions of comparatively longer distances with relatively complete recovery (usually by walking) after each effort. Repetition running is usually concerned with repetitions of distances such as 880 yards to 2 miles with relatively complete recovery between, during which time the heart rate falls below 120 beats/minute. Conversely, interval training includes repetitions of shorter distances (ordinarily 110 to 440 yards) with less than complete recovery after each by jogging a distance equal to the fast run in a time period two to three times as long as required to complete the fast run.

Speed play is a form of training featuring informal fast-slow running, as opposed to the formal fast-slow running in interval training. It involves running preferably, but not necessarily, over natural surfaces such as golf courses, grass, or trails through woods, with emphasis on fast running. Fast and slow interval running, repetition running, sprinting, walking, and continuous fast-running training are informally combined in speed play. This type of training is also known as *fartlek* training.

Interval sprinting is a method of training whereby an athlete alternately sprints about 50 yards and jogs 10 yards for distances up to 3 miles. After the first few sprints, fatigue tends to inhibit the athlete from running at his absolute top speed. Similarly, fatigue causes the athlete to slow his recovery jogging to a very slow rate.

Acceleration sprinting is the gradual acceleration from jogging to striding to sprinting. For example, an athlete may jog 25 yards, stride 50 yards, and sprint 50 yards, followed by 50 yards of walking, then repeat the procedure several times. This type of training emphasizes both speed and endurance, provided enough repetitions are performed to cause endurance overload.

Hollow sprints are two sprints joined by a "hollow" period of recovery jogging. Examples include sprint 50, jog 50, sprint 50, and walk 50 yards for recovery prior to the next repetition; sprint 110, jog 110, sprint 110, and walk 110 yards before the next repetition; sprint 220, jog 220, and walk 220 yards before repeating.

Many of the programs mentioned are a type of *interval training*. Any interval-training program consists of a series of work bouts with a short rest interval between bouts. Astrand and Rodahl found that a work load that could be tolerated continuously for only 9 min could be carried on for an hour when done intermittently.[7] This means that much more total work can be accomplished before fatigue when interval training is used than when continuous training is used.

In order for an interval-training program to continue to be effective over a period of time, the intensity must be increased as endurance is gained so that overload may continue to be applied. In other words, as an athlete becomes better conditioned, he must do more work during each of the training periods to cause additional endurance gains. Interval-training workouts may be varied four different ways: (1) the number of work bouts can be increased; (2) the length of each bout can be increased; (3) the intensity of each bout can be increased; and (4) the rest periods between bouts can be shortened.

The intensity and length of the work interval should be based upon the primary energy system being used in the activity. Sprinters should have short, high-intensity intervals, whereas marathoners may run intervals of 3 miles at race pace or slower. It should be pointed out that the "rest" interval is really not a time to stop all activity, but only a jog or walk period which allows the body to recover somewhat before the next interval begins.

Perhaps the best approach for quantifying the intensity, number of work intervals, and the rest period between each interval is found in the handbook *Computerized Running Training Programs*.[18] This book

Scoring of Classical English Racing Distances

Points	100 Yd	220 Yd	440 Yd	880 Yd	1.00 Mi	2.00 Mi	3.00 Mi	6.00 Mi	10.00 Mi	Marathon
830	9.99	22.2	50.0	1:56.0	4:19.3	9:20.9	14:28.3	30:20.9	52:26	2:27:11
820	10.04	22.3	50.3	1:56.7	4:20.9	9:24.4	14:33.8	30:32.7	52:46	2:28:10
810	10.08	22.4	50.6	1:57.4	4:22.5	9:28.0	14:39.4	30:44.6	53:07	2:29:10
800	10.13	22.6	50.9	1:58.1	4:24.1	9:31.6	14:45.0	30:56.7	53:28	2:30:10
790	10.18	22.7	51.1	1:58.8	4:25.8	9:35.3	14:50.8	31:08.9	53:50	2:31:11
780	10.23	22.8	51.4	1:59.5	4:27.4	9:39.0	14:56.6	31:21.3	54:11	2:32:14
770	10.28	22.9	51.7	2:00.2	4:29.1	9:42.8	15:02.5	31:33.9	54:33	2:33:16
760	10.33	23.0	52.0	2:00.9	4:30.8	9:46.6	15:08.5	31:46.6	54:55	2:34:20
750	10.38	23.1	52.3	2:01.7	4:32.6	9:50.4	15:14.5	31:59.5	55:18	2:35:25
740	10.43	23.2	52.6	2:02.4	4:34.3	9:54.3	15:20.6	32:12.6	55:41	2:36:30
730	10.48	23.4	52.9	2:03.2	4:36.1	9:58.3	15:26.9	32:25.8	56:04	2:37:37
720	10.53	23.5	53.2	2:03.9	4:37.9	10:02.3	15:33.1	32:39.3	56:28	2:38:44
710	10.58	23.6	53.5	2:04.7	4:39.7	10:06.4	15:39.5	32:52.9	56:51	2:39:53
700	10.63	23.7	53.8	2:05.5	4:41.6	10:10.5	15:46.0	33:06.7	57:16	2:41:02
690	10.68	23.8	54.1	2:06.3	4:43.4	10:14.7	15:52.6	33:20.7	57:40	2:42:13
680	10.74	24.0	54.4	2:07.1	4:45.3	10:19.0	15:59.2	33:34.9	58:05	2:43:24
670	10.79	24.1	54.7	2:07.9	4:47.2	10:23.3	16:06.0	33:49.3	58:30	2:44:37
660	10.85	24.2	55.1	2:08.7	4:49.2	10:27.6	16:12.8	34:04.0	58:56	2:45:50
650	10.90	24.4	55.4	2:09.5	4:51.2	10:32.0	16:19.7	34:18.8	59:22	2:47:05
640	10.96	24.5	55.7	2:10.4	4:53.2	10:36.5	16:26.8	34:33.8	59:48	2:48:21
630	11.01	24.6	56.0	2:11.2	4:55.2	10:41.1	16:33.9	34:49.1	1:00:15	2:49:38
620	11.07	24.7	56.4	2:12.1	4:57.2	10:45.7	16:41.2	35:04.6	1:00:42	2:50:56
610	11.12	24.9	56.7	2:13.0	4:59.3	10:50.4	16:48.5	35:20.3	1:01:10	2:52:15
600	11.18	25.0	57.1	2:13.9	5:01.4	10:55.1	16:56.0	35:36.3	1:01:38	2:53:36
590	11.24	25.2	57.4	2:14.8	5:03.6	10:59.9	17:03.6	35:52.5	1:02:06	2:54:58
580	11.30	25.3	57.8	2:15.7	5:05.8	11:04.8	17:11.2	36:09.0	1:02:35	2:56:21
570	11.36	25.4	58.1	2:16.6	5:08.0	11:09.8	17:19.0	36:25.7	1:03:04	2:57:46
560	11.42	25.6	58.5	2:17.5	5:10.2	11:14.8	17:27.0	36:42.7	1:03:34	2:59:11
550	11.48	25.7	58.9	2:18.5	5:12.5	11:20.0	17:35.0	36:59.9	1:04:04	3:00:39
540	11.54	25.9	59.2	2:19.5	5:14.8	11:25.2	17:43.2	37:17.4	1:04:35	3:02:07
530	11.60	26.0	59.6	2:20.4	5:17.1	11:30.4	17:51.5	37:35.2	1:05:06	3:03:38
520	11.67	26.2	1:00.0	2:21.4	5:19.5	11:35.8	17:59.9	37:53.2	1:05:38	3:05:09

Gardner, J. B., and Purdy, J. G.: Computerized Running Training Programs. Los Altos: Tafnews Press, 1970.

contains computerized training tables for any normal level of fitness and allows a wide variety of workouts to be generated for any running event. The book is easy to use and provides the beginning track coach with the information to prescribe individualized training programs for each athlete on his team. The first step is to time the athlete in his best event, and enter the "scoring tables" with that time to get a "point" level for the athlete. Most world-class athletes score between 980 to 1060 points. A typical high school miler may score only 780 points (a 4:27.4 mile) (Table 8–4). Using this information (the number of points scored), you can enter the "pacing" tables, which show various combinations of repetitions and times, as well as the recommended rest intervals between work intervals. Table 8–5 shows the pacing tables for the 780-point miler. If you desire a series of 440s on a given day, you can use eight to nine 440s in 1:03, with a 2- to 3-min jog between. Note that the clock is used to pace the athlete so he can complete the amount of work desired, rather than as a means of increasing the speed of each interval. No athlete could run this workout at full speed.

It is possible to vary the program in many different ways, using any combination of distance, speed, rest, and the like. There is a close correlation between the programs generated in the book, and actual workouts of world-class runners.

It should be emphasized that aerobic conditioning can be accomplished using interval training procedures which have been selected primarily to train other systems (alactacid; lactacid). For example, you desire to develop the aerobic capacity of a group of basketball players while emphasizing the anaerobic energy sources, and at the same time have them practice the skills involved in basketball. You can do this easily by having the players perform a series of high-intensity drills (such as fast-break drills), and still keep their heart rates above 120 beats per minute during the rest period by having them jog back to their starting positions on the basketball floor. You must force the intensity of the drill during the fast-break portion and never allow the heart rate to drop below 120 beats/minute during the recovery portion, for a total period of 15 to 20 min. You can go from drill to drill, but you must not stop the activity and allow the heart rate to drop until the total time has elapsed. Many successful coaches use this technique without realizing why it works.

SPECIFICITY OF TRAINING

Someone has suggested that if an athletic training book were written which was only one page long, it should have as its central theme *specificity of training*. It is important to realize that the body responds to any training program specifically. The long-distance runner needs to run rather than to swim, the tennis player will get little help from

Speed	Reps	Rest	110 Yd	150 Yd	165 Yd	220 Yd	275 Yd	330 Yd	352 Yd	385 Yd	440 Yd	495 Yd
95.0%	0– 1	—	11.0	15.2	16.8	22.8	29.5	37.0	40.1	44.9	53.1	1:01.6
92.5%	1– 2	4– 5 M	11.3	15.6	17.2	23.4	30.3	38.0	41.2	46.1	54.5	1:03.3
90.0%	2– 3	4– 5 M	11.6	16.0	17.7	24.1	31.2	39.0	42.3	47.4	56.0	1:05.1
87.5%	3– 4	3– 4 M	11.9	16.5	18.2	24.8	32.1	40.2	43.5	48.7	57.6	1:06.9
85.0%	4– 5	3– 4 M	12.3	17.0	18.8	25.5	33.0	41.3	44.8	50.2	59.3	1:08.9
82.5%	6– 7	2– 3 M	12.6	17.5	19.3	26.3	34.0	42.6	46.2	51.7	1:01.1	1:11.0
80.0%	8– 9	2– 3 M	13.0	18.0	19.9	27.1	35.1	43.9	47.6	53.3	1:03.0	1:13.2
77.5%	10–12	1– 2 M	13.5	18.6	20.6	28.0	36.2	45.3	49.2	55.0	1:05.1	1:15.6
75.0%	13–15	1– 2 M	13.9	19.2	21.3	28.9	37.4	46.9	50.8	56.9	1:07.3	1:18.1
72.5%	16–18	60–90 S	14.4	19.9	22.0	29.9	38.7	48.5	52.5	58.8	1:09.6	1:20.8
70.0%	19–21	60–90 S	14.9	20.6	22.8	31.0	40.1	50.2	54.4	1:00.9	1:12.1	1:23.7
67.5%	22–24	45–75 S	15.5	21.4	23.6	32.1	41.6	52.1	56.4	1:03.2	1:14.7	1:26.8
65.0%	25–29	45–75 S	16.0	22.2	24.5	33.3	43.2	54.1	58.6	1:05.6	1:17.6	1:30.1
62.5%	30–35	30–60 S	16.7	23.1	25.5	34.7	44.9	56.2	1:00.9	1:08.2	1:20.7	1:33.7
60.0%	36–40	30–60 S	17.4	24.0	26.6	36.1	46.8	58.6	1:03.5	1:11.1	1:24.1	—

Speed	Reps	Rest	550 Yd	660 Yd	880 Yd	1100 Yd	1320 Yd	1.00 Mi	1.25 Mi	1.50 Mi	1.75 Mi	2.00 Mi
95.0%	0– 1	—	1:10.5	1:28.5	2:04.8	2:42.9	3:21.5	4:40.7	6:01.3	7:23.3	8:45.8	10:08.7
92.5%	1– 2	4– 5 M	1:12.4	1:30.9	2:08.2	2:47.3	3:26.9	4:48.3	6:11.1	7:35.2	9:00.0	10:25.1
90.0%	2– 3	4– 5 M	1:14.4	1:33.4	2:11.8	2:51.9	3:32.6	4:56.3	6:21.4	7:47.9	9:15.0	10:42.5
87.5%	3– 4	3– 4 M	1:16.5	1:36.1	2:15.5	2:56.8	3:38.7	5:04.7	6:32.3	8:01.3	9:30.8	11:00.8
85.0%	4– 5	3– 4 M	1:18.8	1:38.9	2:19.5	3:02.0	3:45.2	5:13.7	6:43.8	8:15.4	9:47.6	11:20.3
82.5%	6– 7	2– 3 M	1:21.2	1:41.9	2:23.7	3:07.5	3:52.0	5:23.2	6:56.1	—	—	—
80.0%	8– 9	2– 3 M	1:23.7	1:45.1	2:28.2	3:13.4	3:59.2	5:33.3	—	—	—	—
77.5%	10–12	1– 2 M	1:26.4	1:48.5	2:33.0	3:19.6	4:06.9	—	—	—	—	—
75.0%	13–15	1– 2 M	1:29.3	1:52.1	2:38.1	3:26.3	—	—	—	—	—	—
72.5%	16–18	60–90 S	1:32.4	1:55.9	2:43.6	—	—	—	—	—	—	—
70.0%	19–21	60–90 S	1:35.7	2:00.1	2:49.4	—	—	—	—	—	—	—
67.5%	22–24	45–75 S	1:39.2	2:04.5	—	—	—	—	—	—	—	—
65.0%	25–29	45–75 S	1:43.0	—	—	—	—	—	—	—	—	—
62.5%	30–35	30–60 S	—	—	—	—	—	—	—	—	—	—
60.0%	36–40	30–60 S	—	—	—	—	—	—	—	—	—	—

Gardner, J. B., and Purdy, J. G.: Computerized Running Training Programs. Los Altos: Tafnews Press, 1970.

shooting baskets. Although these examples are fairly obvious, there are still many unanswered questions concerning specificity of training. For instance, the interpretation of literature dealing with weight training has been difficult because of the specific effects of certain programs on subjects. Researchers compare isometric to isotonic programs using a cable tensiometer (static tension) as the criterion measure. It is now known that subjects who train isometrically will show the greatest gains if tested with static devices and those who train isotonically show better gains if tested using the isotonic techniques. This means that a study comparing two different training programs often finds in favor of the program that used a testing method similar to the training method.

Another question being investigated is the effects of slow resistance training for activities requiring high-speed motion or power. For instance, are a series of heavy squats as effective for a football lineman as a series of high-speed isokinetic movements? Research concerning fast-twitch and slow-twitch fibers may lead to the idea that high-speed movements would be much more effective for the development of muscular power than the standard weight-training techniques now used, since slow repetitive movements are associated more with changes in slow-twitch oxidative fibers. One study comparing high-speed techniques with conventional methods reported that although the high-speed training exhibited its greatest improvements when measured with high-speed equipment, high-speed techniques also were at least as effective, and often more effective, even when measured at low limb speeds.[33] Apparently, training at high limb speed increased strength effectively at all limb speeds.

Specificity of training also has been demonstrated in cardiovascular endurance programs. When two groups of men were trained on different apparatus (treadmill vs. bicycle ergometer), the improvement in $\dot{V}O_2$ max for the bicycling group was significantly greater when tested on a bicycle ergometer than when tested on a treadmill.[32] This same principle was demonstrated graphically with identical twins who had both been outstanding swimmers. They were tested some time after one of the twins had stopped competitive training (but had remained active). The $\dot{V}O_2$ max of the highly trained twin was much higher when tested in the swimming flume. However, there was no significant difference between the two when tested on a treadmill.[22]

Subjects who train specific body areas (arms vs. legs) always show greater effects in the trained limbs than in the untrained limbs.[16] These experiments show that specificity of training applies to specific muscle groups also.

When two groups of subjects were trained using either a fast sprint interval or a slower endurance interval, the changes were related to the type of training performed.[15] Both groups made significant $\dot{V}O_2$ max improvements, but the capacity of the ATP-CP systems was much greater in the sprint group, whereas in the endurance group the amount of lactic acid produced during a submaximal exercise decreased. These data are convincing evidence that specificity of training also applies when training the energy systems of the body.

It is clear that the body adapts to the stresses placed upon it in a rather specific manner, and in order to maximize the training effect, one must identify the specific energy systems and movements of the sport or activity and develop training programs for them (see reference 29 for a detailed review of literature concerning specificity of training).

FACTORS THAT INFLUENCE ENDURANCE

The following factors relate to endurance and influence it in different ways.

Pace

The most economical pace is an even rate over the entire distance. In walking, running, swimming, and other locomotive activities, stopping, starting, accelerating, and decelerating are costly in terms of energy. Theoretically a 4-min mile should consist of four 60-sec quarters; however, this may not be feasible because the quarters are influenced by the start and finish of the race and by the necessity of gaining and holding position during the race. The idea of an even pace also has strong application to long-duration games, such as basketball, soccer, tennis, or handball. Playing in "bursts" requires much additional energy and should be avoided when endurance is of prime concern.

Skill

During performance a certain amount of energy is wasted in unnecessary and uncoordinated movements. A skilled individual wastes less energy than the unskilled. For example, an unskilled swimmer may use more than five times as much energy as a skilled person to swim the same distance. Similar comparisons could be made between skilled and unskilled performers in other activities. Repeated practice improves skill and efficiency, and thus influences endurance favorably.

Age

Endurance increases with age to a certain point, after which endurance decreases as age increases. Among trained individuals, maximal endurance usually occurs slightly later than maximal strength; the early 20s among women, and the middle to late 20s among men. Morehouse and Miller state that the ability of boys to perform endurance activities increases steadily to about the age of 20.[31] (With training, endurance will increase beyond this age.) They make these observations about the endurance of children: "The physiological systems of younger children are apparently not as well developed to meet the demands of strenuous exercise as they become when puberty is reached. Children under twelve years of age possess a highly active sympathetic nervous system that predisposes to a high heart rate and an easily depleted capacity to utilize oxygen." They further state that children have a small stroke volume of the heart and consequently a small capacity for increased circulation of blood. These limitations on endurance gradually diminish as the person matures into young adulthood, and endurance reaches its peak potential soon after full physical maturation is achieved.

After maximal endurance is reached, it holds fairly constant for 3 to 5 years, then begins to decline gradually because of several changes that occur in the circulatory and respiratory systems with increased age. Men in their 70s or 80s have lost about one half of their capacity for transforming energy aerobically. The ability to supply blood to active tissues has decreased, and skeletal muscles are weak. Nevertheless, when working within the limits of their ability, many men well advanced in years can carry on work with a lower heart rate and less evidence of fatigue than that exhibited by certain younger men. It should be noted that the loss of endurance at any stage in life can be reduced significantly as a result of training.

Sex

Studies show that up to the beginning of puberty, girls are about equal to boys in endurance. Women reach maximal endurance potential at about the age of 20, whereas men continue to increase until at least the mid 20s.

There is only a slight difference in endurance in moderate exercise, between adult men and women, but the endurance of women in strenuous activities is considerably less than that of men. Morehouse and Miller point out that adult women have only one half the endurance of adult men in running.[31] Limiting factors of endurance among women for vigorous activity are (1) a more rapid heart rate; (2) a small heart with a resultant smaller capacity to deliver blood; (3) smaller chest cavity, resulting in inferior lung capacity; and (4) the blood of women is limited in its oxygen-carrying capacity owing to fewer red blood cells.

Jokl has said this about girls: "Endurance training for girls ought to be initiated prior to the onset of puberty."[23] Training seems to reverse the natural trend toward decline of endurance in untrained girls. Once the effect of training upon performance is established, it can be stabilized over many years. And since sustained practice improves techniques, gains in efficiency may continue long after the establishment of optimal endurance.

Body Type

Physique studies by Cureton show that only swimmers with high mesomorphic characteristics have held world records.[13] A few slightly built ecto-mesomorphic swimmers have achieved high success at the long distances. Cureton also learned that champion runners have slight frames with long and well-muscled legs. Distance runners are typically more slight and less heavily muscled than sprinters.

Morehouse and Miller claim that people of moderate build have the greatest ability to sustain prolonged muscular effort.[31] Sills and Everett, (1953), in a study of the relationship between extreme body types and performance, found that mesomorphs were only slightly better than ectomorphs in endurance tests, and endomorphs were far inferior to the other two body types.[37] Bookwalter's evidence generally supports Sills' findings.[8]

In summary, it can be said that most persons who find success in endurance activities have a high degree of mesomorphy, and are also inclined toward ectomorphy. Individuals of heavier body types (more endomorphy) are inclined to be more successful in activities requiring endurance, such as swimming, rather than in those involving running. This is because in swimming the body weight is not carried by the muscles.

Overweight

Fat lacks the ability to contract; therefore, it does not contribute to performance. In fact, it hinders performance in three ways: (1) fat within the muscles causes friction and contributes to inefficiency in muscle contractions; (2) fat adds dead weight and thereby increases resistance against movement; (3) fatty tissue places an overload on the circulatory system, because it is estimated that 1 pound of fat increases the vascular system by 1 mile (mostly in the form of capillaries).

Temperature

Grose found that endurance is adversely affected by immersion of the arm for 8 min in water at 120° F.[20] Conversely, the effects of cold have proven to be advantageous, until a muscle temperature of 80° F is reached. According to Clark and associates, 80° F appears to be the optimal muscle temperature for endurance, and muscle temperatures below this level produce adverse effects on endurance.[12]

Hyperventilation

Hyperventilation may occur in an athlete either unintentionally or intentionally. It is brought on intentionally by forced deep breathing, which results in a greatly increased exchange of air to the lungs. Hyperventilation results in an appreciable decrease in CO_2 in the circulorespiratory system, but it does not increase the amount of O_2 in the blood, as commonly believed. The amount of oxygen transferred to the blood is not usually limited by the amount entering the lungs, but rather by the available area of contact between the alveoli and the capillary bed and by the carrying capacity of the blood. If the blood is already fully saturated, the excess oxygen in the lungs will be expelled only in normal expiration, because oxygen cannot be stored.

DeVries found that hyperventilation can approximately double breath-holding time.[14] Consequently, it will definitely improve performances where breath holding is important, such as underwater swimming, or crawl-stroke sprinting. But it is not established that hyperventilation is of any measurable value in performances in which breath holding is not involved.

Vital Capacity

Vital capacity, the total amount of air that can be forcibly expired after a complete inspiration, has been used frequently as a measure of adequacy of the respiratory system. Although it measures the approximate capacity of the lungs, recent information indicates it is of little use in predicting ability to perform tasks of endurance. Obviously, other factors are more significant. For example, any limitation of the oxygen delivery system to the cells will reduce the effectiveness of the delivery, regardless of vital capacity.

Probably a large vital capacity is important in intense exercise when there may be a lack of oxygen in the alveoli, but it is of little value when the exercise is less demanding. The main advantage of a large vital capacity is the ability to take in more air per unit of time with fewer, but deeper, inspirations, thus prolonging the onset of fatigue in the respiratory muscles.

SELECTED REFERENCES

1. American College of Sports Medicine: Guidelines for Graded Exercise Testing and Exercise Prescription. Philadelphia: Lea & Febiger, 1975.
2. Astrand, I.: Aeorbic work capacity in men and women with special reference to age. Acta Physiol. Scand., 49(Suppl. 169) 1960.
3. Astrand, I., Astrand, P.-O., Christensen, E. N., and Hedman, R.: Intermittent muscular work. Acta Physiol. Scand., 48, 448, 1960.
4. Astrand, P.-O.: Experimental Studies of Physical Working Capacity in Relation to Sex and Age. Copenhagen: Ejnar Munksgaard, 1952.
5. Astrand, P.-O. : Human physical fitness with special reference to sex and age. Physiol. Rev., 36:307, 1956.
6. Astrand, P.-O., Hallback, J., Hedman, R., and Saltin, B.: Blood lactates after prolonged severe exercise. J. Appl. Physiol., 18:619, 1963.

7. Astrand, P. -O., and Rodahl, K.: *Textbook of Work Physiology.* New York: McGraw-Hill Book Co., 1970.
8. Bookwalter, K. W.: The relationship of body size and shape to physical performance. *Res. Q., 22–23*:271, 1951–52.
9. Bowles, C. J., and Sigerseth, P. O.: Telemetered heart rate responses to pace patterns in the one mile run. *Res. Q., 39*:36, 1968.
10. Carlsten, A., and Grimby, G.: *The Circulatory Response to Muscular Exercise in Man.* Springfield, Ill.: Charles C Thomas, 1966.
11. Christensen, E. H., Hedman, R., and Saltin, B.: Intermittent and continuous running. *Acta Physiol. Scand., 50*:269, 1960.
12. Clark, R. S. J., Hellon, R. F., and Lind, A. R.: The duration of sustained contractions of the human forearm at different muscle temperatures. *J. Physiol., 143*:454, 1958.
13. Cureton, T. K.: *Physical Fitness of Champion Athletes.* Urbana, Ill.: University of Illinois Press, 1951.
14. DeVries, H. A.: *Physiology of Exercise for Physical Education and Athletics,* 2nd ed. Dubuque: Wm. C. Brown Co., 1974.
15. Fox, E.: Differences in metabolic alterations with sprint versus endurance interval training programs. In *Metabolic Adaptations to Prolonged Physical Exercise.* H. Howard and J. Poortmans (Eds.). Basel: Birkhauser Verlag, 1975, pp. 119–126.
16. Fox, E., McKenzie, D., and Cohen, K.: Specificity of training: Metabolic and circulatory responses. *Med. Sci. Sports, 7*:83, 1975.
17. Fox, E. L., Robinson, S., and Wiegman, D. L.: Metabolic energy sources during continuous and interval running. *J. Appl. Physiol., 27*:174, 1969.
18. Gardner, J. B., and Purdy, J. G.: *Computerized Running Training Programs.* Los Altos: Tafnews Press, 1970.
19. Gollnick, P., et al.: Effect of training on enzyme activity and fiber composition of human skeletal muscle. *J. Appl. Physiol., 34*:107–111, 1973.
20. Grose, J. E.: Depression of muscle fatigue curves by heat and cold. *Res. Q., 29*:19, 1958.
21. Hodgkins, I.: Influence of unilateral endurance training on contralateral limbs. *J. Appl. Physiol., 6*:991, 1961.
22. Holmér, I., and Åstrand, P.-O.: Swimming training and maximal oxygen uptake. *J. Appl. Physiol., 33*:510–513, 1972.
23. Jokl, E.: *Physiology of Exercise.* Springfield, Ill.: Charles C Thomas, 1964.
24. Karlson, J., Nordesjö, L., Jorfeldt, L., and Saltin, B.: Muscle lactate, ATP, and CP levels during exercise after physical training in men. *J. Appl. Physiol., 33*:199–203, 1972.
25. Karvonen, M. J.: Effects of vigorous exercise on the heart. In *Work and the Heart.* F. F. Rosenbaum and E. L. Belnap (Eds.). New York: Paul B. Hoeber, Inc., 1959.
26. Keul, J. Doll, E., Keppler, D., and Reindell, H.; Interval training and Anaerobe Energiebereitstellung. *Sportarzt Sportmid., 12*:493, 1967.
27. Knuttgen, H. G.: Oxygen debt, lactate, pyruvate and excess lactate after muscular work. *J. Appl. Physiol., 17*:639, 1962.
28. Mathew, D. K., and Fox, E. L.: *The Physiological Basis of Physical Education and Athletics.* Philadelphia: W. B. Saunders Co., 1976, p. 242.
29. McCafferty, W. B., and Horvath, S. M.: Specificity of exercise and specificity of training: A subcellular review. *Res. Q., 48*:358–371, 1977.
30. Milesis, C. A., et al.: Effects of different deviations of physical training on cardio-respiratory function, body composition, and serum lipids. *Res. Q., 47*:716–725, 1976.

31. Morehouse, L. E., and Miller, A. T.: *Physiology of Exercise*, 7th ed. St. Louis: C. V. Mosby Co., 1976.
32. Pechar, G., et al.: Specificity of cardio-respiratory adaptation to bicycle and treadmill training. *J. Appl. Physiol., 36*:753–756, 1974.
33. Pipes, T. V., and Wilmore, J. H.: Isokinetic vs. isotonic strength training in adult men. *Med. Sci. Sports, 7*:262–274, 1975.
34. Ricci, B.: *Physiological Basis of Human Performance*. Philadelphia, Lea & Febiger, 1967.
35. Saltin, B.: Aerobic work capacity and circulation at exercise in man. *Acta Physiol. Scand., 62*(Suppl. 230), 1964.
36. Saltin, B., and Astrand, P.-O.: Maximal oxygen uptake in athletes. *J. Appl. Physiol., 23*:353, 1967.
37. Sills, F. D., and Everett, P. W.: The relationship of extreme somatotypes to performances in motor and strength tests. *Res. Q., 24*:223, 1953.

Chapter 9
Power, Speed, and Reaction Time

The first section of this chapter deals with the power/work relationship and is designed to help the reader understand the logic of emphasizing power as an important characteristic of athletic performance. The chapter continues with a discussion of the different aspects of speed and how it can be improved. Reaction time is then discussed in terms of its importance and how to improve this valuable characteristic.

POWER-WORK RELATIONSHIP

The term *work* has often been employed to describe the amount of energy expended. Work (W) is equal to force (F) times distance (D), and the formula is written:

$$W = FD$$

Work can be calculated easily by knowing the amount of force that is needed to overcome the resistance and the distance that the motion travels. This means that if a person does an exercise against 100 lb of resistance through a range of motion of 2 feet, he accomplishes 200 foot-pounds of work.

This concept of work involves motion and without motion no work occurs. Because of this, work as an estimate of the energy expended is quite unreliable in some cases, because much energy can be expended through isometric contractions but no motion is involved. For example, if a person contracted the leg extensor muscles for 10 sec against an immovable resistance, a significant amount of energy would be expended, but the amount of work accomplished would be zero. Because of this, the definition of work and the utilization of its formula have become somewhat useless to physiologists.

Furthermore, the calculation of work does not take into consideration the time element of the expenditure of energy, which is important in both performance and conditioning for performance. If a person lifted a 200-lb weight through a 3-foot range of motion at a slow rate, and another lifted 200-lb weight through the same range of motion at a rapid rate, the amount of work accomplished would be the same. But certainly the amount of energy expended would not be the same. If the two different speeds of exercise were used in training, the training results would certainly not be the same.

To give another example, suppose one person sprinted for 100 yd and another jogged for 100 yd and each weighed 100 lb. According to the formula, each one would accomplish 30,000 foot-pounds of work (100 lb × 300 ft), but in actual fact, the one who sprinted the distance would expend much more energy than the one who jogged. The dilemma of work not including the element of time provides good reason to place greater emphasis on the concept of *power* and less emphasis on the concept of *work*.

Power is the rate of accomplishing work; therefore, it includes the time element. Maximal power (sometimes called explosive power) results from the optimal combination of *strength* and *speed*. If two individuals each lifted 200 lb a distance of 3 ft, but one is able to do it with twice as much speed as the other, then he would demonstrate twice as much power, although they both would accomplish the same amount of work. Likewise, if the two individuals were to move at the same speed, but one worked against twice as much resistance as the other, then he would demonstrate twice as much power. When expressed in a formula:

$$\text{Power} = \text{Force (strength)} \times \text{Velocity (speed)}$$

It may also be written:

$$\text{Power} = \frac{\text{Force} \times \text{Distance}}{\text{Time}} \text{ or } \frac{\text{Work}}{\text{Time}}$$

These formulae point out that when maximal power is demonstrated, maximal force is applied as rapidly as possible. For use by physiologists and athletic specialists, the term *power* is actually more valid and more useful than the term *work*.

Significance of Power

Maximal power is demonstrated in athletic performances by the ability to project an object or the body through space, or by the ability to put an object into rapid motion. Power produces momentum, and momentum becomes the striking force when contact is made. Thus, power has many applications in a variety of athletic events. In *projecting an object* the object might be thrown, kicked, or struck, and the *power* is determined by the combination of *force* and *speed*. For example, if a baseball batter applies more force to the bat at a faster rate than usual, the bat will accelerate faster and will have greater velocity (and thus greater momentum) when it strikes the ball. Another consideration in this example is the weight of the bat the player can handle effectively. A more powerful person can accelerate a heavier bat at a faster speed than a less powerful individual, and the heavier bat has greater momentum because mass is an element in momentum. A batter who is lacking in the force element of power cannot accelerate a heavy bat effectively.

A similar analysis can be made of the football punt. At the moment foot contact is broken, the football is moving at a given speed (final velocity). The final velocity is determined by the *amount* of force and the *speed* of the force applied to the ball.

Probably putting the shot depends as much on true power as any athletic activity. If the angle of projection is constant, then the distance the shot will travel is related directly to its final velocity (velocity at moment of release). Thus, the prime objective of the shot putter is to have the shot moving as fast as possible. To achieve this he must apply *maximal force* at *maximal speed* over *maximal distance* (the longer the distance of force application, the longer the shot can be accelerated and the greater will be the final velocity). If the distance of force application is constant, the amount and speed of the force applied are fundamental to success.

Sprint running is dependent largely upon power because it is essentially a series of body projections, alternating from the two legs. The rate of these projections is dependent upon the combination of force and speed of muscle contractions. Power plays an even more prominent role in sprinting during the acceleration phase than during the remaining phase of the sprint. When one considers the prevalence of running acceleration and sprinting, along with jumping, throwing, kicking, and striking in athletic performances, the significance of power becomes apparent.

Numerous other examples of the importance of power could be given in a variety of maximum-effort throwing, kicking, and striking activities where the amount of impetus given to the object is fundamental to a successful performance.

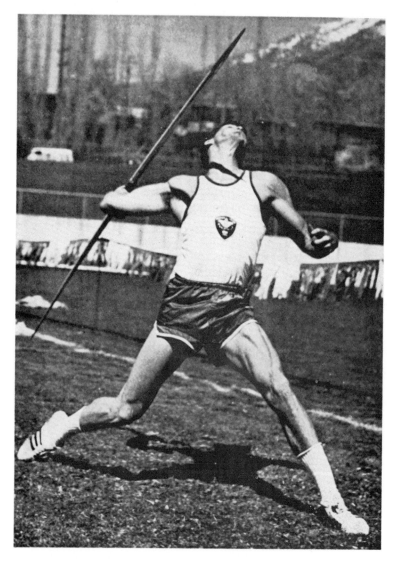

Figure 9–1. The javelin throw is a power event in which the resistance (javelin) is relatively light. Thus, speed is the primary factor of power in this instance.

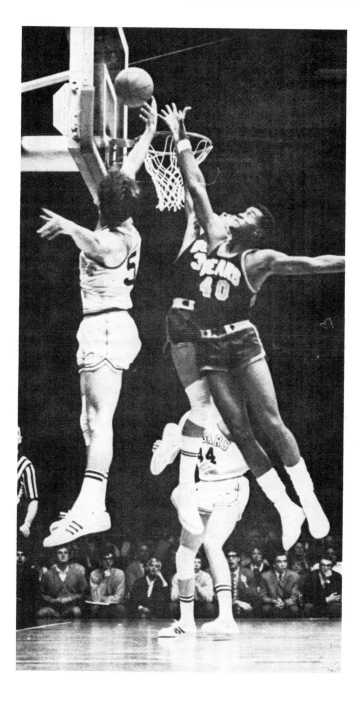

Figure 9–2. Jumping, which is involved in many activities,
depends directly on leg power.

Even though power always involves a combination of the components strength (force) and speed, different kinds of performances often require more emphasis on one component than on the other. Power events involving light resistance place emphasis on speed, whereas performances against heavy resistance depend more upon strength. For example, consider the unique throwing event known as the 35-lb weight throw sometimes included in track meets. In this event, speed is not a great limitation, because even a strong person is unable to contract the muscles with great speed against the resistance of the 35-lb weight.

Speed is of greater relative importance in putting the 16-lb shot, but strength is still the prominent component of power because the resistance is still relatively heavy. In throwing the discus, speed contributes more and strength less than in putting the shot. Throwing a javelin depends even more on speed and less on strength, and throwing a fast pitch in baseball depends almost entirely on the speed component.

So in power performances there are those that depend greatly upon speed, and those that depend greatly upon force. Between the two extremes are numerous performances that require different amounts of emphasis on speed or force. It is always the right combination of these two components that produces the best result in terms of power.

Increasing Power

Since power consists of the components of force and velocity, it can be increased by increasing strength or by increasing the speed of muscle contraction, or by improving both of these components. Usually the best approach for increasing power is to increase strength.

THE STRENGTH COMPONENT OF POWER. The guidelines for increasing strength are found in Chapter 7. Several research studies have produced evidence that increasing the strength of the leg extensor muscles through weight-training programs has a consistent, positive effect on vertical jumping ability, which is a measure of power. Isotonic strength exercises have proven to be highly effective in bringing about this change, whereas isometric exercises produce a positive but lesser result.[6]

Practical experience and observation support the claim that performances in many power events have been vastly improved during the past couple of decades as a result of emphasis placed on strength training. Let us consider, for example, the shot put event wherein no one in history had ever exceeded the 60-foot mark a little more than 2 decades ago. Since then, the 70-ft mark has been exceeded several times and dozens of athletes exceed 60 ft annually. There are other contributing factors to this remarkable improvement, but probably the emphasis on strength training has had more influence on this power event than any other single factor.

It is less apparent but certainly true that top level basketball players are significantly better jumpers than the players of 2 decades ago. Football players are harder hitters, sprinters are faster at accelerating, and the explosive portions of many other performances have been improved as a result of strength-training programs. Realistically, an athlete cannot be expected to compete favorably in explosive power events these days unless his training program involves effective strength-improvement procedures.

THE SPEED COMPONENT OF POWER.   The key to improving the speed component of power is to increase the contractile speed of the muscles that cause the movement (agonistic muscles). This can best be accomplished by increasing the strength, as described previously. The other ways to increase the speed component are to improve the coordination of muscles, warm them up before use, and work on the efficiency of movement.

COORDINATION.   Improved coordination of muscles (skill) can increase speed of movement because, as the several mover muscles become better coordinated, they can cooperatively overcome external resistance with greater speed. Furthermore, when muscles are well coordinated, the contractual force of one muscle (or group of muscles) better matches the peak velocity of the previous force; consequently, the second force is more effective. The antagonistic muscles often relax more slowly than the agonistic muscles contract; thus ability to relax antagonistic muscles often may be an important factor in movement speed. If increased speed is desired, the specific movements involved in the performance should be practiced at rates equal to or exceeding those used in performance.

WARM-UP.   Hill found that speed of contraction can be increased approximately 20% by raising body temperature 2° C, and speed of contraction is diminished significantly by a reduction in temperature of 10° C.[10] The truth of this claim lacks sufficient evidence, but it is clearly established that increased body temperature does improve rate of contraction to some degree. Apparently, such increase is due mostly to decreased viscosity in the muscles. A considerable amount of exercise is required to raise body temperature a measurable amount, and this is one argument in favor of warm-up.

MUSCLE EFFICIENCY.   The efficiency of muscle contraction can be increased by training, and this may result in increased contractile speed. For example, if fatty tissue within a muscle is eliminated, or if viscosity is reduced, the result is greater efficiency and faster contraction. If flexibility of antagonistic muscles is inadequate, then increased flexibility will cause less resistance to movement, resulting in greater

184 Conditioning Guidelines

speed. Also, reducing neural inhibitions as a result of training will allow the performer to call voluntarily upon greater numbers of available motor units. The more motor units involved, the more quickly the resistance can be overcome.

SPEED

There are different forms of speed: (1) speed of movement of body segments, (2) running acceleration speed, and (3) maximal running speed. Because of these different forms of speed, it is difficult to clearly label a person "fast" or "slow."

Speed of movement is highly specific to regions of the body. For example, an individual with fast arm movements may have slow leg movements. In fact, this kind of specificity extends, to some degree, even to specific movements. As explained in the previous chapter, some persons have fast leg movements, which contribute to their running speed, but are not capable of developing fast arm and hand movements as needed in boxing, ball handling skills, and the like.

Running speed can be discussed in terms of two factors: *rate* of acceleration and *maximal velocity*. The first factor is related to how fast a person can increase his rate of speed. This is the most important consideration in speed for distances of 20 to 30 yd, and it is important in short sprints, and in court and field games in which moving quickly from one locaton to another is an advantage, and when getting away from an opponent is important. On the other hand, for distances greater than 20 to 30 yd, maximal running speed is more important than acceleration speed. Possessing a high level of both forms of running speed is often a great advantage.

These two factors of running speed are not as highly related as some persons think. Some individuals are slow starters with fast maximal speed, whereas others are fast starters with relatively slow maximal speed. Indeed, a person may be proficient in football, basketball, or tennis, in which quick acceleration is important, and be only about average speed in the 100-meter or 200-meter sprint, and vice versa.

Two other aspects of running speed are *average speed* and *final speed*. A runner who is attempting to cover a given distance in the shortest time possible, such as the mile run, is concerned with the fastest average speed over the entire distance. Acceleration speed and sprint speed are relatively unimportant in such instances. Conversely, in jumping for horizontal distance, average speed is of no real value, whereas final speed (speed at the moment of takeoff) is of utmost importance.

Significance of Speed

Running speed is an athletic event in itself and at the same time is important in numerous other sports. Speed, mostly in the form of

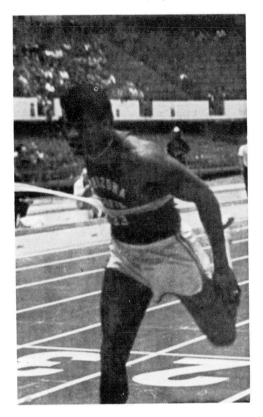

Figure 9–3.   Sprint champion breaking the tape. (Robinson, C. F., Jensen, C. R., James, S. W., and Hirschi, W. M.: *Modern Techniques of Track and Field.* Philadelphia: Lea & Febiger, 1974, page 54.)

acceleration speed, is an important factor in almost all court and field games, and it can make the difference in whether a performer is able to gain an advantage over his opponent.

Both the offensive and defensive phases of the game of basketball provide good examples of the significance of fast acceleration speed. Fast acceleration can enable a player to compete better against his opponent in all phases of floor play. Acceleration speed, as well as top running speed, is important on fast-break plays covering the length of the floor. Similar examples of the importance of acceleration speed can be seen in other court games such as tennis, badminton, and handball.

Speed is equally important in field games, and here a better balance of acceleration speed and top running speed is often an advantage, because large playing fields afford the opportunity for all-out running. Football, soccer, rugby, baseball, and lacrosse are excellent examples of

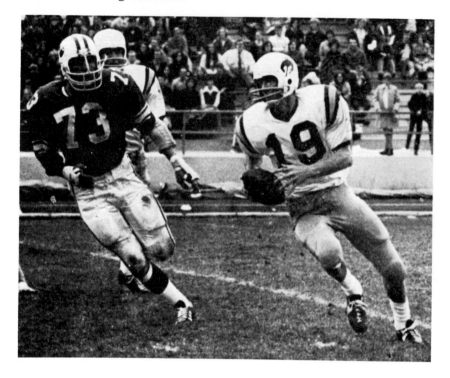

Figure 9-4. Field running in football depends greatly on fast acceleration and running maneuverability (agility).

field games in which both acceleration speed and running speed are basic to success.

Movement speed of specific body parts is particularly important in hand and arm movements, as exemplified in combative sports and in ball-handling skills. Often, only a small increase in speed of the kind that applies to the performance can improve an athlete's effectiveness a considerable amount.

How to Increase Speed

Speed is basically a result of rapid application of force to a mass. In human movements, the body or segments of it represent the mass; the force is caused by muscle contractions. If the force is greater than the resistance, then movement occurs, and as the force becomes proportionately greater, the speed with which the mass moves increases. This general idea is explained by Newton's second law, which in essence means that the rate at which an object accelerates is directly proportional to the force causing it.

In speed there are both *positive* and *negative* forces acting. The positive forces are caused by muscle contractions, and the negative forces are caused by friction, air resistance, gravity, and inertia. DeVries has calculated that in running, a person might have negative forces equal to 3.45 horsepower (hp).[7] He determined the forces as coming from the following: (1) gravity, 0.1 hp; (2) velocity changes, 0.5 hp; (3) accelaration of limbs, 1.68 hp; (4) deceleration of limbs, 0.67 hp; and (5) air resistance, 0.5 hp. This means that in order to maintain a constant speed the runner would need to provide a propelling force of 3.45 hp. Of course, it must be recognized that this is only an illustration which does not accurately represent all cases. As the running speed is increased, the resisting forces are likewise increased, which means that proportionately more propelling force is needed to maintain a faster speed. Speed can be increased by either decreasing the negative forces or increasing the positive forces.

REDUCING THE NEGATIVE FORCES.   Some of the negative forces tend to be constant, whereas others are variable. *Gravity* is represented by the mass (weight) and is constant, except when weight is gained or lost. *Velocity changes* are variable and can be controlled rather easily. Velocity changes waste energy and influence overall speed in a negative way. The negative effects of *acceleration and deceleration of limbs* can be controlled only partially. Unnecessary movements can be eliminated, and the efficiency of the necessary movements often can be improved. *Air (or water) resistance* can sometimes be reduced by altering the body's position. For example, cyclers, skiers, and skaters perform in a semiflexed position to reduce the body surface in the direction of movement, and thus reduce the air resistance. Likewise, swimmers present the smallest surface area possible in the direction of movement in order to meet minimal water resistance.

The theoretical square law has significant meaning when the negative effects of air and water reistance are considered. The law means that when a body's velocity is increased, the air or water resistance increases by the square. This means that if the velocity is doubled, the resistance would increase by four.

Each kind of speed event offers slightly different possibilities for reducing the negative forces. The coach and athlete should carefully analyze each case separately to determine what can be done to reduce negative effects to a minimum.

INCREASING THE POSITIVE FORCES.   Under this topic we should consider (1) intrinsic speed of muscle contractions; (2) the amount of force muscles can apply against the resistance; (3) coordination; and (4) the leverage involved in the movements. Each of these factors is discussed separately.

It is true that the *speed of muscle contraction* is inherent in the muscle tissue. Different muscles contract at different rates even when they are detached from the body and stimulated artificially. The rate of muscle contraction can be increased a limited amount by repeated practice of fast movements. Such practice over an extended period will improve innervation to the muscles and also increase the efficiency of the muscles themselves. The speed of movement is directly proportional to the speed of contraction of the mover muscles; therefore, if the contractile rate is increased by 5%, the speed of movement would increase by the same percentage, if other factors remain constant.

Movement usually involves working against some resistance, even if the resistance is only the weight of the body segment. Because of this, *contractile force* can influence the rate of movement. As the muscles become stronger, the external resistance has less retarding effect on speed. Where resistance is light, it is doubtful that contractile force is a significant factor in speed, but as the resistance becomes greater, contractile force has a larger influence. Whitney and Smith found that regardless of the kind of strengthening exercises used, increasing the strength of muscles involved in a particular task makes it possible to perform the movement faster.[24]

Improvement in *coordination* can increase the speed of specific movements, because as the several mover (agonistic) muscles become better coordinated, they can cooperatively overcome the external resistance faster. Also, as the agonists and antagonists become better coordinated, the antagonists furnish less resistance to the contractile effects of the agonists (reciprocal inhibition is involved here). This is of utmost importance because, by reducing tension in the antagonists, speed is improved and the onset of fatigue is postponed.

Not only is it important to coordinate the muscles involved in a movement, but it is also important to coordinate the several specific movements that contribute to overall speed. This is demonstrated well in the baseball throw (or other throws) in which each successive movement builds on previous movements, and if all of the movements are put together in correct sequence and timing, the final velocity of the ball is equal to the sum of the velocities of the contributing movements. (This idea relates to the principle of summation of forces.) Other examples are speed swimming and speed running, in which the arms and legs move simultaneously, and the movements must be well coordinated in order to achieve maximal speed.

In motor performances the body functions as a *system of levers*, and often the leverage can be improved. It is known that if the angular velocity at the joint remains constant, then the speed at the end of the lever is directly proportional to the lever's length. This means that if lever A is twice as long as lever B, and if both levers rotate about their fulcrums (joints) at the same angular velocity (expressed in degrees/

second), then the end of lever A will move twice as fast as lever B, because it is twice as long. Thus, speed can sometimes be influenced by voluntarily adjusting body levers to their optimal length. This is demonstrated in the overarm throw, wherein the hand passes high above the shoulder. If the lever is purposely shortened, causing the hand to pass close to the shoulder, the speed the ball travels is reduced proportionately. Other examples of the influence of leverage on speed could be related to baseball batting, the discus throw, or hammer throw. To achieve the greatest speed, the best combination of angular velocity and lever length must be attained. Incidentally, angular velocity is determined by how fast the muscles can overcome the external resistance.

To summarize, the following facts have been pointed out: (1) Speed of muscle contraction can be increased a limited amount by training with repeated fast movements. (2) Speed of movement against a significant resistance can be increased by increasing the ability to apply force (strength) against the resistance. This method is ineffective against light resistance, but it becomes progressively more effective as the resistance is increased. (3) Speed can be increased by improving the coordination of the various muscles involved in each movement and by improving the coordination of the various movements involved in the skill. (4) Speed can be increased by employing the optimal combination of angular velocity and length of the levers involved.

SPECIAL CONSIDERATIONS IN RUNNING SPEED.   Speed is determined by the length of stride and frequency (speed) of stride. In order to increase running speed, one or both of these factors must be increased. Length of stride is dependent primarily upon leg length and leg power. Leg speed (frequency) is mostly dependent upon speed of muscle contractions and neuromuscular coordination.

Sprinting is essentially a power performance. It depends on one's ability to project one's body forcefully and rapidly from alternate feet. Top speed is developed relatively early in life, about the age of 21 for men and 18 for women, and it is a trait that can be improved only a limited amount through training. Traditionally, it has been thought that there are three possibilities for increasing speed: (1) increase the power (force × velocity) of the leg extensor muscles, thus causing more propelling force; (2) practice running at top speed to improve the specific coordinations involved; and (3) correction of errors in running mechanics.

Slater-Hammel shed additional light on the subject when he demonstrated that the rate of leg alternation in sprinting ranges from 3.10 to 4.85 per sec among different individuals, and in cycling it ranges from 5.5 to 7.1 per sec.[16] This illustrates that maximal leg alternation is not used in sprinting, and it indicates that the rate of alternation is probably not the limiting factor. Other research has demonstrated that the length of stride, rather than the rate of alternation of the leg, is the main limitation in sprinting. It is known that length of stride can be increased by increasing leg power, which is the ability to apply more force rapidly, and thereby to project the body faster and farther with each stride.

Factors That Influence Speed

Several factors influence speed, among which are:

MUSCLE LENGTH. Physiologists generally agree that a muscle fiber that is twice as long as another fiber can shorten twice as much in the same time, provided the intrinsic properties of the two fibers are the same. This means that muscles with long fibers have speed advantages over muscles with short fibers. Further, it is explained in the section on power that muscles whose fibers run parallel to the longitudinal axis of the muscle have speed advantages over muscles whose fibers are diagonal to the longitudinal axis.

FORCE AND ACCELERATION. According to Newton's second law of motion, acceleration of a body is proportional to the force causing it. This means that if the accelerating force is doubled, the rate of acceleration also will double (except for the effects of the resistance, which vary with the theoretical square law). Thus, a sprinter increases acceleration by increasing the force he applies against the surface on which he runs, and a swimmer achieves increased acceleration by increasing the force of the kick and stroke against the water (in the correct direction).

With regard to acceleration, it must be realized that muscle contractions provide the force, and more forceful contractions expend more energy. The energy cost of a contraction varies with the cube of the speed of contraction. If muscle A contracts twice as fast as muscle B, then its energy cost is 8 times as great as that of muscle B. If muscle A contracts 3 times as fast as muscle B, its energy cost is 27 times as great as that of muscle B. This fact has much application in determining the rate at which a performer should accelerate, especially in endurance activities.

EFFECTS OF THE THEORETICAL SQUARE LAW. This law has to do with the negative or retarding forces. The law states that air and water resistance vary approximately with the square of the velocity, meaning that if the velocity at which a body travels is increased by 2 the air or water resistance against it will increase by 4; if velocity is increased by 4, the resistance will increase by 16. Thus, if a swimmer pulls his arm through the water at a rate of 5 ft/second, he meets a given amount of water resistance, which he uses to propel him forward. If the rate of pull is increased to 10 ft/second, the resistance is increased four times, resulting in four times as much propulsive force from the stroke. But, four times the propulsive force will not increase the swimmer's speed through the water by four times, because the water's resistance against him also increases with the square of his velocity, meaning that as he moves faster he meets proportionately more resistance.

SPEED-FORCE RELATIONSHIP.   It has been shown through research that the force available from a muscle contraction decreases as the rate of shortening increases. A muscle can contract with its greatest force at zero speed (isometric contraction). Likewise, a muscle can contract with its greatest speed when it applies zero force (no resistance). In other words, as a muscle applies more force against resistance, it contracts with proportionately less speed, and as it contracts with greater speed, it can overcome proportionately less resistance.

AGE AND SEX.   Generally, men increase in all aspects of speed until about the age of 21 years. Peak speed remains approximately constant for 3 to 4 years, after which speed tends to decrease at a gradual but steady rate. Women reach maximal speed at a younger age than men, about 18 years.

Records of sports events involving running and swimming speed indicate that women have about 85% as much speed as men. Limited research supports the claim that speed of body segments is also about 85% as fast in women as in men. This difference between men and women might be accounted for by differences in strength, because strength influences the speed of movement against resistance.

TEMPERATURE.   Researchers have found that the contractile speed of muscles of animals as well as those of humans is increased as a result of raising the muscle temperature. Such changes may be brought about in humans by diathermy or other deep heat treatment, but warming the muscles through the use of a well planned warm-up exercise routine is the most effective and the surest way to improve speed by increased temperature (see Warm-up in Chapter 15).

BODY TYPE.   It is difficult to relate movement speed of a specific body part to body type except to say that obese individuals tend to lack speed of movement, and this is probably due to (1) the friction caused by fat molecules within the muscles, and (2) the extra weight caused by fat which must be overcome in movement. Running speed favors persons of medium size with medium-light builds. They would be characterized as meso-ectomorphs. However, there are many individual exceptions to this statement in terms of both acceleration speed and running speed.

STRENGTH.   Strength and speed are only mildly related when light resistance is involved, but when speed movements against heavy resistance are needed, then strength becomes more of a contributor. An abundance of research supports the idea that increased strength does not detract from speed as some have claimed, and it often has a positive influence on speed, with the influence becoming greater as the resistance is increased. There is some evidence that strength developed dynamically makes a better contribution to speed than strength developed statically.

FLEXIBILITY. It is known that restricted (less than normal) dynamic flexibility in the hip and thigh region can retard running speed, because it increases the resistance provided by the antagonistic muscles toward the end of the range of motion. However, there is no evidence that speed will be improved by increasing flexibility beyond a reasonable or normal amount.

DOMINANT FACTORS IN SPEED UNDER VARIOUS CONDITIONS. There are several considerations under this topic: (1) In *lightly loaded and simple* movements, intrinsic speed of the muscles, which depends on physicochemical and biochemical properties, is probably the main limitation on movement speed. Neuromuscular coordination and strength are secondary limitations under such conditions. (2) In *lightly loaded, complex* movements, it is likely that coordination of the various muscles and of the different movements sets the limits on speed. (3) In *heavily loaded and complex* movements, coordination and strength are the dominant factors which influence speed.

BODY MECHANICS AND RUNNING SPEED. Photographic analysis has shown that effective sprint running is characterized by a high knee lift, a long running stride, and placement of the feet on a line beneath the runner's center of gravity. It is important in running that the propelling forces be directed properly and efficiently. Specifically, the leg movements should be straight forward and backward, the arm and shoulder movements should be directed to pull the body optimally in the desired direction, and the angle of projection should be optimum in order to achieve maximal speed.

An example of negative effects of incorrect mechanics can be seen when the feet are turned outward. If this is done, there are three undesired results: (1) Approximately 1 inch is lost on each stride because the foot covers less distance in the direction of movement. In a 100-yd dash this would result in a loss of about 50 inches. (2) Part of the propelling force is lost from the four smaller toes of each foot, thus reducing the total propelling force. (3) The propelling forces from the feet tend to be diagonal instead of straight forward, so the forces are misdirected. Other forms of incorrect running mechanics have different effects but similar results on running speed.

REACTION TIME

Reaction time relates to, but is different from, reflex time, movement time, and response time. It is the interval between a stimulus and the initiation of movement. Teichner has divided reaction time into four phases:[21] (1) the onset of the stimulus; (2) the first latency period, during which the receptor process occurs; (3) the second latency period, involving the central transmission of the sensory impulses to the motor fibers (thought time); and (4) the delay involved in the motor process preceding contraction of the muscles. Tripp defines reaction time as being a human time lag consisting of (1) a sense time (receiving of the stimulus), (2) a decision time (thought time), and (3) a movement time (initiation of movement).[22]

Reflex time is a shortened reaction time wherein the thought or decision-making phase is eliminated. In a reflex the impulses travel through the sensory nerves, across the reflex arc, and through motor nerves to the muscles. (The reflex arc relays messages directly from sensory to motor nerves.)

There are two kinds of reflexes, innate and conditioned. An *innate (inborn) reflex* is a predictable response to a given stimulus which is accomplished below the level of conscious control. Such reflexes must originate in the afferent (sensory) system, and the efferent (motor) response will often occur simultaneous to the time the person becomes consciously aware of the stimulus. If the person is aware of the stimulus, the reflex response may occur without interference, or it may be consciously inhibited or intensified. Learned reflexes (not innate) are called *conditioned reflexes.* If the performer learns to respond automatically in the same manner to the same stimulus, this is a conditioned reflex. A conscious movement can be superimposed on a conditioned reflex the same as on an innate reflex. (For more detailed information about reflexes, refer to Chapter 2.)

Movement time starts where reaction time ends. It is the time that elapses between the beginning of a movement and its completion.

Response time is a combination of reaction time and movement time. It is the total time that elapses from the onset of the stimulus until the act is completed.

Significance of Reaction Time

The speed with which an indiviudual can react in a competitive situation is of great interest to those concerned with physical education and athletic performance. For example, this factor partly determines how successful a basketball player or a soccer player can be on defense. When the offensive player makes his move, the difference between a slow and a fast reaction by the defensive player can determine his success or failure. Both offensive and defensive players are often hindered by slow reactions because they are not able to demonstrate the quickness necessary to outmaneuver their opponents. Similar examples could be stated in connection with tennis, badminton, football,

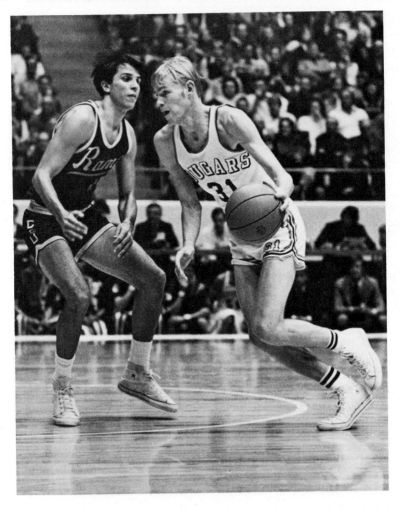

Figure 9–5. In both offensive and defensive play in basketball, reaction time is important because it strongly influences whether a player can out-maneuver his opponent.

and several other court and field games. Further, reaction time is of obvious importance in all combative activities.

In running and swimming races, a difference in speed of reaction to the pistol shot can result in several feet gained or lost. On such slim margins hang the fruits of victory in closely fought contests. Even small improvements in reaction time may produce significant results in performance in which quick reactions are essential.

How to Improve Reaction Time

Reaction time in specific movements will improve as a result of extensive practice of those movements. Tripp claims that practice reduces decision time by eliminating incorrect decisions and enables the correct decision to be made more efficiently.[22]

If an act is practiced enough, a conditioned reflex may develop. For example, a sprinter might develop a conditioned reflex to a pistol shot. A boxer might develop conditioned reflexes which cause him to automatically respond in specific ways to movements made by his opponent. Similar examples could be given in connection with numerous other performances.

There is no evidence that a person's basic reaction time can be improved significantly by any method other than actual practice of the particular act, placing emphasis on quickness. Improvements tend to be specific rather than general, meaning that improved reaction time in one act will not guarantee improved reactions in another act, or in body movements in general. It has been theorized that mental practice of a movement may improve reaction time, but this idea has not been substantiated by research.

Factors That Influence Reaction Time

Several factors influence reaction time in different ways. Some of the more important factors are:

AGE AND SEX.   The correlation of age and reaction time has received considerable attention. Karpovich states that reaction time is slow in young children and gradually improves with age, reaching its maximum at the college age level.[11] Henry and Whitley found that maximal reaction time had not been fully reached at high school age.[8] Teichner believes that reaction time improves to about the age of 30, after which the latency period grows longer; but even at the age of 60 reaction time is faster than at the age of 10.[21] This conclusion was supported by Tripp, who indicates that recent studies show little slowing of reaction time prior to the age of 60.[22]

Regarding sex differences, Teichner[21] and Tripp[22] agree that men react slightly faster than women. In a study of the reaction time of limb movements of men and women, it was found that reactions are slower in women, but the difference is slight. The difference can probably be attributed to the fact that men practice activities requiring fast reactions more than women.

READINESS TO ACT.   It is reasonable to assume that reaction time is influenced by the degree an individual is ready to react. Based on a study of track sprinters, Pierson concluded that imagining or anticipating an act prepares the muscles for movement before the stimulus triggers a response.[15] In a study concerning the effects of muscle stretch, tension, and relaxation upon reaction time, Smith found that subjects produced a reaction time 7% faster if the muscles were in a state of tension as opposed to being relaxed.[18] Studies on the effects of preliminary muscular tension on reaction latency show that the latency period is shortened as a result of tension.

INFLUENCE OF PREPARATORY SIGNALS.   According to Teichner, reaction time is improved if a preparatory signal is given prior to the stimulus.[21] Such signal causes a performer to concentrate on the stimulus, and to prepare his muscles for a quick response once the stimulus is given. Practical experience also supports this claim.

INFLUENCE OF INTENSITY OF STIMULUS.   An increase in the intensity of visual, auditory, thermal, and pain stimuli produces improvements in reaction time. Baumeister and associates, in a study involving both normal and mentally retarded subjects, found that both groups reacted more quickly when the stimulus was intensified, with the retarded profiting more from increased intensity.[3] Morehouse and Miller believe there is a limit of intensifying the stimuli beyond which increased intensity will not speed up reaction time, and may even slow it down.[14] The validity of this belief is questionable, and deserves additional research.

INFLUENCE OF NUMBERS OF RECEPTORS STIMULATED.   The greater the number of receptors stimulated, the shorter is the latency period, and thus the shorter the reaction time. It has been found that simultaneous combinations of light, sound, and shock produce improved reaction times. Morehouse and Miller believe that reaction time is slowed by stimuli that are too complicated, intermittent distracting noises, and sound signals that vary in pitch and loudness.[14] They believe that easily perceived stimuli produce faster reaction times. There is some evidence that the presentation of two stimuli in close succession causes a delayed response to the second stimulus.

ATHLETES vs. NONATHLETES.   Karpovich[11] and Morehouse and Miller[14] claim that athletes in high-level competition have faster reactions than nonathletes, and sprinters have faster reactions than distance runners. It is believed that faster reactions in athletes are probably due partly to the training they have received, but it is reasonable to assume that training does not account for all the differences.

DIET.   In a study of the effects of breakfast upon reaction time, Tuttle and associates discovered that a light breakfast resulted in a shorter reaction time than a breakfast consisting of coffee only, and that coffee only produced a shorter reaction time than a heavy breakfast.[23] Subjects who went without breakfast were found to have slower reactions.

Information is lacking about the effects of the total diet on reaction time. It is doubtful that any relationship exists, provided the diet is conducive to good health. A survey of literature by Teichner showed that coffee and Benzedrine slowed reactions in subjects who were awakened just prior to testing.[21] Alcohol consistently slows reaction time under all circumstances. Smoking has been found to slow reaction time when the stimulus is in the form of a visual signal.

EFFECTS OF FATIGUE ON REACTION TIME.   Physiological fatigue lengthens reaction time; however, Keller found that it takes a considerable amount of fatigue to slow reactions measurably.[12] Several experiments show that lack of sleep has little effect on reaction time when the subjects are concentrating on the stimulus.

EFFECTS OF WEIGHT TRAINING.   Baer and Gersten, in a study of the effects of various exercise programs on reaction time, found that high-resistance isotonic contractions produced a 13% improvement in reaction time, and that high-resistance isometric contractions produced improvement in reactions by 6%.[1] Low-resistance exercises produced no change in reaction time. There is no substantial evidence contradicting the results of this research. However, the topic deserves additional study.

SPECIFICITY OF REACTION TIME.   An interesting question is whether reaction time is highly specific to a body part or a movement, or whether it tends to be general. The research on this topic indicates a high degree of specificity by limb and by movement. Thus, an individual may be quick in reacting with his arms, but relatively slow with his legs. Also, he may be fast in reacting with certain arm movements and slower in other arm movements. Conversely, even though there is a high degree of specificity, there is still a general component that enables a person to be labeled either fast or slow in his reactions.

RELATIONSHIP OF REACTION TIME TO MOVEMENT TIME.   Another interesting question is whether movement time can be predicted from reaction time. The research on this topic fails to demonstrate a relationship between these two factors. Henry[9] and Smith[19] concluded that individual differences in ability to react quickly and ability to move fast are almost entirely unrelated.

SELECTED REFERENCES

1. Baer, A. D., and Gersten, G.: Effects of various exercise programs of isometric tension, endurance and reaction time in the human. Arch. Phys. Med. Rehabil., 36:495, 1955.
2. Ball, J. R., Rich, G. Q., and Wallis, E. L.: Effects of isometric training on vertical jumping. Res. Q., 35:213, 1964.
3. Baumeister, A., Hawkins, W., and Kellas, G.: The interactive effects of stimulus intensity and intelligence upon reaction time. Am. J. Ment. Defic., 69:530, 1965.
4. Berger, R. A., and Henderson, J. M.: Relationship of power to static and dynamic strength. Res. Q., 37:9, 1966.

5. Clarke, D. H., and Glines, D.: Relationships of reaction, movement and completion times to motor strength, anthropometric and maturity measures of 13-year-old boys. *Res. Q., 33*:194, 1962.
6. Considine, W. J., and Sullivan, W. J.: Relationship of selected tests of leg strength and leg power on college men. *Res. Q., 4*:4, 1973.
7. DeVries, H. A.: *Physiology of Exercise for Physical Education and Athletics*, 2nd ed. Dubuque: Wm. C. Brown Co., 1974.
8. Henry, F. M., and Whitley, J. D.: Relationships between individual differences in strength, speed and mass in an arm movement. *Res. Q., 31*:24, 1960.
9. Henry, F.M.: Stimulus complexity, movement complexity, age and sex in relation to reaction latency and speed in limb movements. *Res. Q., 32*:353, 1961.
10. Hill, A. V.: The design of muscles. *Br. Med. Bull., 12*:165, 1956.
11. Karpovich, P. V.: *Physiology of Muscular Activity*, 7th ed. Philadelphia: W. B. Saunders Co., 1971.
12. Keller, D. T.: Effect of strenuous physical activity upon reaction time. *Res. Q., 40*:332, 1969.
13. McClements, L. E.: Power relative to strength of leg and thigh muscles. *Res. Q., 37*:71, 1966.
14. Morehouse, L. E., and Miller, A. T.: *Physiology of Exercise*, 7th ed. St. Louis: C. V. Mosby Co., 1976.
15. Pierson, W. R.: Note concerning the focus of attention in the sprint start. *Physical Educator, 20*:119, 1963.
16. Slater-Hammel, A. T.: Comparison of reaction time measures to a visual stimulus and arm movement. *Res. Q., 26*:470, 1955.
17. Smith, L. E.: Specificity of individual differences of relationship between forearm strength and speed of forearm flexion. *Res. Q., 40*:191, 1969.
18. Smith, L. E.; Influence of strength training on pre-tensed and free arm speed. *Res. Q., 35*:554, 1964.
19. Smith, L. E.: Reaction time and movement in four large muscle movements. *Res. Q., 32*:88, 1961.
20. Start, K. B., et al.: A factorial investigation of power, speed, isometric strength, and anthropometric measure in the lower limb. *Res. Q., 37*:553, 1966.
21. Teichner, W. H.: Recent studies of simple reaction time. *Psychol. Bull., 51*:128, 1954.
22. Tripp, R. S.: How fast can you react? *Science Digest, 57*:50, 1965.
23. Tuttle, W. W., et al.: Effects of altered breakfast habits on physiological response. *J. Appl. Physiol., 11*:545, 1947.
24. Whitley, J. D., and Smith, L. E.: Influence of three different training programs on strength and speed of a limb movement. *Res. Q., 37*:142, 1966.

Chapter 10
Agility and Flexibility

Few characteristics are more important than agility in a variety of athletic activities. It is one of the most prominent factors in general athletic ability because it has great influence on the precision and quickness with which a person can handle his body.

Flexibility, which involves range of motion, is also important in certain kinds of performances, but it is relatively unimportant in other performances.

AGILITY

Agility is often represented by the terms "maneuverability," "mobility," and "shiftiness." It is the ability to change direction of the body and its parts rapidly. Agility is a combination of several athletic traits, including reaction time, speed of movement, coordination, power, and strength. It is demonstrated in such movements as dodging, zigzag running, stopping and starting, and changing body positions quickly.

Agility is both general and specific. Examples of general agility (or total body agility) are as follows: a football running back who eludes would-be tacklers by shifting and dodging while he runs; a soccer player who cleverly maneuvers the ball past his opponents as he zigzags down the field; a basketball player who darts past his opponents, then stops quickly to leap into the air for a shot; a trampoline performer who shifts his body quickly from one position to another as he does a complex routine; or a skier who gracefully zigzags down a slope continually shifting his body parts to maintain balance and to maneuver. *Specific agility* may be demonstrated in the rapid maneuverability of the hands and arms, as in playing a piano. Some athletes have "good hands," or "quick hands," meaning their hands and arms are highly maneuverable, which enables them to handle a ball or another object with unusual proficiency.

Significance of Agility

Agility is important in all activities involving quick changes in positions of the body and its parts. Fast starts and stops and quick changes in direction are fundamental to good performance in practically all *court games*, such as basketball, tennis, badminton, and volleyball, and in many *field games*, such as soccer, football, speedball, and baseball. These games require running agility. Gymnastics and diving also depend largely upon rapid body movements and quick changes in body position. Skiing, figure skating, and certain forms of dance require rapid adjustments in position and quick changes in direction. Conversely, some activities do not depend on agility to any large degree. Examples are track-and-field events, and swimming.

The importance of agility in athletic performances can be summarized by saying that in certain activities it is fundamental to good performance, and may even be the most important single characteristic, whereas in certain other activities agility is practically noncontributory. In the majority of activities, performance will improve with increased agility.

How to Increase Agility

Agility, general or specific, can be improved by betterment of the athletic components that constitute it. *Coordination* involved in the specific movements is by far the most important component of agility. If a person is poorly coordinated (awkward), he will lack agility regardless of the other traits he possesses. Therefore, great emphasis should be placed on developing coordination in the movement patterns essential to the given performance. The specifics of how to increase coordination are discussed in Chapter 11.

Improvement of the other components of agility offer limited but worthwhile opportunities. The procedures for improving the components are discussed in detail in other chapters. Therefore, only the application of the components to agility is discussed here.

Some people lack enough *strength* to control the inertia of the body in motion effectively. For example, great leg strength is needed to abruptly stop or change the direction of a 200-lb body in motion at 20 mph. Thus, it is apparent that increased strength, at least to a rather high level, will contribute to maneuverability of the body. *Power,*

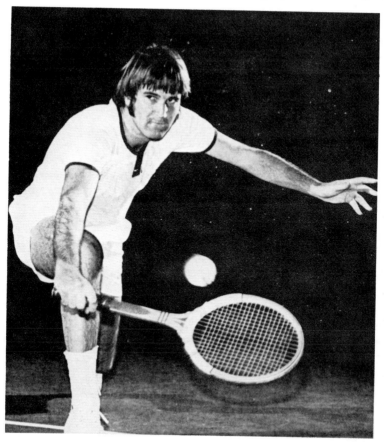

Figure 10–1.   A tennis player must be agile in order to cover the court effectively against a skilled opponent.

which is demonstrated in projecting the body, is an important contributor to agility, because in the absence of adequate power the body cannot be projected rapidly in any direction, nor can it be accelerated rapidly. Fast *reaction time* is essential in game situations wherein a performer must respond quickly to an external stimulus with an act of agility. For example, athletes must often react to immediate game situations, to the moves made by opponents, or to signals given by teammates. Slow reactions detract from one's maneuverability, whereas improved reaction time enhances agility. In addition to fast reactions, an agile performer displays *fast movements*, which often enable him to outmaneuver his opponents. A normal amount of *flexibility* is essential to full ranges of motion and to smooth, graceful, and effective movement. However, it seems doubtful that more than normal flexibility would improve agility.

Even though the components mentioned form the basis for agility and have potential for improving agility, it should be recognized that the best way to improve agility in specific movement patterns is to practice the patterns correctly over and over, and to do so at high speeds. This approach emphasizes the development of specific coordinations, the prime component of agility, and at the same time contributes to some of the other components.

Factors That Influence Agility

Several factors relate to agility in different ways. Points of information about the different factors are:

SOMATOTYPE.   Tall and lanky persons tend to lack agility, as do obese or pear-shaped individuals. Conversely, persons of medium height or shorter who are well muscled tend to be highly maneuverable. To relate to somatotypes, it can be said that mesomorphs and meso-ectomorphs tend to be fairly agile, whereas ectomorphs and endomorphs tend to be less agile. However, there are exceptions to this rule.

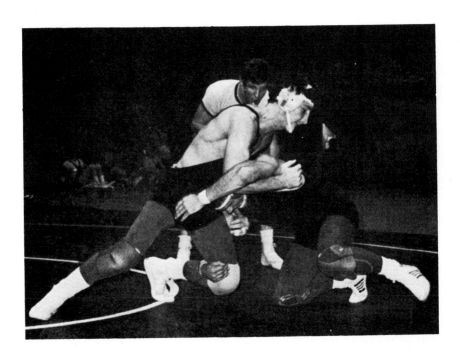

Figure 10–2.   Agility is fundamental to excellence in wrestling.

AGE AND SEX.   Young children increase steadily in agility to about the age of 12, when they enter the "awkward years" of fast growth. During this period of about 3 years, their agility tends not to increase and may even decrease. After the rapid growth period is over, agility increases once again at a rather steady rate until maturity is reached. Then after a few years it begins to diminish.

Boys are only slightly more agile than girls during the years before puberty. After puberty boys increase in agility to a level somewhat higher than that of girls.

OVERWEIGHT.   Excess weight detracts directly and significantly from agility. It increases the inertia of the body and its parts, and it reduces the speed of muscle contraction, thereby causing changes in direction to be less rapid.

FATIGUE.   Fatigue detracts from agility, because fatigue has a diminishing effect on the components of agility, such as strength, reaction time, speed of movement, and power. Especially, fatigue causes a loss of coordination.

FLEXIBILITY AND RANGE OF MOTION

Flexibility is expressed by the range of motion in a given joint or combination of joints. It is influenced by three factors: (1) the bone and ligament structure of the joint; (2) the amount of bulk surrounding the joint; and (3) the extensibility of muscles whose tendons cross the joint. The third factor is of greatest concern to those seeking to increase flexibility.

The *first* factor is well illustrated in the elbow and knee joints. Because of their bone and ligament structure, these joints are unable to extend beyond approximately 180°. Nearly every joint has limitations because of its bone structure. An example of the *second* factor is the restriction of elbow flexion by the mass of the biceps muscle. If the biceps were doubled in size, the range of motion would be reduced considerably. The *third* factor is best illustrated by attempting to flex at the hips and lower back to place the hands flat on the floor. In order to do this, the muscles and connective tissues in the backs of the legs and lower back must possess sufficient extensibility.

Inactivity causes muscles and connective tissues to lose their normal extensibility, and thus reduces flexibility. Inactivity also may contribute to accumulation of body fat, which may further restrict flexibility.

There are two kinds of flexibility, passive and dynamic. *Passive* flexibility is demonstrated by the range of movement that occurs in a joint when the muscles are relaxed and the body part is moved by another person. *Dynamic* flexibility is demonstrated by the range of movement that can occur in a joint as a result of contractions of the muscles which control the joint. Obviously, dynamic flexibility is of greater concern in performance than passive flexibility.

Significance of Flexibility

Therapists and movement experts claim that lack of flexibility is one of the frequent causes of improper movement. When ungainly movement is observed, especially in walking and running, flexibility should be one of the first things to check.

Flexibility is involved in many motor patterns, and its inadequate development may be regarded as another possible deterrent to achievement in certain sports. There is no set standard as to the amount of flexibility a person should possess. This depends on the activities in which he desires to participate. Most activities require no more than normal (or average) flexibility. But a few activities are directly dependent upon an unusual degree of flexibility in certain joints. Gymnastics, diving, hurdling, modern dance, and ballet all require great flexibility in certain body regions in order to demonstrate *good form*. On the other hand, there is no evidence that more than average flexibility will improve performance in such activities as basketball, tennis, volleyball, and golf. Some experts claim that in rough-and-tumble games like football, soccer, and rugby, better-than-average flexibility will reduce the likelihood of injury. But this idea is based only on observation and judgment and is not supported by research. Conversely, other experts claim that too much flexibility may make a joint injury-prone because it reduces the stability of the joint, and the joint is more likely to be too far out of alignment when it receives stress.

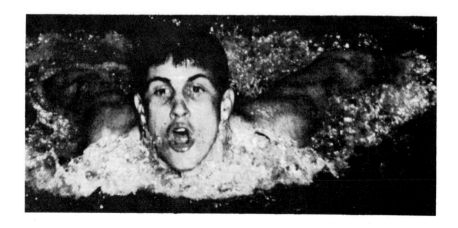

Figure 10–3. The butterfly stroke requires a high degree of flexibility in the shoulder region.

Cureton found that competitive swimmers have a large amount of flexibility in the ankle joint and in trunk flexion and extension.[1] Other studies support the idea that ankle flexibility is important in swimming. Cureton also reported that the Danish Exhibition Gymnastics Team scored higher than any group ever measured by him in trunk flexion and extension.

Research has shown little or no relationship between flexibility of the body appendages and performance in sports. Conversely, significant relationships have been shown between the flexibility of the trunk and hips and performance in several activities.

From research and practical experience, it can be concluded that a normal amount of flexibility throughout the body is desirable in all athletic performances, and some activities demand large degrees of flexibility in specific body regions. By seriously analyzing the task to be accomplished, the coach or athlete can determine which body regions need additional flexibility.

How to Increase Flexibility

Flexibility can be improved on an immediate or a long-range basis. For *immediate* improvement, flexibility can be increased a limited amount by preparatory stretching exercises. DeVries found that prior to warm-up antagonistic muscles relax slowly and imcompletely when the agonists contract, and thus retard free movement and accurate coordination.[2] Warm-up exercises cause the antagonists to relax more completely, and the movements become smoother and better coordinated. Slow-stretch exercises during which the antagonistic muscles are stretched and consciously relaxed for several seconds are the most effective for immediate improvement in flexibility.

To consider *long-range* improvement in flexibility, recall the previous statement that flexibility is limited by three factors: (1) bone structure; (2) amount of bulk surrounding the joints; and (3) the extensibility of the muscles whose tendons cross the joint. The first factor is constant. The second factor offers some potential for improvement of flexibility in some individuals. Overweight persons can increase flexibility throughout the body by losing weight. Take, for example, the person who is unable to touch his hands to the floor because of too much bulk in the abdominal region. For nearly all athletic performers, however, the third factor is the one that offers significant potential for improvement.

Two forms of exercises have been used to stretch muscles and connective tissues, *ballistic* (bobbing) and *slow-tension* (static stretching). Flexibility can be increased effectively with either method, but the slow-tension method is recommended because it has these advantages: (1) there is less danger of exceeding the limits of extensibility of the tissues, which would cause injury and soreness; (2) this method does not activate the stretch reflex; and (3) it provides the opportunity to relax the antagonistic muscles consciously and allow them to s-t-r-e-t-c-h.

Logan and Egstrom[8] and DeVries[2] conducted separate studies which support the claim that flexibility at the hip and lower back can be increased significantly with either ballistic or slow-tension exercises. The subjects who performed ballistic exercises experienced soreness, but those who did slow-tension stretching suffered no soreness. Hansen studied the effectiveness of only ballistic stretching and reported favorable results.[4]

Slow-tension exercises can be done either passively (muscles are consciously relaxed while another person moves the body segment) or actively (movement is caused by muscle contraction). Passive exercises are useful in therapy, but are less desirable than active exercises in athletic conditioning.

The specific recommended procedure for improving flexibility is as follows: Go through the movement slowly until the muscles and connective tissues stretch far enough to experience the "stretch pain." Hold the position for 8 to 10 sec; while doing so, consciously relax the antagonistic muscles, allowing them to stretch as freely as possible. Repeat this procedure five or six times for each movement in which greater flexibility is desired. The best results are accomplished when stretching is done daily.

Dynamic stretching is preferred over passive stretching because flexibility from dynamic stretching has more application to performance. The objective of dynamic stretching is to increase the range through which the body part can move by its own force. Dynamic stretching involves difficult coordinations because the agonistic muscles must contract while the antagonists experience almost complete relaxation. Changes brought about by stretching exercises persist for a considerable period of time (several weeks) after stretching is discontinued. A sizable percentage of the increased flexibility will be retained for as long as 8 to 10 weeks.

Factors That Influence Flexibility

Several factors influence the amount of flexibility that can be attained and the rate at which it can be developed.

STRETCH REFLEX.   When a muscle is stretched suddenly, it automatically responds, owing to the stretch reflex, with a contraction which varies with the suddenness and intensity of the stretch.

The stretch reflex is primarily a postural reflex, and it is essential in maintaining an erect position. An obvious example of it occurs when one falls asleep while sitting and the head nods (neck flexes), causing

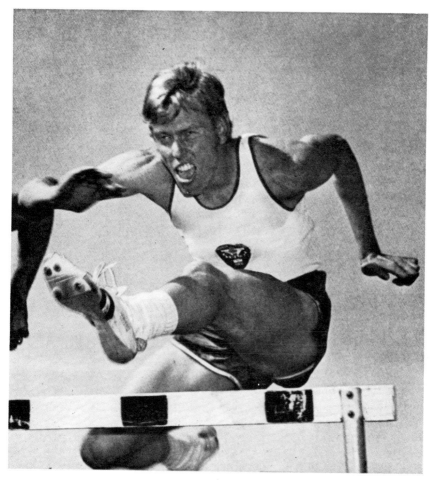

Figure 10–4.   Good hurdling form depends on an unusual amount of
flexibility in the hip and trunk region.

the neck extensor muscles to be stretched suddenly. The stretch reflex
responds, returning the head to the erect position with a jerk. The
stretch reflex also aids in contractions during voluntary movements.
Examples are the dip just prior to the thrust in the vertical jump, or the
backward movement of the arms and shoulders just prior to the forward
action in baseball batting.

The reflex results from a volley of impulses which are automatically
discharged from within the muscle spindles when the muscle is
stretched suddenly. Conversely, slow stretching does not activate the
stretch reflex, and this is one of the arguments for using slow-tension

exercises for increasing flexibility. Walker found that the amount of tension for a given amount of stretch is more than doubled by a quick stretch as compared to a slow stretch, when the degree of the stretch is the same.[10]

WEIGHT TRAINING. Numerous researchers have obtained evidence that weight training does not have harmful effects on flexibility when done properly. Massey and Chaudet point out that weight training tends to increase flexibility in the body regions that are exercised through the range of motion, but it may reduce flexibility in the unexercised regions (static contractions occur in those regions) or in regions where the exercise is done through short ranges.[9] Gardner studied the effects of both isotonic and isometric strength training and found that neither program had detrimental effects on flexibility.[3] It was found that selected weight lifters in the 1976 Olympics ranked second in flexibility only to gymnasts among the several groups of athletes tested. The available evidence clearly supports the idea that if weight training is done through broad ranges of motion, it will not contribute to loss of flexibility.

BODY TYPE AND PROPORTION. Research has shown a low relationship between flexibility and somatotype. Neck, hip, and trunk flexion show the highest relationship, with flexibility steadily decreasing in these movements with increased endomorphic characteristics.[5-7] Body fat, as measured by skinfold calipers, shows a negative correlation with flexibility. The amount of muscle tissue is apparently unrelated to flexibility unless muscle bulk actually interferes with completion of the movement.

No consistent relationship has been shown between flexibility and length of the arms, trunk, and legs. Those who have extremely long arm and trunk measurements in relation to their legs have an advantage in the toe-touching tests, but this tells nothing except the weakness of that particular test.

ACTIVITY LEVEL. Inactivity causes muscles and connective tissues to lose their normal extensibility. Complete inactivity, as when a broken limb is in a cast, results in great loss of flexibility. Inactivity also may contribute to accumulation of body fat which may further restrict flexibility. Conversely, regular activity tends to maintain normal flexibility, and unusual amounts of flexibility can be developed with specific exercises.

SPECIFICITY OF FLEXIBILITY. Research results have established that flexibility tends to be highly specific to a particular movement, meaning that a person might have large ranges of motion in some movements and rank below normal in other movements. This is determined primarily by the extensibility of the muscles and connective tissues surrounding the particular joint, and it is influenced directly by the kind and amount of use the body part receives.

AGE AND SEX.   The greatest flexibility is usually achieved during the early elementary school years, and it never again reaches that level. Numerous test results indicate that elementary school children gradually become less flexible until they are 11 or 12 years old. Then they tend to increase slowly in flexibility until young adulthood. From that point on, flexibility gradually decreases with age. There is sufficient evidence to indicate that elementary school girls are more flexible than boys. Practical experience and observation would indicate that this difference continues throughout life.

TEMPERATURE.   Wright and Johns found that by warming a body region to 113° F dynamic flexibility increased about 20%, whereas cooling to 65° F resulted in decreases of 10 to 20%.[11] It is believed that increasing body temperature through exercise increases the extensibility of muscles and connective tissues, thus increasing flexibility temporarily. Further, it is believed that this increased extensibility will reduce the chances of injury to the tissues.

SELECTED REFERENCES

1. Cureton, T. K.: Flexibility as an aspect of physical fitness. *Res. Q.*, 12:381, 1941.
2. DeVries, H. A.: Evaluation of static stretching procedures for improvement of flexibility. *Res. Q.*, 33:222, 1962.
3. Gardner, G. W.: Flexibility Changes as a Result of Isometric and Isotonic Exercise Over a Limited Range of Motion. Unpublished doctoral dissertation. Los Angeles: University of Southern California, 1963.
4. Hansen, T. W.: Selected Effects of Stretching on Flexibility. Unpublished master's thesis. Los Angeles: University of California, 1962.
5. Harvey, V. P., and Scott, G. D.: Reliability of a measure of forward flexibility and its relation to physical dimensions of college women. *Res. Q.*, 38:28, 1967.
6. Laubach, L. L., and McConville, J. T.: Relationships between flexibility, anthropometry and the somatotype of college man. *Res. Q.*, 37:241, 1966.
7. Laubach, L. L., and McConville, J. T.: Muscle strength, flexibility and body size of adult males. *Res. Q.*, 37:384, 1966.
8. Logan, G. A., and Egstrom, G. H.: Effects of slow and fast stretching on the sacro-femoral angle. *J. Assoc. Phys. Ment. Rehabil.*, 15:85, 1961.
9. Massey, B. H., and Chaudet, N. L.: Effects of systematic heavy resistance exercises on range of joint movement in young male adults. *Res. Q.*, 27:41, 1956.
10. Walker, S. M.: Delay of twitch relaxation induced by stress and stress relaxation. *J. Appl. Physiol.*, 16:801, 1961.
11. Wright, V., and Johns, R. J.: Physical factors concerned with the stiffness of normal and diseased joints. *Johns Hopkins Hosp. Bull.*, 106:215, 1960.

Chapter 11
Development of Neuromuscular Skill

The functions of the nervous system as it relates to muscle use were discussed in Chapter 2. We suggest the reader study that chapter before turning attention to this chapter, which deals specifically with concepts associated with the development of skill.

Skill is the ability to perform a combination of specific movements smoothly and effectively. It is the coordination of all the different muscles involved, whether they are agonists, antagonists, neutralizers, or stabilizers. In other words, skill is the ability to use the correct muscles at the correct time, with the exact force necessary to perform the desired movements in the proper sequence and timing.

Coordinated movements occur as a result of muscle contractions, and muscles contract only in response to nerve impulses. Therefore, coordinated movement occurs if nerve impulses reach the proper muscles at the correct time.

Even though skill is a result of the teamwork of the nervous and muscular systems, it is primarily a function of the nervous system, since the muscles contract at specified times and with certain amounts of force as dictated by nerve impulses. Of course, some conditions of the muscles themselves, such as strength and speed of contraction, influence skill. But even these factors are partially determined by the functioning of the nervous system.

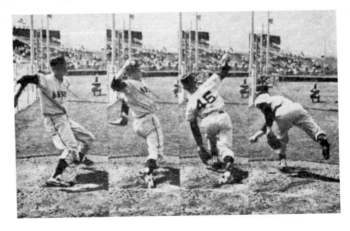

Figure 11-1. Pitching with speed and accuracy is a real test of skill. (Athletic J., pp. 56–57, January, 1968.)

Significance of Skill

Effective performance requires sufficient amounts of several physiological traits, such as strength, speed, endurance, agility, and flexibility, but athletes possessing lesser amounts of these traits often outperform their stronger and faster opponents because of well-coordinated neuromuscular patterns (specific skills). The excellent athlete has an abundance of all the physiological traits mentioned, combined with the exact neuromuscular control needed to assure success. Some performance experts claim that skill is the most important single factor in performance.

Each activity requires certain specific skills. For example, a soccer player must be able to dribble, pass, screen, dodge, and kick effectively. A football player must be proficient at blocking, tackling, and handling the ball. Each of the other sports has its own set of specific skills. Regardless of the other traits a person might possess, he will not be an effective tennis player until he learns the skills that are specific to tennis, and he will not swim well until he develops the specific skills of swimming. The development of specific skills is one of the greatest concerns of the coach and teacher.

How to Increase Skill

Most athletic performances include several specific skills, and each skill involves a combination of movements. An effective and systematic approach to improving performance requires analysis of the performance in order to determine what skills are involved. Then a program is designed to improve those skills. For example, basketball is composed of such skills as running, rebounding, jumping, dodging, dribbling, passing, and catching. Basketball performance may be improved by enhancing one or more of these skills. The problem, then, is to identify the specific skills in a performance and to employ effective techniques to improve them.

Essentially, skill improvement involves (1) determining the correct mechanics and (2) practicing the skill repeatedly many times. The skill must be practiced *correctly* until the movement patterns become effective and efficient. As a result of such practice, the performer will also increase his skill by improving judgment of speed, distance, and time, and by developing insight into the various circumstances of the performance.

Several categories of basic skills require different emphasis. Skills are logically divided into (1) accuracy skills, (2) power skills, and (3) maneuverability skills.

Examples of *accuracy skills* are putting in golf, shooting in basketball, target shooting, and bowling. These skills often do not involve fast or vigorous movements, but require great concentration and much practice of fine muscle coordinations. Under competitive conditions, some accuracy skills are performed at high speed. Slowing down the performance during practice will aid in analyzing the mechanics of the skill and improving the movement patterns. But for best results, accuracy skills should be practiced extensively at the same speed and intensity as they will be performed in competition.

In addition to being dependent upon neuromuscular coordination, accuracy skills also are dependent upon judgment of speed, distance, and time. For example, such judgments are important to a football player when he throws downfield to a running receiver. The passer must be able to judge the distance to the receiver and the speed at which he is moving, then throw the ball so it will meet the receiver. In shooting a basketball, the player must correctly judge his distance from the basket, then be able to put the ball where he judges it should go. If a post man passes to a guard cutting in for a lay-up, the passer must correctly judge the speed of the guard. When the guard lays up the shot, he must correctly judge his speed and the rebound angle of the ball. Many other examples could be given of activities in which judgments of speed, distance, and time must be made frequently in order to enhance accuracy skills.

Among the *power skills* are football blocking, putting the shot, long jumping, sprint swimming, and sprint running. These skills are performed with great speed and force (power). In developing power skills, the emphasis is on neuromuscular coordinations which result in fast and forceful movements. Some skills combine accuracy and power.

Examples are pitching a baseball, batting a baseball, kicking a football field goal, and boxing.

Maneuverability skills include gymnastic performances, skiing, court games such as tennis, basketball, and badminton, and field games such as soccer, football, and rugby. In developing these skills, the emphasis is on agility (quick change of direction and body position). In some cases, mobility skills are best improved by practicing the specific movement patterns over and over at increasingly faster speeds and with more precision. In others, mobility skills can be increased a limited amount by increasing some of the contributing elements such as strength, speed of movement, and reaction time of the specific movements.

NERVOUS SYSTEM INVOLVEMENT. In general, the lower the involvement is in the central nervous system (CNS), the more gross, primitive, and stereotyped the movement will be. For example, a walking or running stride can probably be repeated over and over with the involvement of only the cerebellum, brain stem, and spinal cord. But if an abrupt change of direction or speed is required, the more involved coordinations and judgments would probably require the involvement of the higher centers such as the cerebral cortex and/or the thalamus.

It has been postulated that, as skill develops, the innervation is relegated to lower centers of the CNS. The pathways of impulses within the cerebrum develop ruts by repeatedly traveling the same paths, and these ruts allow faster impulse travel with fewer detours and fewer errors. The performance of the act then requires less conscious consideration to keep the impulses on the proper course.

It is generally agreed that highly skillful acts are accomplished with little conscious thought, except for the thought needed to begin the act. Consequently, highly skillful acts are mostly *conditioned reflexes*. For example, we can perform the skill of walking while we are occupied in deep thought or conversation. Actually, we may walk more skillfully under these conditions than if we concentrate on the movements. The movements involved in walking result from conditioned reflexes. During active contests, it is often necessary for the performer to concentrate on external cues, and any preoccupation with specific body movements will destroy his effectiveness. In such cases, although the general idea of the desired response is conveyed by the cerebrum, lower centers of the central nervous system work out the details.

In the final analysis, the resulting movements are dependent upon three factors: (1) which neurons conduct impulse volleys, (2) the frequencies of the impulses, and (3) exactly when these impulses reach the muscle fibers. An important related factor is which muscles are prevented from contracting because of neural inhibition.

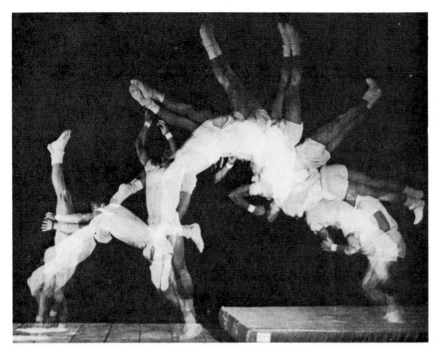

Figure 11–2. Gymnast doing a back somersault with a full twist in a layout position, preceded by a back somersault and other movements in the routine. This complex performance requires a high level of strength, power, and neuromuscular coordination. (From *Applied Kinesiology: The Scientific Study of Human Performance* by Jensen and Schultz, page 4. Copyright © 1977 by McGraw-Hill, Inc. Used with permission of McGraw-Hill Book Company.)

As a certain skill is developed, its specific movements tend to become less variable and more exact, because the selected patterns of impulses become duplicated more easily. This is because the impulse volleys tend to follow previously established pathways within the nervous system. As stated previously, the impulses are conducted along the paths of least resistance. Nerve pathway possibilities are inherited, but it is use that determines the development of the pathways. As certain synapses are used repeatedly, their thresholds are lowered, and the chance of repeating that pattern under like conditions is increased. Conversely, it is difficult to blaze new pathways for the same act once the pathways have been established. Like walking through deep grass, the more often a certain path is taken, the deeper the pathway becomes. Paths not used often tend to become obscure, but they are not completely eliminated.

When one begins to learn a skill, many pathways are possible. But gradually, pathways that have resulted in successful performances are selected, and the other pathways are rejected. The more often a pathway is repeated, the more firmly ingrained the pattern becomes and the more difficult it is to avoid. Gradually the path is used with greater ease and smoothness, and superfluous movements are eliminated. Unproductive paths are rejected, and the act becomes "skillful."

Certain obstacles exist such as the following: (1) Conditions, both of the internal and external environments, are never exactly the same from one time to the next. (2) Most skills are complex enough to involve several joints and many muscles, and even though the skill may appear correct, variations in only a few movements may detract from success. (3) The performer may incorrectly judge his performance as successful and continue to perform incorrectly. For instance, a youngster may throw with the wrong foot forward and assume this is the correct procedure since he achieves a degree of success. Or a young basketball player who is a head taller than his opposition may use an undesirable shooting technique with much success until he meets an opponent of equal height.

INSTRUCTIONAL TECHNIQUES.   In theory, skill development is a simple matter, but in actuality it is difficult. *The key is repetition*, but it is necessary to repeat the skill pattern *correctly*. Otherwise, lack of skill or incorrect technique will result.

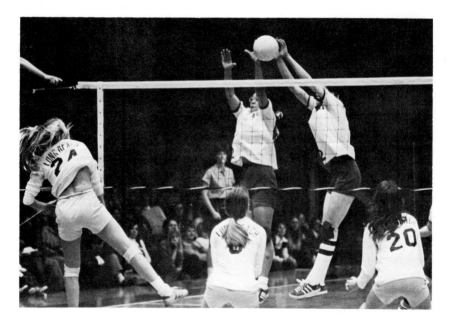

Figure 11–3.   Power volleyball has developed into a highly skilled game.

In order to ensure correct practice, the learner must know what is correct. This means his practice must be preceded by information about the correct technique. The information may be obtained from *instruction* by one who knows correct technique, from *reading, watching film,* or *observing a skilled performer.* Once the learner understands the elements of correct technique and has had some opportunity to practice the skill, *error detection and correction* become an effective tool for the instructor. As the learner practices the skill over and over, the instructor detects imperfections and prescribes methods for correcting them. Bit by bit, as a result of practice and correction, the skill is perfected.

A key role of the teacher or coach is to recognize incorrect techniques and prescribe drills which will cause improvement. The younger the performer, the easier, quicker, and more precise will be his development, assuming his nervous system has matured adequately to develop the skill in question.

FROM BASIC TO REFINED SKILLS. The acquisition of refined skills necessitates prior learning of gross skill patterns (basic skills). Highly refined skills are usually only slight modifications of basic patterns. For example, if a child learns a basic throwing pattern by throwing objects of all sorts under a variety of conditions, the addition of a forearm rotation and a wrist snap in the direction of the little finger can result in a curve ball. Similarly, once a tennis player has learned the basic tennis strokes, he can add slight modifications which result in spin (english) on the ball. In golf, the basic stroke patterns are learned rather quickly, but the refinement of them and the learning of stroke variations require much time and practice. In every athletic activity there is a set of basic skills, and there are refinements and variations of the basic skills which make the difference between *mediocrity* and *excellence.*

Factors That Influence Skill

Several factors relate to skill and influence its development. Among the factors are the following:

RECIPROCAL INHIBITION. The inhibition, or blocking, of nerve impulses to muscles in opposition (antagonistic) to a desired movement is of utmost importance to the efficiency of that movement. It appears that the antagonistic muscles are automatically inhibited. Thus, one may wonder why it should even be discussed. It must be recognized that with the practice of a movement, the inhibition of the antagonistic muscles becomes quicker and more complete. Obviously, antagonistic tension interferes with the effectiveness of a performance, and by reducing tension, effectiveness is increased, and the onset of fatigue is postponed.

Anxiety or other emotional involvement can limit the effectiveness of reciprocal inhibition. Thus, such heightened emotions tend to hinder performances in which fine muscle coordinations are required. Golf is an activity that is adversely affected by anxiety. Another example is a basketball player who misses a crucial free throw when the pressure is on. Conversely, activities not requiring a high degree of fine muscle control may benefit from heightened emotions. For example, the performance of a football lineman or a shot-putter may be enhanced by anxiety. But if the football player must handle the ball, his performance is likely to suffer. Many so-called "sophomore mistakes" are attributable to the inability to contend with emotional stress because it has a detrimental effect on refined neuromuscular coordinations.

STRENGTH AND ENDURANCE. The exhibition of strength is a skill in itself because it requires correct muscle involvement and coordination of a number of muscles in different roles: agonists, antagonists, stabilizers, and neutralizers. Dynamic strength requires more coordination than static strength, and total body strength movements require more coordination than strength movements of specific body segments. It is questionable whether the development of strength has any direct influence on specific skills. However, research by Berger and Blaschke supports the idea that strength contributes to general motor ability and that dynamic strength contributes more than static strength.[1]

Endurance makes a contribution to skill in performances in which fatigue is a consideration. It is known that refined coordinations are adversely affected by the onset of fatigue. Baseball pitchers lose their control, golfers make more mistakes, and basketball players shoot lower percentages when fatigue becomes excessive. Thus, endurance contributes to skill in long-duration performances.

MENTAL PRACTICE. Research results support the idea that skill can be increased through mental practice. In the strict sense, mental practice means concentrated thought about the movement patterns involved. However, some researchers have included in the defnition of mental practice the viewing of films and demonstrations and other nonmanual activities which clarify the mental image of the performance. Stebbins,[6] Egstrom,[2] Oxendine,[4] and Phipps and Morehouse,[5] all obtained evidence that skill can be increased within certain limits by mental practice, either in the form of mental concentration or other nonmanual techniques.

PROPRIOCEPTION. Awareness of body position is determined by a variety of sensory inputs to the central nervous system. The organs of balance in the inner ear, vision, and pressures applied to the surface of the body all help to provide information about position of the body and its segments. The muscles and joints are provided with special organs to sense position and tension in the muscles and in the joints. All this sensory information about body movement and position is termed *proprioception,* and can be classified into two general areas: vestibular and kinesthetic.

Vestibular Reception. Vestibular receptors are found in the nonauditory area of the inner ear. The most important system involves three small fluid-filled canals called the *semicircular canals.* These canals are especially sensitive to acceleration, deceleration, and rotation, which cause the fluid in the canals to displace small hairlike organs called *cristae.* The movement of the cristae is transmitted to the brain, causing the awareness of the movement.

Two other systems in the inner ear are the *utricle,* which provides the body with information concerning the sense of body position, and the *saccule,* which is involved in sensory perception of vibrations.

Kinesthetic Reception. Kinesthetic sense (muscle sense) is an important factor in skill because it provides information concerning positions and movements of body segments or limbs. Because of this sense, a person while his eyes are closed can touch his fingers together in front of his face, or can place a spoon to his mouth while looking out the window. Likewise, a golfer is able to swing a club correctly without taking his eyes off the ball, and a basketball player can concentrate his sight on the basket and perform a jump shot with awareness of the positions and movements of all his body parts. A baseball batter can concentrate on the baseball and still be aware of the position of the bat. This "muscle sense," or kinesthetic sense, involves mainly the following receptors: (1) the muscle spindles, (2) the Golgi tendon organs, (3) the pacinian corpuscles, and (4) free nerve endings.

SELECTED REFERENCES

1. Berger, R. A., and Blaschke, L. A.: Comparison of relationships between motor ability and static and dynamic strength. *Res. Q., 38*:144, 1967.
2. Egstrom, G. H.: Effects of an emphasis on conceptualizing techniques during early learning of a gross motor skill. *Res. Q., 35*:472, 1964.
3. Jensen, C. R., and Schultz, G. W.: *Applied Kinesiology,* 2nd ed. New York: McGraw-Hill Book Co., 1977.
4. Oxendine, J. B.: Effect of mental and physical practice on the learning of three motor skills. *Res. Q., 40*:755, 1969.
5. Phipps, S. J., and Morehouse, C. A.: Effects of mental practice on the acquisition of motor skills of varied difficulty. *Res. Q., 40*:773, 1969.
6. Stebbins, R. J.: A comparison of the effects of physical and mental practice in learning a motor skill. *Res. Q., 39*:714, 1968.

Chapter 12
Training Considerations for Women

There has been an abundance of research in recent years concerning women in sport. It seems clear from these data that women are physiologically similar to men, and that training programs that work for men will also work for women. The existing differences are those of magnitude not basic physiological function. The enzyme systems and cellular control mechanisms are the same in both men and women.

The purpose of this chapter is to discuss both the similarities and differences in performance which can be expected by those who work with women athletes.

STRENGTH

There is no doubt that men are generally stronger than women. Men also are generally larger than women. This fact accounts for much of the difference in the absolute strength. There is also a difference among the basic muscle groups. For example, women are weaker than men in absolute strength of all the major muscle groups. However, this difference is greatest in the muscles of the chest, arms, and shoulders, and least in muscles of the legs. It is difficult to determine if these differences would be less apparent if boys and girls had the same activity profile as they developed.

When strength is expressed in terms of total body weight, the differences mentioned previously still exist, but are not so great. When expressed in terms of lean body mass, women are actually stronger in flexor and extensor muscles at the hips.[9]

There seems to be no basic difference in the quality of muscle in men and women. In other words, the amount of force exerted by muscle cross-sectional area is about 4 to 6 kg/cm^2 in both sexes.[3]

Effects of Strength Training

Most women are concerned about the effects of strength-training programs on muscle size. Large, bulging biceps would not be particularly attractive. The truth is women can make fine strength gains with little or no hypertrophy.[6] Strength training does yield muscular hypertrophy in men, but not in women. Apparently, muscular hypertrophy is regulated by the hormone testosterone, which is found in much higher levels in men than in women. The results of strength-training programs for women have been delightful. Not only have strength gains occurred, but the subjects have often lost girth in areas where girth loss is desirable.[8]

Weight-training programs for women often have led to a significant loss of relative and total body fat, usually with a similar gain in lean body mass.[6]

Programs for strength development of women have been similar to those reported for strength training of men. There seems to be no reason to use special programs for developing strength in women, and results should be similar in terms of percentage of increase.

ENDURANCE

There is a definite and significant difference in aerobic capacity between men and women of about 15% to 25%. This difference is not apparent in young children, but begins to show up after the size difference becomes a factor during young adulthood. The difference in aerobic capacity (VO$_2$ max) is not so great when expressed in milliliter/kilogram/minute, and is even smaller if expressed in milliliter/kilograms of *lean body tissue*/minute,[1] or in milliliters/kilogram of active tissue mass/minute. However, since oxidative capacity must support the total body weight in most athletic events, the expressions which make the difference between men and women smaller are really not very meaningful. The truth is that women cannot really expect to compete evenly with men in activities requiring aerobic energy sources.

The decreased aerobic capacity can at least partially be accounted for. Women have not only less hemoglobin but also a lower total blood volume per body mass and a smaller total heart volume than do men.[4]

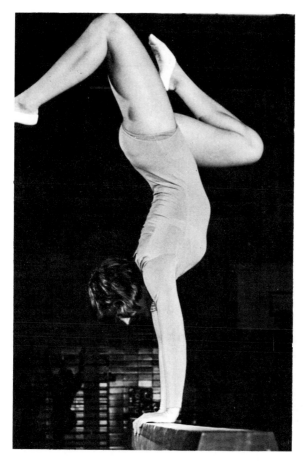

Figure 12–1. Women's gymnastics has gained world recognition through effective television coverage. It requires vigorous training and exact discipline.

Although maximal heart rates are similar in men and women, the amount of blood pumped per beat (stroke volume) is smaller in women, which yields a smaller cardiac output. Although not as important, women's vital capacity and maximal ventilation volumes also are lower in relation to their size. As always, corrections for body size reduce the differences, but do not completely eliminate them.

The total ATP and CP available for rapid energy usage is found in the same concentration in men and women. However, since women have relatively less muscle than men, they have a smaller total supply. Surprisingly, there is little difference in power measurements made using the Margaria-Kalamen power test.[5]

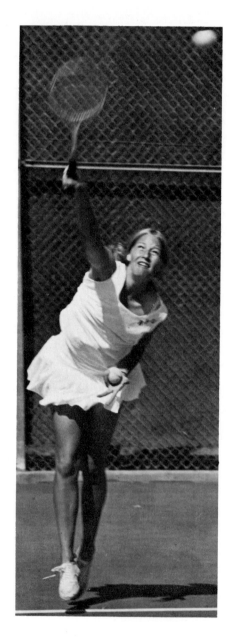

Figure 12–2. A hard serve by a highly skilled woman tennis player.

Women are not able to develop blood lactic acid levels to the same extent as men,[2] and are at their greatest disadvantage in events requiring high lactate development such as the 400-meter run. This difference may decrease as more women begin to compete in events of this type.

Effects of Endurance Training

The changes in the cardiovascular system associated with endurance-type activities in women are similar to those reported in men for many years. Seven weeks of training two times per week for 30 min yielded an increase in $\dot{V}O_2$ max of 34.8 ml/kilogram/minute to 44.2 ml/kilogram/minute. This was accomplished primarily by an increase in stroke volume which resulted in a larger cardiac output.[5] There were no significant changes in maximal heart rate or in a-v O_2 diff. It should be noted that significant changes occurred in maximal lactate production.

Of course, any submaximal exercise would yield a lower heart rate as the stroke volume increased, and lactate production would decrease if the original submaximal exercise was near the anaerobic threshold.

Females can also expect a decrease in relative fat following endurance training. They may also experience a small increase in lean body mass.[7]

BODY DIFFERENCES

Two differences besides height and weight should be noted in a comparative discussion of men and women.

BODY COMPOSITION.   The average college-age woman has more body fat than the college-age male (22% to 26% vs. 12% to 16%). Whether these differences are genetic or environmental is not known at this time. The higher level of estrogen is surely responsible for at least part of this difference. It should be pointed out, however, that well-trained women distance runners often have less than 10% fat on their bodies. It should also be pointed out that the increased relative fat is an advantage in some events. The greater body fat tends to decrease the total cost of swimming by 10% to 20%.

It seems that the average female could decrease the percentage of fat easily and without harm by engaging in activities requiring large energy outputs on a regular basis.

PELVIC WIDTH.   The width of the female hip is similar to that of the male even though the width of other bones and structures are about 10% less in the female. This may increase the amount of pelvic shift to keep the center of gravity aligned during running. Many successful women sprinters seem to have narrow hips.

GYNECOLOGICAL FACTORS

The question of whether to exercise during the menstrual cycle often arises. Apparently, exercise does not significantly affect menstrual disorders. Dysmenorrhea is probably neither aggravated nor relieved by activity. There have been reports of complete absence of menstruation in females who train for long-distance running. These women run from 70 to 100 miles/week and have extremely low levels of body fat. The absence of menstruation may be related to the low level of fat, since this same problem has been reported in chronically underweight subjects.[10]

Performance during actual menstrual flow seems to be an individual matter with much variability, depending on the performer. Many female athletes report no difference in performance and should be encouraged to train and compete without worry. Surely, no female athlete should be forced to train or compete during menstruation if she has discovered some negative side effects from doing so.

Injuries to the female reproductive organs seem to be rather rare. The breasts are the most vulnerable and should be protected during contact sports. It also may be wise for female water-skiers to wear rubber wet suits during competition or training to avoid forceful entry of water into the vagina, which could lead to several complications.

In general, female athletes have fewer complications with pregnancy and childbirth than do normal nonathletic women. Some have even competed in international meets during early pregnancy. However, untrained females should not be encouraged to increase their activity level significantly *during* pregnancy. There is evidence that the baby's oxygen supply may be somewhat impaired by unaccustomed activity levels of the mother during pregnancy.

SELECTED REFERENCES

1. Drinkwater, B.: Physiological responses of women to exercise. In *Exercise and Sports Sciences Review*, Vol. 1. J. Wilmore, Ed. New York: Academic Press, 1973.
2. Drinkwater, B., Horvath, S., and Wells, C.: Aeorbic power of females, ages 10 to 68. *J. Gerontol.*, 30:385–394, 1975.
3. Ikai, M., and Fukunager, T.: Calculation of muscle strength per unit cross-sectional area of human muscle by means of ultrasonic measurements. Part 2. *Angew. Physiol.*, 26:26–32, 1968.
4. Kjellberg, S., Rudhe, U., and Sjostrand, T.: The amount of hemoglobin and the blood volume in relation to the pulse rate and cardiac volume during rest. *Acta Physiol. Scand.*, 19:136–145, 1949.
5. Mathews, D. K., and Fox, E. L.: The *Physiological Basis of Physical Education and Athletics*. Philadelphia: W. B. Saunders Co., 1976.
6. Mayhew, J., and Gross, P.: Body composition changes in young women with high resistance weight training. *Res. Q.*, 45:433–440, 1974.
7. Moody, D., et al.: The effects of a jogging program on the body composition of normal and obese high school girls. *Med. Sci. Sports*, 4:210–213, 1972.

8. Price, S.: The Effects of Weight Training on Strength, Endurance, Girth, and Body Composition in College Women. Unpublished master's thesis. Provo: Brigham Young University, 1974.
9. Wilmore, J.: Alterations in strength, body composition and anthropometric measurements consequent to a 10-week weight training program. *Med. Sci. Sport*, 6:133–138, 1974.
10. Wilmore, J. H.: *Athletic Training and Physical Fitness*. Boston: Allyn and Bacon, Inc., 1976.

Chapter 13
Training Considerations for Adults

This chapter is presented because of the increased interest in training by adults. Many of these adults never competed in their school years, but have become interested in competition or increased fitness levels as they have grown older. Others are concerned about preventive programs to protect themselves from cardiovascular disease. In either case, it is important to know the techniques and principles of training for these groups.

TRAINING FOR COMPETITION

The concepts of training discussed previously in this text apply equally well for the adult who is interested in high level competition. These men should be encouraged to train with great energy, using programs described previously to improve the systems involved in the activity of their choice.

Adults interested only in cross-country running competition (road races or marathon) should initially follow the instructions in the section "Training for Fitness." After they have reached a moderate level of fitness, they can begin to use the techniques of interval or computerized training to complete their training regimen.

TRAINING FOR FITNESS

Most adults will be interested in exercise for health maintenance and cardiovascular disease prevention and will be content to reach a healthy level of cardiovascular fitness for that purpose alone.

Since some situations could be dangerous for adults beginning exercise programs, the following guidelines have been suggested by the American College of Sports Medicine:[1]

1. Adults under 35 years of age with no known coronary heart disease risk factors nor previous history of cardiovascular disease may begin an exercise program safely without special medical clearance. However, if they have not had a medical examination during the past two years or if they have any questions concerning their health status, they should see their physician prior to beginning their program.

2. Adults 35 years old or older should be advised to have a medical evaluation prior to any major increase in activity level, especially if they have a history of cardiovascular disease or a combination of cardiovascular risk factors.

Any questons concerning the safety of exercise for an adult should be referred to his physician.

Developing a Program

Four basic principles apply to all programs involving cardiovascular endurance for adults: (1) type of activity, (2) intensity of activity, (3) duration of activity, and (4) frequency of activity.

TYPE OF ACTIVITY. Any activity that uses the large muscle groups of the body (primarily the large muscles of the hips and legs) and is rhythmic and continuous in nature will cause the desired changes in cardiovascular fitness to occur. Good examples of these activities are walking, jogging, bicycling, swimming, cross-country skiing, and rope jumping. Activities of a straining nature (such as weight lifting), activities that use only the small muscles of the arms (such as push-ups), or activities that are not continuous (such as golf) will be ineffective in causing the right kind of change to occur.

Certain competitive activities such as handball, racquetball, and tennis are appropriate if played with enough vigor to keep the heart rate in the training zone for the entire workout. However, it is difficult to use these activities properly until proficiency in applying the principles of exercise training has been gained.

The decision concerning the activities to use depends on the availability of facilities (such as a pool or track), and on special health problems (such as arthritic knees or sore ankles). Activities should be rewarding, pleasant, and fun as long as they meet the requirements stated. Remember, the activity must allow a large return of blood to the heart to be effective.

Warm-up and Cool Down. Regardless of the activity chosen for a cardiovascular endurance program, the activity must always include warm-up and cool-down periods. Warming up helps open the blood vessels in the muscles and helps stretch the tendons and ligaments so that injury will not occur so easily. The heart increases its rate gradually, the lungs begin to move the air in and out, and the whole metabolic system prepares itself for the workout ahead.

An interesting study that rather conclusively proves the need of warm-up for adults was conducted. Forty-four normal men (ages 21 to 52 years) were tested on two different occasions with and without a warm-up. In the second test (without a warm-up) 31 (70%) of the men developed abnormal changes on the ECG during the exercises.[2]

Cooling down is even more important than warming up. During aerobic exercise, the large muscles of the legs provide a real boost to the circulating blood to help it get back to the heart. This is done by the action of the muscles on the large veins of the leg. Each time the leg muscles contract, blood is forced up the veins toward the heart. As the muscles relax, blood fills the veins but is not allowed to go backward because of the valves in the vein. Cooling down allows the venous pump to continue to work until the need for blood decreases and the heart can take care of the load by itself.

Many problems with postcardiac patients occur 5 to 10 min after exercise. These problems can be minimized by careful cooling-down procedures which allow the body systems to revert to normal slowly. Cooling down also helps the muscles to rid themselves of the waste products of metabolism more effectively.

INTENSITY OF ACTIVITY. Exercise intensity refers to the vigorousness of exercise. Much research has been done to determine how much exercise is needed to cause cardiovascular changes to occur. Researchers have found that changes in cardiovascular fitness are directly related to the intensity of the training load; therefore, intensity is one of the major factors influencing response to training. Of course, the more intense the exercise, the better will be the training effect. Athletes often train .at or near maximal intensity for long periods of time. Athletes also can run 4-min miles and perform other feats which cannot be accomplished by the average person. The average person can get a fine training effect at a much lower intensity of performance than the athlete and *should* train at this lower intensity for safety and comfort. The question, then, is how intense should activity be for the average person?

Most exercise physiologists agree that the physiological and biochemical changes associated with training occur at about 70% of the individual's maximal aerobic capacity, whereas intensities of less than 60% are not nearly as efficient.[1,5] These same experts also have warned adults against exceeding 90% of their maximal aerobic capacity, even

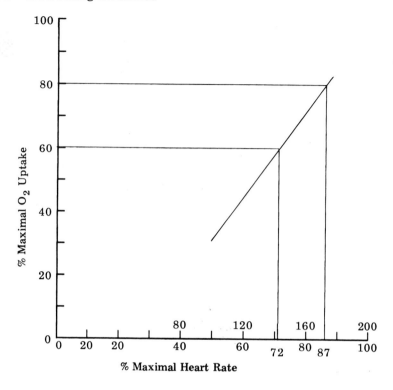

Figure 13–1.   Relationship between percent of maximal oxygen uptake and percent of maximal heart rate. (Fisher, A. G.: *Your Heart Rate—Key to Real Fitness.* Provo: Brigham Young University Press, 1976, page 10.)

during peak exercise effort. They recommend that most adults work at an intensity somewhere between 60% and 80% of their maximal aerobic capacity for safe, effective training. These levels can be estimated by using heart rate as a guide. Research has shown the heart rate, expressed as *percent of maximal heart rate*, bears a significant relationship to *percent of maximal aerobic capacity*. This relationship is shown in Figure 13–1. Note that 60% maximal aerobic capacity is related to 72% maximal heart rate, and that 80% maximal aerobic capacity is related to 87% maximal heart rate. This means that the proper intensity for training is between 72% and 87% of the maximal heart rate.

Maximal heart rate can be predicted using the formula[4]

$$220 - Age = Maximal\ heart\ rate$$

Of course, the predicted value may vary somewhat among adults. However, with this information, the approximate training heart-rate range for a person of any age can be computed by multiplying the predicted maximal heart rate by the recommended heart-rate percentage for effective training (between 72% and 87%). This is called the *training zone*. Using the training zone will allow almost anyone to regulate the intensity of his or her own exercise program effectively and safely, and will result in a fine aerobic training effect (Fig. 13–2).

For example, the training zone for a 40-year-old man was computed by multiplying his maximal heart rate (180 beats/minute) by 72% and 87%. His training heart rate is between 130 beats/minute (72%) and 157 beats/minute (87%).

How to Monitor Heart Rate.   Heart rate must be monitored during exercise for the best results and should be counted during the first 10 sec following exercise. Several locations can be used to monitor this pulse; the carotid artery on each side of the voice box, the radial artery at the base of the thumb on either arm, or at the temple in front of the ear. A problem exists in counting the pulse at the carotid artery.

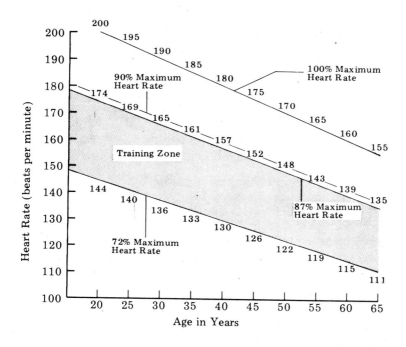

Figure 13–2.   Training heart rate for different ages. (Fisher, A. G.: *Your Heart Rate—Key to Real Fitness.* Provo: Brigham Young University Press, 1976, page 11.)

Because of the carotid sinus reflex, palpation of this artery sometimes causes the pulse to slow and may yield an inaccurate count.[6] Either of the other two areas may be used successfully, and with a little practice will give an accurate indication of intensity.

One of the most difficult things to learn is how to count the pulse during exercise. Research has shown that pulse rate immediately after exercise will be similar to that during exercise.

A person using jogging as his type of exercise would slow down to a walk, and immediately count his pulse for 10 sec. Figure 13–3 shows training heart rate expressed in 10-sec counts. For example, a 40-year-old man would use a 21 to 22 count in 10 sec (130 beats/minute) for the low end of the exercise zone and a 26 count in 10 sec (156 beats/minute) for the high. This simplifies the counting task and is an effective way to use heart rate information during exercise.

The proper intensity of exercise can be determined by simple trial and error. If an exercise bout results in a heart rate that is below the training heart rate, increase the speed or intensity of the next bout; if the heart rate is above the training heart rate, decrease the intensity of the next bout.

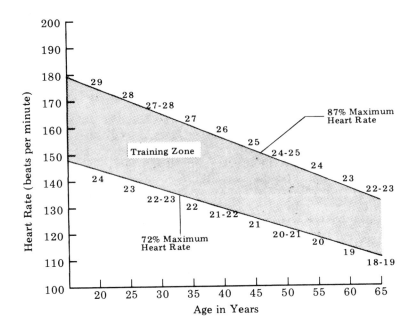

Figure 13–3.   Training heart rate expressed in 10-sec count. (Fisher, A. G.: *Your Heart Rate—Key to Real Fitness.* Provo: Brigham Young University Press, 1976, page 13.)

One of the great advantages of this type of program is that it allows exercise in many varied and different conditions with minimal danger. The heart rate will accurately reflect the stress level on the body and allow an adult to exercise safely in the heat or at altitude. The speed of the activity may decrease, but the training effect will still be the same and the exercise will be safe.

This principle works the other way too. As the cardiovascular system becomes more efficient, work will become easier and the tempo of the activity will necessarily increase to maintain the training heart rate. By using the training heart rate, there is an automatic compensation for this increased fitness. Training by heart rate has many advantages over training by time and distance.

DURATION OF EXERCISE. The principle of duration is easily understood and is critical to the training effect received from any activity. It is inversely related to the intensity of the activity. The more intense the activity, the shorter the duration can be. The less intense the activity, the longer the duration should be. The absolute minimal duration is about 5 min, and is effective only if the exercise is extremely intense. Anyone who desires a good training effect without danger should exercise in the training zone for 15 to 25 min daily. Exercise in the lower part of the training zone (72% to 75%) should be extended to 20 or 25 min. Research seems to indicate that trained adults enjoy working at between 80% and 85% of their maximal heart rate. If they are forced to work at a higher level (90%), they tend to decrease their intensity to about 80% to 85%. If they are asked to work more slowly, they increase to a slightly higher level. Everyone should probably begin at the lower part of the zone and work harder as training occurs.

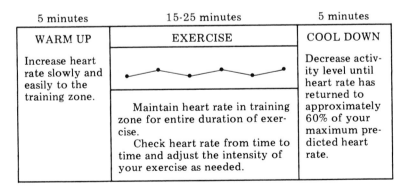

5 minutes	15-25 minutes	5 minutes
WARM UP	EXERCISE	COOL DOWN
Increase heart rate slowly and easily to the training zone.	Maintain heart rate in training zone for entire duration of exercise. Check heart rate from time to time and adjust the intensity of your exercise as needed.	Decrease activity level until heart rate has returned to approximately 60% of your maximum predicted heart rate.

Figure 13–4. Example of steady state exercise program. (Fisher, A. G.: *Your Heart Rate—Key to Real Fitness.* Provo: Brigham Young University Press, 1976, page 15.)

Figure 13–4 is a graphic representation of a typical workout. The exercise period should always begin with a warm-up and end with a cool-down period.

Interval training can be used with certain exercises such as rope jumping in which the work load is so intense that the heart rate may reach maximal if not broken by short rest periods (Fig. 13–5).

Remember that the key to any training program is to stay in the training zone for the entire duration of the exercise. It really does not matter if the heart rate varies, but it must stay in the training zone. This is crucial. The aerobic system does not train well if the proper intensity is not maintained for 15 to 20 min/workout.

FREQUENCY OF ACTIVITY. Frequency of exercise is related to the intensity of exercise as well as its duration. Research indicates that four workouts per week are better than three, and that five are even better than four. Similar training effects can be obtained from three workouts a week *by increasing the duration of each workout by 5 to 10 min.* These sessions should be scheduled on alternate days. Two workouts a week are not effective for training the cardiovascular system even though they will maintain a level of fitness once it has been reached.

Adults should be encouraged to begin and progress slowly. Those who have been extremely inactive should ignore the intensity principle for the first few weeks and exercise at a low intensity for the required duration. After several weeks, the heart rate can be checked and the intensity increased to the low level of the training zone. Later, as

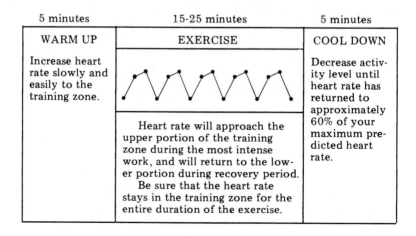

Figure 13–5. Example of interval training exercise program. (Fisher, A. G.: *Your Heart Rate—Key to Real Fitness.* Provo: Brigham Young University Press, 1976, page 16.)

changes in fitness occur, the heart rate will naturally move up to the higher side of the training zone, and exercise will become more effective.

Possible Physical Problems

Certain physical problems such as sore muscles, shin splints, and side ache sometimes occur as the result of exercise. These problems are not serious and can usually be taken care of at home using fairly simple remedies.

Adults who experience any abnormal heart action such as irregular, fluttering, or skipping pulse, sudden rapid heart rate, sudden slowing of the pulse during exercise, or pain or pressure in the chest, arms, or throat should *cool down and stop exercise immediately*. These conditions may or may not be dangerous, but they should be checked by a physician prior to resuming exercise.

Those who get dizzy or lightheaded, or feel sudden uncoordination or confusion, should *stop exercising immediately and lie down or put their head between their legs until the symptoms pass*. These symptoms should also be checked by a physician prior to resumption of exercise.

SELECTED REFERENCES

1. American College of Sports Medicine: *Guidelines for Graded Exercise Testing and Exercise Prescription*. Philadelphia: Lea & Febiger, 1975.
2. Barnard, A. J., et al.: Cardiovascular response to sudden strenuous exercise on heart rate, blood pressure and ECG. *J. Appl. Physiol.*, 34:833, 1973.
3. Fisher, A. G.: *Your Heart Rate—Key to Real Fitness*. Provo: Brigham Young University Press, 1976.
4. Fox, S. M., Naughton, J. P., and Haskell, W. L.: Physical activity and the prevention of coronary heart disease. *Ann. Clin. Res.*, 3:404–432, 1971.
5. Hellerstein, H. K., et al.: Principles of exercise prescription. In *Exercise Testing and Exercise Training in Coronary Heart Disease*. J. P. Naughton and H. K. Hellerstein (Eds.). New York: Academic Press, 1973.
6. White, J. R.: EKG changes using carotid artery for heart rate monitoring. *Med. Sci. Sports*, 9:88–94, 1977.

PART III
FACTORS AFFECTING CONDITIONING AND PERFORMANCE

In addition to the traits that are basic to performance (discussed in Part II), there are numerous other influencing factors. Part III presents information to help the athlete and coach deal effectively with these other factors.

Chapter 14 deals with nutrition and the effects of the consumption of various substances. Chapter 15 describes important procedures relative to training and preparation for performance. Chapter 16 covers the influences of altitude and atmosphere and water pressure on performance. The psychological implications of both training and performance are covered in Chapter 17.

Nutrition, Ergogenic Aids, and Training Malpractices

Nutrition, ergogenic aids, and training malpractices are elements in the preparation for performance which deserve special attention. Coaches and athletes need to know how to deal effectively with these influencing factors.

NUTRITION

Competitive athletes constantly seek methods of improving their conditioning and performance. As a result, many athletes seem to be influenced easily by the success of others whose training regimes may have included special dietary substances. But it is a fact that the nutritional requirements of the athlete are not much different from those of anyone else. There is no scientific evidence that athletic performance can be improved by modifying a basically sound and nutritious diet. Conversely, an athlete's state of conditioning can be affected negatively if his diet is less than optimal. Thus, a sound diet is important in athletic conditioning and competition.

There is such great variety of nutritious foods that many different combinations can result in a sound diet, but the best diet for one athlete may not be the best for another. Individual differences exist in persons' tastes as well as in their enzyme systems, which are so necessary for digestion and absorption of foods. Thus, "one man's meat may be another man's poison."

In a brief statement, the best that can be said about the diet of athletes is that it should be well balanced and nutritious, sufficient in quantity to maintain normal body weight, and composed of foods that are satisfying and not disrupting. Such a diet need not be supplemented with "fad foods," and it is doubtful whether food supplements such as vitamins, wheat germ, and so forth are of additional value. On the other hand, if the diet is not sound in content, then properly selected food supplements may be beneficial.

Quantity of Food

The total daily energy requirement for an active athlete may range from 3000 to 7000 cal, depending upon his size, condition, and the amount of work he performs. As the athlete works harder in his training, he consumes more calories and must have a proportionate increase in food. He must consume enough food to meet his energy demands and maintain his desired body weight. If he eats less than this amount, he will burn body tissues to make up the deficit, and approach "staleness" more readily. If he consumes more food than he needs, he will add fatty tissue, with its accompanying mechanical and endurance disadvantages. The best indicator of whether an athlete is consuming the correct amount of food is his body fat. He should be near normal weight for his body build, not too fat and not too lean. However, the degree of thinness that is desirable relates to the athletic event. For example, wrestlers and distance runners must be relatively fat-free, whereas football and baseball players normally can carry more fatty tissue without detrimental effects.

Proportion of Different Foods

There has been much debate over the correct proportion of *carbohydrates, fats,* and *protein* the athlete's diet should contain. It is known that the human body prefers to burn carbohydrates for energy during muscular activity, although it is also capable of utilizing fats or protein.

One liter of oxygen yields 5 Kcal when carbohydrates are used and 4.7 Kcal when fats are utilized. Because the burning of carbohydrates yields more kilocalories/liter of oxygen, it has been concluded that a person might be as much as 10% more efficient on a high-carbohydrate diet than on a high-fat diet. Studies show that endurance diminishes on a high-fat diet as compared to a high-carbohydrate diet. Astrand indicates that endurance activities require well-stocked glycogen reserves, which result from a high-carbohydrate diet.[3] He found that after a normal mixed diet and with an initial glycogen content of 1.75 gm/100 gm of muscle, a workload of 75% of maximal oxygen uptake could be tolerated for 114 min (nine subjects). After 3 days of a diet consisting entirely of fat and protein, the glycogen concentration fell to

0.63 gm/100 gm of muscle. The standard work load could be maintained only for 57 min. After 3 days of carbohydrate-rich diet, the glycogen content was higher: 3.51 gm/100 gm of muscle, and the time on the same level of work (75% load) could be continued for 167 min. What the subject could do for less than an hour on a fat and protein diet, he could do for over 2½ hours when an abundance of carbohydrate was included in the diet for 3 days.

Even though carbohydrates produce energy more efficiently than fats, the exclusion of fats from the diet is not recommended. Aside from the important vitamins and essential fatty acids in fats, there appears to be a fat-contained factor that is necessary for the normal metabolism of carbohydrates. Fat has a high-energy value, even though the burning of it requires more oxygen. The prime value of fat is that it contains fat-soluble vitamins A, D, E, and K, and the essential fatty acids which cannot be synthesized by the body. Provided these dietary requirements are met, fat in itself is not an essential food. There is accumulating evidence that too much fat contributes to the formation of high levels of cholesterol, a factor in arteriosclerosis.

Protein is needed mainly for building new body tissue. Only under conditions of starvation, when the carbohydrate and fat stores have been depleted, is the protein of body tissue consumed for energy. The protein molecule is made up of long chains of amino acids. These acids, sometimes known as "tissue-building stones," are absorbed from the intestines and sent throughout the body, where their important functions of repair and formation of tissues are initiated. During athletic training there is an increase of muscle tissue; thus, additional protein is required for the formation of new capillaries, connective tissue, and sarcoplasm.

Pizzo tested college swimmers during morning practice sessions under three conditions: (1) with no breakfast or nutrition for a 12-hour period, (2) with a regular breakfast, and (3) with a fluid diet supplement high in simple sugars.[23] Toward the end of the experiment, significantly higher nitrogen levels were discovered in the urine of those swimmers having had no nutrition before practice. This indicates a higher metabolism of protein, and means that possibly the muscles were using body protein for fuel.

Morehouse and Miller made the following generalizations relative to the proportions of foodstuff:[19] (1) a diet of 700 gm of carbohydrates, 150 gm of fats, and 100 gm of protein, plus adequate minerals and vitamins daily for long-duration events; and (2) 350 to 411 gm of carbohydrates, 100 to 300 gm of fats, and 210 gm of protein, mostly meat, for athletes in speed and power events.

When the available information is transposed into percentages, it appears that the athlete's typical diet should consist of about 65%

carbohydrates, 20% fats, and 15% protein. If one of the training objectives is to increase strength and muscle mass, the percentage of protein should be increased to as much as 20%, with a proportional decrease in fats.

Principal Sources of Carbohydrates, Fats, and Protein

No ordinary food is all carbohydrate, fat, or protein, but many foods are predominantly of one type. The following are some principal sources of the three food types:

Carbohydrates
Grain and cereal products—breads, cornbread, grain cereals
Vegetables—corn, potatoes, beans, rice
Fruits—bananas, grape juice
Sugars—honey, candies, jams and jellies
Pastries—pies and cakes

Fats
Certain meats—pork, mutton, goose, bacon (influenced by the fatness of the meat)
Certain fish—salmon
Nuts—pecans, almonds, peanuts
Cooking fats—animal fats and vegetable oils
Margarine, butter, lard
Mayonnaise, salad dressing
Whole milk

Proteins
Meat—beef (pot roast, steak, tongue), lamb chops
Fish—tuna, white, sword, smoked, cod, blue, cat, trout
Fowl—chicken, turkey
Milk—skim, powdered
Cheese
Eggs
Soybeans
Dried yeast

Quality of Protein

The quality of the protein is as important as the quantity. All protein food breaks down to form amino acids, and these acids form the building blocks for synthesis which results in the proteins found in body tissue. Of the 23 amino acids normally present in animal protein, only 13 can be synthesized in the cells. The other 10 must be supplied in the diet, and they are called the *essential amino acids*. Supplying these acids is no problem for those who eat meat, fish, and other animal products. Regular consumption of "complete protein foods" such as milk, eggs, fish, and meat solves this problem quite easily. For those who do not eat animal products, the problem is more complicated.

Reports stating that vegetarians have greater endurance than meat eaters should be discounted, because there is no scientific evidence to support the idea that vegetarians are superior in any respect. Indications are that unless vegetarians eat a well-rounded diet of a variety of foods they are likely to suffer from some aspect of malnutrition. However, vegetarians can get along satisfactorily if they use a variety of vegetables and fruits to assure an adequate supply of the *essential amino acids*.

Carbohydrates and Short-term Activity

Many athletes depend upon a high-carbohydrate diet and sugar supplements for quick energy. However, research indicates that unusually high-carbohydrate diets are of great value only to athletes who compete in long-term endurance events. Most sports require short bursts of activity and intermittent rest periods, and for participants in these sports unusually high-carbohydrate diets offer only limited physiological benefit.

Carbohydrates are stored in the form of glycogen in the liver and muscles where they present a readily available source of energy for muscular work. However, the practice of using sugar and other concentrated carbohydrates as pre-event supplements for quick energy generally has not been substantiated in the literature for athletes involved in performances of short duration. Fowler pointed to several research studies that showed no effect on performance from the ingestion of sugar as a pre-exercise supplement.[13] Bergstrom and Hultman found that in a well-trained athlete the size of the glycogen store is not a limiting factor in *short duration*, high-intensity exercise, provided the store is not subnormal at the beginning of exercise.[5] In fact, excessive quantities of sugar ingested just prior to competition may be detrimental to performance, because sugars tend to draw fluid into the gastrointestinal tract from other parts of the body and possibly hasten dehydration.[10]

Carbohydrates and Long-term Activity

According to Astrand, an athlete on a normal diet has only enough glycogen to perform heavy exercise for about 90 min before exhausting his glycogen store.[3] This finding has been substantiated by others, namely, Bogert and associates,[6] Bergstrom and Hultman,[5] and Darden.[11] Thus, in events such as marathon running, long-distance cross-country skiing, walking, cycling, and swimming, *loading* the diet with carbohydrates seems important.

Because of the discovery that endurance is related directly to the amount of glycogen stores in the muscles and liver, interest has been generated to determine whether such stores can be increased through dietary alterations. It was observed that in long-term physical activity, the practice of increasing carbohydrates in the diet several days before the event significantly enhanced the ability of the performers to sustain high-intensity exercise. However, such a diet is only effective when it is combined with other procedures. *First*, the athlete must exercise to exhaustion approximately 1 week prior to the event in order to deplete the muscle glycogen stores. *Then* the athlete must continue to keep the muscle glycogen content low by consuming a low-carbohydrate diet for 3 days. *Thereafter*, the athlete must shift to a high-carbohydrate diet until the time of competition.[16] As a result of this regime, the glycogen concentration in the muscles is increased two to three times that of normal. This procedure has been labeled *glycogen overshoot* or *carbohydrate loading*.

Slovic attempted to determine the efficiency of this diet among marathon runners, and found that the diet made little or no difference in the runners' performances during the first half of the run (60 to 75 min), but marked improvement during the last half and especially over the last quarter of the run was noted among those who were *carbohydrate loaded* as compared to those who were not.[26]

Carbohydrate loading has already become quite popular among marathon runners. For example, it was found that in the 1976 Trails End Marathon in Oregon, over 50% of those who finished in 3 hours or less had followed this diet. The practice of carbohydrate loading will undoubtedly spread to participants in other long-duration endurance events, and it will become the topic of additional research in the future.

One of the major dangers with carbohydrate overloading is possible overconfidence in its potential. It is important to emphasize that the diet has been found effective only for participants in certain athletic events, namely, those involving continuous exercise for an hour or more. It has not established that beneficial results can be expected in athletes in such sports as football, basketball, or track events in which the bouts of continuous exercise are of relatively short duration.

Even when this dietary procedure is used by long-term endurance athletes, it may not be entirely satisfactory. Some athletes find that training during the diet period is unpleasant, and it also has been suggested that the indiscriminate use of the technique may deprive the body of essential nutrients found in other kinds of foods. Further, a weight gain is a usual occurrence, since with the increase of glycogen, water is drawn into the muscles. When glycogen stores are filled to maximum, the amount of water in the tissues can result in feelings of heaviness or stiffness.

Nelson expressed a special concern about the retention of increased fluid caused by the diet, when he noted that the cardiac muscle is not exempt from excess glycogen and increased water deposits.[20] Olsson and Saltin observed that athletes seem to build a tolerance to the diet, and it loses some of its effectiveness if it is used too frequently and without adequate intervals between administrations.[22] Other limitations and potential side effects of carbohydrate loading have not yet been studied thoroughly. It will take a few more years of experimentation and experience to learn all that we need to know about its effectiveness and the side effects which accompany it.

Effects of Fasting

The American Medical Association is opposed to "crash diets" for athletes. Its opposition is based on the idea that repeated periods of starvation and/or dehydration produce essentially the same pathological conditions that natural famine and voluntary sustained food restrictions have produced. On the other hand, many wrestling and boxing coaches believe that rapid weight reductions of as much as 7% of the body's weight are harmless and may actually aid performance. The two positions are not as incompatible as they might seem. The medical opinion relates to general health, and the coaches' opinion to immediate effects upon performance.

Small weight losses (5% of initial weight) from starvation do not cause appreciable changes in performance. On the other hand, from medical research, it must be concluded that submitting to several days of dehydration and/or acute starvation in order to "make weight" is inadvisable, especially for young persons who are not physically mature.

An underfed person cannot sustain hard work as long as a well-fed one, because a substandard diet causes a reduction in the performance of the physiological systems, especially those systems that deliver oxygen and remove metabolic wastes. Another argument against excessive starving is the fact that as the demand for energy exceeds the supply, body tissue is consumed (use of body tissue protein). The depletion of body tissue impairs the functions of the organs of which the tissue is a part. Furthermore, physical efficiency is lower when body tissue rather than stored energy is used as fuel.

It has been shown that after repetitive periods of fasting, individuals can tolerate fasting better. The blood sugar level remains higher, and motor speed and coordination deteriorate less readily. But the body never truly adjusts to long periods of fasting. Often associated with this practice is voluntary dehydration and salt deprivation. In turn, the resulting dehydration leads to impairment of circulatory functions. The result is diminished physiological efficiency and reduced ability for enduring vigorous athletic performance. This tends to offset any advantage gained in competing in a lower body weight classification. Continuation of the "starvation" process over an entire season by a youthful competitor could affect his normal growth.

Some Facts and Fallacies about Diets

1. *Does honey consumed in large quantities prior to competition produce any special benefits?*

   Honey contains two sugars—glucose and fructose. These are the same main forms of sugar contained in table sugar. Both honey and table sugar are digested quickly, making their glucose readily available to the body. However, honey is not significantly superior to other sweets, even though its heavy promotors have successfully sold the idea that it is. When taken in *excessive* quantities, honey, glucose, dextrose, sugar cubes, or similar sweets can be mildly detrimental, because they tend to draw fluids from other body parts into the gastrointestinal tract. This fluid drain may increase the possibility of dehydration during endurance events when sweat loss is excessive. A few persons react unfavorably to excessive intake of sugars, and they develop stomach cramps, nausea, and diarrhea.

   There is no reason not to consume a moderate amount of honey or other sugar-containing products prior to competition or at intervals during long sessions of competition, but it should not be assumed that honey possesses miraculous properties for athletic performance, and possible detrimental effects should be watched for closely.

2. *Should athletes restrict their intake of fats, fried foods, and oily dressing?*

   Most fats, whether in the form of butter, margarine, salad dressings, shortenings, or the natural fats contained in meat or other natural sources, are digested at about the same slow rate. Upon entering the intestinal tract, fats cause release of the hormone enterogastrone which retards the stomach's emptying. Thus, when emptying time is important, as it is following the pre-contest meal, the athlete's fat intake should be limited. On the other hand, it is important to recognize that the body requires a certain amount of fat in order to function properly. Fats carry the fat-soluble vitamins A, E, D, and K, as well as the fatty acid linoleic, which is an essential nutrient. Fats provide calories in concentrated form and give food more taste.

   The athlete's diet should contain a normal amount of fat but not so much that it causes overweight or replaces the essential amount of carbohydrate or protein. Only small amounts of fat should be consumed during the day of competition

3. *Which kind of nutrients does the body prefer for energy?*

It has already been stated that the body prefers carbohydrates for the production of energy, because carbohydrates can be converted to energy more efficiently than fats or protein. The more strenuous the exercise in relation to the capacity of the involved muscles, the greater is the relative energy yield from carbohydrates. A high-carbohydrate diet shifts the metabolism toward a high-energy release level, and improves the capacity for prolonged heavy work.

4. *Is the ingestion of large amounts of protein essential to an athlete who is involved in vigorous training?*

Some coaches and athletes believe that vigorous activity produces extra wear on the muscles, and thereby increases the need for protein, and this idea has been promoted heavily by distributors of protein supplements. A leading manufacturer of protein recently reported a monthly production of over 1,000,000 protein pills. There has been substantial research done on this topic over a long period, and the research indicates no scientific evidence for the popular theory that athletes engaging in strenuous activity require *massive* amounts of protein-rich foods. The National Research Council on Nutrition has stated that 1 gm/day of protein per 2.2 lb of body weight is sufficient for both athletes and nonathletes. For body builders or weight lifters who want to gain muscle mass rapidly, a small amount of additional protein per day might be helpful. However, any amount beyond an additional 15 to 20 gm/day would result in unproductive overloading of the system with protein.

In studies on rats, evidence has been obtained that extensive amounts of protein supplements may produce tissue damage by causing the various organs to overwork and hypertrophy. In order to metabolize and excrete the large increases in amino acids, the liver and kidneys of the rats became enlarged. Even though it cannot be concluded that the same condition would result in humans, we must accept it as a real possibility. The fact is that a well-balanced diet will provide most persons, including most athletes, the amount of protein they need, and only a small amount of protein supplement will suffice for those who are on special muscle-building programs.

5. *Is there truth to the claim that certain foods offer a psychological advantage?*

Almost any aspect of training, including which side of the bed the competitor gets up on, might produce a psychological benefit. Whenever an athlete approaching maximal performance sincerely believes a certain substance or procedure will

provide a special benefit, then possibly it will. Most procedures
that an athlete believes in strongly are important to his psychological readiness.

6. *Does milk in the diet adversely affect athletic performance?*

   Research done on this topic during the last decade shows that
   milk neither is hard to digest nor contains a large amount of fat.
   If it were acid forming as some have claimed, doctors would not
   recommend it to patients with stomach ulcers. The fact is that
   milk has no ingredients that are harmful in the diet of athletes,
   including a moderate amount of milk in the precompetition
   meal. However, milk should not be overemphasized to the
   extent that it contributes to dietary imbalance.

7. *Does cooking or freezing destroy some of the nutritional value
   of vegetables and fruits?*

   Some nutritionists claim that quick-frozen fruits and vegetables have more nutritional value than fresh foods, because they
   are generally processed immediately after picking and before
   oxidation and dehydration can adversely affect the nutrients.
   There are variables of time here that can easily influence the
   answer, so it is not possible to make a clear conclusion that
   frozen fruits and vegetables are either more or less nutritional
   than unfrozen ones.

   Cooking affects the nutritional value of different foods in
   different ways. For example, the vitamin C in tomatoes is water
   soluble and heat labile. Cooking washes out and destroys some
   of it. A raw tomato has considerable more vitamin C than a
   cooked one. Conversely, vitamin A is fat soluble and locked into
   the vegetables' cell walls. These walls are broken down more
   easily by cooking than by chewing. A cup of diced carrots
   properly cooked provides more than three times the amount of
   usable vitamin A than a cup of raw carrots does.

   Much of the vitamin content of canned vegetables passes into
   the cooking liquid, which is often drained and discarded rather
   than consumed. To conserve the vitamins, canned vegetables
   should be heated in a small amount of the liquid that comes
   from the can, and the rest of the juice should be used in a soup
   or stew. However, aside from a few exceptions, it is true that
   vegetables and fruits contain more nutrients when raw than
   when cooked, and a diet ought to include a variety of fresh
   fruits and vegetables.

8. *Are there certain fad foods that produce special benefits for
   athletes preparing for competition?*

   Some fad foods, such as sunflower seeds, kelp, raw meat,
   blackstrap molasses, and other such substances, are sometimes
   claimed to have miraculous properties for improving perfor-

mance. Typically, when these foods are tested scientifically, it turns out that the consumer performs well in spite of and not because of the particular food. In rare cases when a person is sincerely dedicated to the value of the food, a psychological effect may be present. But, aside from possible psychological effects, there is no evidence that such foods have special value.

Diet Guidelines

Fifty or more nutrients work together in the body, and all are important. From these nutrients the body synthesizes about 10,000 different compounds. A lack of any one kind of nutrient might result in the underproduction of dozens of essential compounds. Similarly, the addition of large amounts of any one or two nutrients might have an upsetting effect. Thus, the athlete should subscribe to a well-balanced diet composed of a wide variety of wholesome and nutritious foods. *Well-balanced* infers a daily diet of two or more servings from the meat or meat equivalent (animal products) groups, 2 cups of milk for adults and 4 for teenagers, four servings from the bread/cereals group, and four or more servings of fruits and vegetables (Fig. 14–1).

The hardworking athlete will naturally need to consume more calories than the nonathlete, but these should be balanced calories from all of the four basic food groups. Exceptions can be made with respect to *carbohydrate loading* for long-endurance events. In short, the kinds of foods in the athlete's diet should not differ markedly from those in the diet of any other healthy individual.

Here are some summary guidelines that would be valuable for anybody, but are especially useful to athletes preparing for competition.

1. Foods ingested prior to competition should be easy to digest and contribute to raising the level of stored glycogen. The best foods to accomplish this are complex (nonrefined) carbohydrates. (There is a section in the next chapter about the precompetition meal.)

2. Foods in their natural state should be emphasized, and refined and processed foods should be avoided. In spite of all the claims made by those involved in profit making, there is still no reliable evidence that processed and refined foods are as useful and safe for consumption as are natural foods.

3. Most foods contain more nutritional value when raw than when cooked. For health reasons, certain foods must be cooked, but it is always an advantage to emphasize natural grains and raw fruits and vegetables in the diet.

4. Selection of a wide variety of wholesome foods from the four basic food categories will assure a balanced diet (Fig. 14–1).

5. Overeating and undereating should be avoided. The tendency

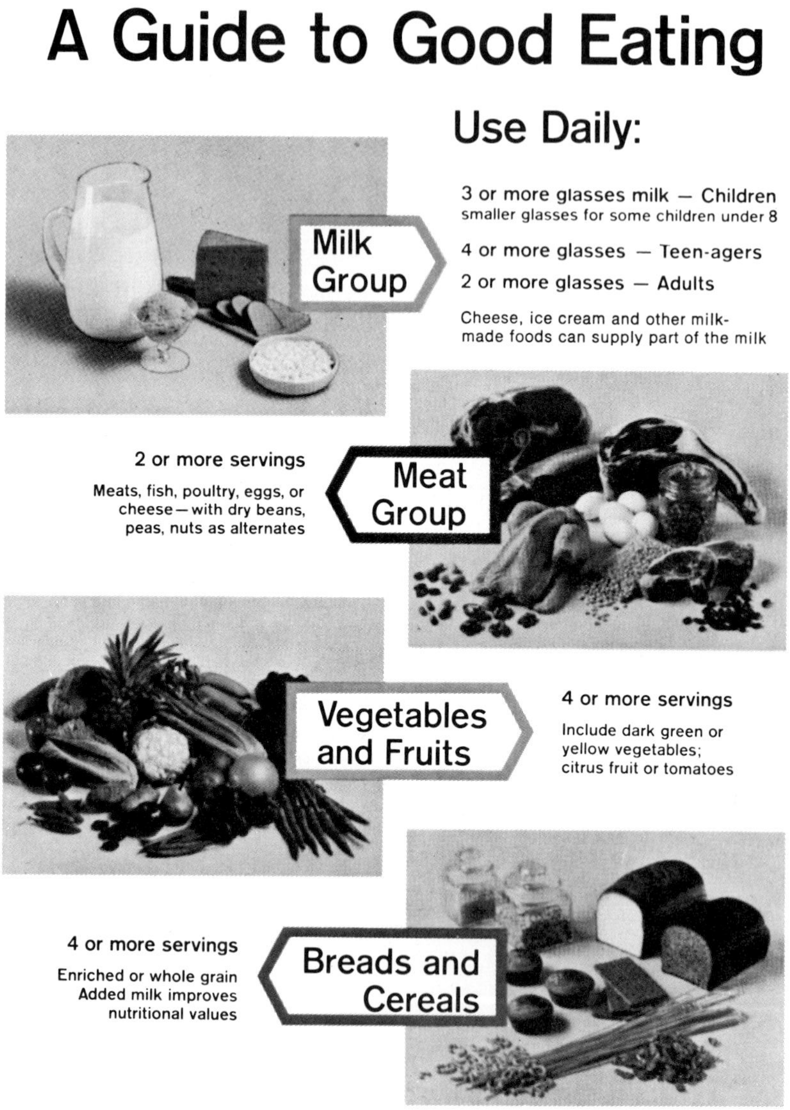

A Guide to Good Eating

Use Daily:

Milk Group

3 or more glasses milk — Children
smaller glasses for some children under 8

4 or more glasses — Teen-agers

2 or more glasses — Adults

Cheese, ice cream and other milk-made foods can supply part of the milk

Meat Group

2 or more servings

Meats, fish, poultry, eggs, or cheese — with dry beans, peas, nuts as alternates

Vegetables and Fruits

4 or more servings

Include dark green or yellow vegetables; citrus fruit or tomatoes

Breads and Cereals

4 or more servings

Enriched or whole grain
Added milk improves nutritional values

Figure 14–1. Four basic food groups. (Courtesy of National Dairy Council.)

of most people in America, including some athletes, is to overeat. This places unnecessary stress on the digestive and elimination processes, and it often results in overweight.

6. The overuse of food supplements of any kind should be shunned. To some persons, certain food supplements can be valuable, but the need for supplements is highly individualized and related directly to the individual's diet. If an athlete is on a well-balanced diet, there is no justification for large doses of any food supplement unless prescribed by a physician for medical reasons.

7. Good sound judgment and common sense relative to diet should be demonstrated by every athlete and every coach. This will lead to a diet which incorporates these guide lines and which avoids dietary deficiencies, excesses, or extremes.

POTENTIAL ERGOGENIC AIDS

Many athletes contend that their success is due in part to consumption of certain substances which might be termed *ergogenic aids*. Fortunately, numerous useful research studies have been reported on this topic. However, some of them must be interpreted with caution, because much of the research has been done either by or under the auspices of companies that market the products in question.

Vitamins

At one time it was believed that the requirements for vitamins increased more rapidly than the increase in metabolism caused by increased exercise, but recent research shows that vitamin needs increase in about the same proportion as does metabolism. This would suggest that ingestion of larger amounts of food as daily work levels increase automatically provides the needed increases in vitamins.

Van Huss recorded favorable results in the recovery rate of laboratory animals which had received vitamin C before exercising, compared with those animals that received no supplements.[27] Counsilman stated that "all research seems to indicate an increasing need for vitamin C during the stress of a training program."[8] He further pointed out that vitamin C cannot be stored in the body, and moderate excesses are harmless and will be excreted.

Conversely, it has been found that excessive vitamin C supplementation contributes to destruction of natural vitamin C sources in the body, and this can contribute to malnutrition after the supplementation is discontinued. Rhead and Schrauzer found that the vitamin C level in blood of persons who consumed 5 gm of vitamin C per day were no different from the levels in blood of those who ate a similar diet but took no vitamin C.[24] This suggests that the increased rate of destruction of natural vitamin C produced by the supplementation counteracted the effect of the supplementation itself. Further, Herbert and Jacob found that excessive doses of vitamin C taken with food destroys vitamin B_{12}.

Information from the American Medical Association's Division of Foods and Nutrition indicates that a balanced diet is still the best method of obtaining adequate vitamins. Vitamins should be obtained from their natural sources rather than from purified synthetic sources. Too much long-term vitamin supplementation can eventually create an unnatural adaptation—dependence on vitamins from unnatural sources. An athlete on a well-rounded diet probably needs no vitamin supplements. But if the diet is not sound then supplementary vitamins might be beneficial to both athletes and nonathletes.

Other Food Supplements

MINERALS. Like vitamins, there is no scientific evidence that the need for minerals is increased any more than the need for food in general as a result of increased exercise. An adequate supply of minerals apparently is present in a well-balanced diet, but if the diet is not well balanced, then mineral supplements might prove beneficial.

WHEAT GERM. Wheat germ is a rather complete food composed of a large number of nutrients. For this reason, some persons have reasoned that regular consumption of wheat germ will assist in overcoming deficiencies in the diet. This reasoning is based on the assumption that the diet does have some deficiencies. Cureton states; "Studies at the University of Illinois Physical Fitness Research Laboratory indicate that wheat germ, or its derivative wheat germ oil, aids those who consume it under proper conditions over a long period of time to enable the body to build up its glycogen (muscle fuel) reserve."[9] There is some indication that wheat germ contributes to low cholesterol levels, and low cholesterol has been associated with superior physical fitness. There is no evidence that harmful effects will result from consuming a reasonable amount of wheat germ on a regular basis.

GLYCINE. There has been some interest among athletes in the use of glycine (aminoacetic acid) to increase muscular power and endurance. Gelatin, which averages about 25% glycine, has been widely sold for this purpose. The basic idea behind this has been to promote endogenous creatine formation, presumably to enhance the supply of phosphocreatine in the muscles. This idea is not substantiated by research results. However, there is no evidence that the consumption of a reasonable amount of glycine is harmful in the training diet.

ALKALIZERS. During high levels of work, the body depends heavily upon anaerobic processes to provide energy for muscular contraction. The by-product from these processes, lactic acid, must be buffered by the blood to prevent a severe decrease in blood pH. This buffering action depends mainly upon the blood alkaline reserve. Early researchers found that the blood pH could be raised (become more alkaline) by the ingestion of alkaline salts. They theorized that if the blood was more alkaline before work, more lactic acid would be required to cause the pH to decrease to an intolerable level. Researchers have found evidence that would tend to support this theory. However, the theory seems to apply only to moderately trained subjects. Highly trained runners are not improved by the ingestion of these salts.

Oxygen Inhalation

Oxygen inhalation has proved to be of little value in athletes, whether oxygen is administered before, during, or after performance. Experiments show that oxygen breathed *before* a contest has little effect, because oxygen cannot be stored successfully by the body. Any increase in oxygen saturation in the blood or lungs is quickly diluted by atmospheric air when the athlete begins his performance. Oxygen breathed *after* the contest does not seem to speed up the elimination of anaerobic by-products, so is of little value. Increasing the supply of oxygen *during* work does increase the maximal oxygen uptake and reduces pulmonary ventilation, so it would be of some help for activities requiring a high-energy yield. But oxygen equipment is heavy and awkward and could not be used during performance, even if the procedure were acceptable.

Anabolic Steroids

The use of anabolic steroids by athletes attempting to develop high strength levels has become quite common. Anabolic steroids have been used clinically for some time for treatment of osteoporosis, fracture healing, burns, protein tissue building, myotrophy, muscular dystrophy, and so forth, because they increase nitrogen retention in the form of protein synthesis, and because they decrease the rate of catabolism of amino acids. Because of their effects on clinical patients, it would seem that steroids should stimulate muscle growth and strength increases in normal subjects.

The changes in muscle strength, body weight, and lean body mass of athletes who have used anabolic steroids are probably greater than many would hope and less than others would think, and there is apparently a wide range of individual responses to these drugs. Lamb did a careful review of the research on this topic, and found that there was about an equal number of studies which furnished evidence in favor and not in favor of administration of anabolic steroids as an aid to increasing strength.[18] He found that the differences in the research results related to several associated factors, such as the psychological conditioning of the subjects, the level of protein in the diet, the level of dosage, the duration of the experiment, and individual reactions to the drug. Even though some of the studies did not furnish evidence in favor of anabolic steroids for building of strength, none reported negative results.

Johnson and O'Shea found that strength, body weight, oxygen uptake, and blood nitrogen retention were significantly increased in healthy subjects who were administered anabolic steroids in connection with strength training.[17] Fowler reported no effects of steroids on strength.[14] Casner reported no significant increases in strength from the steroid treatment.[7] Ariel and Saville noted psychological enhancement of performance by those who took steroids in connection with their training. In another study, Ariel found that steroids combined with strength training produced favorable effects on the development of strength.[1]

When all of the objective evidence is considered, along with the mass of testimonial evidence, it would appear that steroids administered for 3 to 6 weeks often contribute to extra gains in strength, body weight, and lean body mass, if the recipients participate simultaneously in a program of intensive strength training. Some strength specialists advocate a protein-rich diet along with the training. Why the strength training and high-protein diet are necessary for effectiveness has not been answered satisfactorily.

The potential detrimental effects of steroids have long been a legitimate concern. Possible sterilization and retardation of long bone growth have been the most prevalently suggested side effects. Fortunately, the newer synthetic steroids seem to be less dangerous in terms of potential side effects, but this should not cause one to conclude that prolonged use of high dosages will not be detrimental. It is hard to believe that such powerful drugs will not have damaging effects with long-term or indiscriminate use. Therefore, until proof is given that such effects will not occur, there seems to be no good argument for regularizing the use of anabolic steroids in athletic training. Steroids should be used only for special reasons and then under the supervision of a qualified physician.

Blood Doping

In essence, blood doping means the infusion of blood, either whole blood or packed red blood cells, into an athlete before competition. The athlete's own blood, which was withdrawn several weeks before the injection, may be used. His body will regenerate new blood cells to restore normal hemoglobin levels after withdrawal of the blood.

The theory underlying blood doping is based on a possible increase in the blood's oxygen-carrying capacity. DeVries states that of the three main factors governing maximal oxygen uptake (external respiration, gas transportation, and tissue respiration), the available evidence suggests that gas transportation by the blood stream is the main limiting factor.[12] Shepherd indicates that maximal oxygen uptake is normally limited by physiological rather than by biochemical processes, and he thinks that overall conduction of oxygen can be augmented by an increase in blood hemoglobin or increased cardiac output, or both.[25]

Even though blood doping seems logical, research does not clearly support the technique as being valuable in athletic performance. Woods studied the effects of blood reinfusion (blood doping) in 16 university men.[29] With concealed methods, a pint of blood was drawn from half the subjects and then reinjected 17 days later to increase the concentration of red blood cells. Work capacity was measured by treadmill tests, and it was found that the blood reinfusion did not contribute to increased work capacity.

Of the several other studies that have been done on this topic, the results are conflicting. Unfortunately, most of the studies have involved submaximal work by the subjects, and this really does not prove much of anything. Of the studies involving maximal work, the results have been inconsistent. Therefore, it must be concluded that at this time sufficient research evidence does not exist to support the claim that blood doping will increase either work efficiency or maximal work capacity. It is a topic that will undoubtedly receive additional attention from researchers during the next decade, and it will certainly be interesting to keep abreast of the new findings.

TRAINING MALPRACTICES

Frequently the difference between winning and losing in athletics is a half stride, a fraction of a second, or a near miss. Incorrect training practices can often cause this difference. Even champions who violate training often could do better if they were free of such malpractices. One of the most common malpractices is the use of alcohol.

Alcohol

Alcohol has long been on the athlete's taboo list, but strict enforcement is difficult because many "social drinkers" argue that moderate drinking is unlikely to affect general health or life span. The coach should resist such logic because drinking can have a direct negative effect upon performance, and from moderate drinking it is only a short glass to heavy or program drinking. Let us look at the use of alcohol as it relates to athletes. (1) Alcohol is not a stimulant, as some believe, but a narcotic which suppresses body functions. It provides a temporary sense of well-being, but in reality it serves as a depressant to both mind and body. (2) It increases fatigue by slowing the removal of lactic acid from the cells. (3) It seriously interferes with the functioning of the nervous system, slowing reaction time and reducing coordination. (4) It affects the cerebral portion of the brain which controls thoughts and actions, causing the person to be less coherent and less responsive than normal. (5) It interferes with both voluntary and involuntary reflexes. (6) Habitual use leads to poor eating patterns and eventual malnutrition. (7) It often is associated with loss of sleep and normal inhibitions, both of which are vital to athletes.

Strong alcoholic drinks are undoubtedly detrimental to both conditioning and performance. Since there are no points in favor of alcohol, athletes should refrain from its use, and coaches ought to enforce prohibition for their athletes and themselves.

Nicotine

According to the American Medical Association's Committee on Medical Aspects of Sports, an aspiring athlete should not smoke, or he should quit if he has already started. The AMA drew the following important conclusions: (1) Carbon monoxide from smoking may be absorbed in the blood, thereby temporarily reducing the blood's oxygen-carrying capacity. (2) Habitual smoking on an empty stomach can cause digestive disturbances and distress. (3) Continued smoking sometimes affects the nervous system, producing irritability. (4) Smoking over a period of time causes constriction of the blood vessels, thus contributing to reduced circulatory capacity. (5) Inhalation of smoke induces chronic coughing, renders the throat more susceptible to infections, and restricts the exchange of oxygen and carbon dioxide in the tiny air sacs of the lungs.

One of the immediate and temporary effects of nicotine is the constriction of blood vessels, which raises blood pressure and increases the heart rate. These conditions have negative effects on performance, particularly of the strenuous type. Smoking inhibits the flow of gastric juices and postpones the onset of hunger pains, thus interfering with normal nutritional patterns.

The relationship between cigarette smoking and lung cancer cannot be ignored. Statistics show that a heavy smoker is 42 times as likely to develop the disease as is a nonsmoker.

Since there is no evidence of positive effects from smoking, and since there is much evidence to the contrary, the wise coach will vigorously enforce a no smoking rule.

Narcotics

According to the common usage of the term, there are three classes of narcotics: opium and its derivatives, cocaine, and marijuana. There is strong support for the addition of alcohol to the list. Opium and its derivatives (morphine, heroin, and codeine) relieve pain and produce a false sense of well-being. They suppress the central nervous system and induce sleep. (They may cause temporary excitement of the nervous system but this soon wears off.) A large dose of these drugs will suppress the respiratory function and may cause death. Heroin, the most commonly used of the opium drugs, is an illegal product having no medical uses. Seventy-five percent of all confirmed addicts use heroin.

Cocaine is a powerful, quick-acting drug capable of producing strong addiction. Unlike most narcotics which act as depressants, a moderate dose of cocaine stimulates the central nervous system, accelerating respiratory and circulatory rates. When taken in excess, cocaine can produce psychotic symptoms of peculiar sensations of creatures crawling on the skin, commonly referred to as "cocaine bugs."

Marijuana is a relatively mild intoxicating drug to which some persons become psychologically addicted. Records show that its use leads to the use of the more harmful drugs. This alone is sufficient reason to require avoidance of the use of this drug.

After careful evaluation of the evidence, it must be concluded that there are no arguments in favor of athletes using narcotics, and there are strong arguments against their use by persons in general and especially in athletes.

Caffeine

Caffeine is the alkaloid consumed daily by millions of individuals in coffee, tea, and cola. It is a mild stimulant, and moderate intakes of caffeinated beverages are apparently harmless. But it should be kept in mind that caffeine is a toxic drug. If even a small amount is injected into the blood stream, it can prove fatal. When injected into a muscle, it causes temporary paralysis, and when injected directly into the brain, a single drop can cause severe convulsions. Fortunately, since the caffeine in drinks is diffused into the blood stream and then to the kidneys for excretion, these severe toxic effects never occur.

Caffeine mostly affects the blood vessels, heart, and nervous system. A mild dose may cause general vasoconstriction with simultaneous dilation of the coronary artery, increase the contractile force of the heart, and increase the heart rate. Mild doses also may cause an increase in metabolic rate, up to 25%, stimulate the central nervous system, and accelerate the respiratory rate. Small doses may act beneficially upon the psychic processes for a short time.

The research that has been done shows conflicting results about whether caffeinated drinks will increase work output and postpone the onset of fatigue. At this point, the answer to this question is nonconclusive. However, exercise physiologists and other conditioning experts generally agree that caffeinated beverages are not ergogenic aids. They also agree that moderate consumption of such beverages has no detrimental effects on conditioning and performance, provided it does not interfere with a well-balanced diet and adequate sleep.

Sedatives

Sedatives generally reduce nervous system activity, produce a state of relaxation, and depress the actions of the vital organs. They are basically sleep-producing drugs. The most commonly used of this group are *barbiturates*, of which there are at least 20 different drugs. Under proper medical supervision, the barbiturates serve a useful medical purpose. However, to use these drugs indiscriminately as an easy, quick method of reducing conscious activity of the brain is unwise. The danger in using barbiturates indiscriminately lies both in development of a dependency upon them and in the possibility of overdosage. There is no argument in favor of using sedatives in connection with athletes except under medical supervision.

Amphetamines

Amphetamines (trade names: Benzedrine, Dexedrine, Desamine, and Methedrine) produce effects similar to those caused by the activity of the sympathetic nervous system. In most persons, the immediate effect is an increase in alertness and faster reactions. Because of the stimulating effect of amphetamines, there has been some interest in determining whether athletic performance can be improved by their use. Medically speaking, the practice of using stimulating drugs for performance purposes is not recommended. However, no legal restrictions exist for the use of mildly stimulating drugs. The best evidence presently available indicates that amphetamines do not produce superior performance, but do tend to cause the participant to perceive that he is performing well.

SELECTED REFERENCES

1. Ariel, G. B.: The effects of anabolic steroids upon skeletal muscle contraction force. *J. Sports Med.*, 15:187–190, 1975.
2. Ariel, G. B., and Saville, G.: Anabolic steroids: Physiological effects of placebos. *Med. Sci. Sports*, 4:124–126, 1972.
3. Astrand, P.-O.: Something old and something new—very new. *Nutrition Today*, 4:9, 1968.
4. Astrand, P.-O. and Rodahl, K.: *Textbook of Work Physiology.* New York: McGraw-Hill Book Co., 1970.
5. Bergstrom, A. B., and Hultman, E.: Nutrition for maximal sports performance. *J.A.M.A.*, 221:999–1006, 1972.
6. Bogert, L. J., Bridges, G. M., and Calloway, D. H.: *Nutrition and Physical Fitness.* Philadelphia: W. B. Saunders Co., 1973.

7. Casner, S. W., Early, R. G., and Carlson, B. R.: Anabolic steroid effects on body composition in normal young men. *J. Sports Med.*, 11:98–103, 1971.
8. Counsilman, J.: *The Science of Swimming.* Englewood Cliffs, N.J.: Prentice-Hall, Inc., 1968.
9. Cureton, T. K.: What about the wheat germ? *Scholastic Coach*, 24:30, 1959.
10. Darden, E.: Nutrition and athletic performance. *Scholastic Coach*, 42:88, 1972.
11. Darden, E.: Olympic athletes view vitamins and victories. *J. Home Econ.*, 65:8–11, 1973.
12. DeVries, H. A.: *Physiology of Exercise for Physical Education and Athletics*, 2nd ed. Dubuque: Wm. C. Brown Co., 1974.
13. Fowler, W. M.: The facts about ergogenic aids and sports performance. *J. Health, Phys. Educ. Rec.*, 40:37–42, 1969.
14. Fowler, W. M., Jr., Gardner, G. W., and Egstrom, G. H.: Effect of an anabolic steroid on physical performance of young men. *J. Appl. Physiol.*, 20:1038–1040, 1965.
15. Herbert, V., and Jacob, E.: Destruction of vitamin B in ascorbic acid. *J.A.M.A.*, 230:241–242, 1974.
16. Hyman, M.: Glycogen stores and increased stamina. *The Athletic Coach*, 6:24–26, 1972.
17. Johnson, L. C., and O'Shea, J. P.: Anabolic steroid: Effects on strength development. *Science*, 164:957–959, 1969.
18. Lamb, D. R.: Androgens in exercise. *Med. Sci. Sports*, 8:1, 1975.
19. Morehouse, L. E., and Miller, A. T.: *Physiology of Exercise*, 7th ed. St. Louis: C. V. Mosby Co., 1976.
20. Nelson, R. A.: Exceptional Nutritional Needs of the Athlete. Paper presented at the 15th National Conference on the Medical Aspects of Sports. Anaheim, California, December 1, 1973.
21. Nelson, R. A.: What should athletes eat? Unmixing folly and facts. *The Physician in Sportsmedicine*, 3:67–72, 1975.
22. Olsson, K., and Saltin, B.: Diet and fluids in training and competition. *Scand. J. Rehabil. Med.*, 3:31–38, 1971.
23. Pizzo, A.: Unpublished research on the influence that different pre-workout breakfasts have on blood sugar levels of competitive swimmers. Bloomington, Ind.: Indiana University, 1961.
24. Rhead, W. J., and Schrauzer, G. N.: Risks of long-term ascorbic acid overdosage. *Nutr. Rev.*, 29:262–263, 1971.
25. Shepherd, R. L.: *Frontiers of Fitness*, Springfield, Ill., Charles C Thomas, 1971.
26. Slovic, P.: Eating away precious minutes. *Runners World*, 9:34–35, 1974.
27. Van Huss, W. D.: What made the Russians run? *Nutrition Today*, 1:20, 1966.
28. Williams, M. H.: Blood doping—does it really help athletes? *The Physician and Sportsmedicine*, 3:52–56, 1975.
29. Woods, M. C.: Effects of Blood Reinfusion on Work Capacity. Unpublished study, University of Utah, 1977.

Chapter 15

Procedures Related to Preparation and Performance

This chapter is composed of valuable information on such interesting topics as (1) the procedures that an athlete should follow prior to and after competition, (2) the effects of warm-up on performance and injury, (3) problems and procedures associated with making weight in certain athletic activities, (4) dangers of dehydration and heat injuries, (5) prevention and care of muscle soreness, and (6) off-season conditioning procedures.

COMPETITION PROCEDURES

The guidelines for precompetition procedures are rather simple and well substantiated.

1. The food eaten during the 24 hours prior to competition should be high in carbohydrates in order to build a good supply of glycogen. To help conserve the glycogen supply, extensive heavy work should be avoided during this period, and only moderate work is advised for as long as 48 hours prior to strenuous competition.

2. During the 24 hours before competition, large amounts of fatty foods and other slow-digesting foods should be avoided. Also to

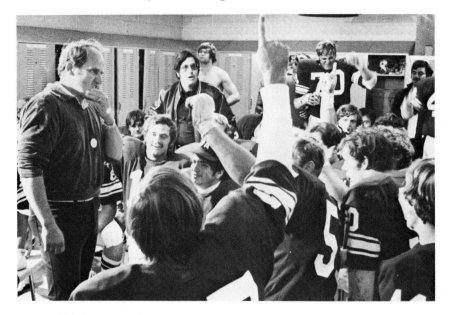

Figure 15–1. The coach is attempting to put the finishing touch on the team members' preparation for the game at a pregame meeting.

be avoided are heavily spiced foods and foods that tend to cause indigestion.

3. The training sessions during the 2 days prior to competition should emphasize strategy and the fine points of the skills involved in the performance, in order to "sharpen" the performer.

4. Slightly more than the normal amount of rest during the 48 hours before competition is recommended so the performer will feel fully rested and ready to compete. However, excessive rest or any other significant deviation from the normal living routine is not advised.

5. The competitor should occupy himself in pursuits that are interesting and relaxing, which tend to keep him from becoming too anxious about the upcoming competition. Emotional involvement over a period of several hours is fatiguing and should be avoided.

6. As much as possible, without violating basically sound practices, an athlete should do those things that cause him to feel that he is "ready" for the competition.

7. Deviations from these procedures will occur if the athlete participates in *"carbohydrate loading,"* a unique preparatory

procedure for long-duration endurance events described in the previous chapter.

Precompetition Meal

Concern over the precompetition meal has existed for many centuries. Records indicate that athletes of ancient times swallowed powdered lions' teeth to make themselves strong, and some ate lean meat both before and after competition, believing it would build muscle mass, and thereby help them perform better. Through the ages much confusion and many misconceptions have existed relative to premeet meals, and even today there is much disagreement about this matter.

There are two aspects to the precompetition meal: *physiological* and *psychological*. From the *physiological* standpoint, the content, quantity, and timing are all important factors. *Psychologically,* the performer must feel that the meal was "right" to prepare him for his best effort.

The content of the precompetition meal will influence the time it should be eaten. In turn, the timing of the meal will influence its content. The idea is to have the athlete well nourished with an abundance of carbohydrates in the diet, and yet have his stomach empty or near-empty when the performance begins. When vigorous exercise is performed while the stomach is full, the inspiratory descent of the diaphragm may be impaired. It is also conceivable that in some persons a full stomach may encroach upon the action of the heart during heavy exercise. The consequent restriction of blood flow through the heart would reduce endurance. Further, digestion requires the blood supply and the energy needed for the performance. Also, food that is still in the stomach has not been digested, and therefore it does not contribute to glycogen stores for use in performance.

The following guides should be helpful. Even when these guides are followed, adequate flexibility remains as to the exact content of the meal.

1. A substantial (but not large) meal should be eaten 3 to 4 hours before competition. A *small* amount of fast-digesting carbohydrates may be eaten without harm as close as 1 hour before competition.
2. The precompetition meal, and also the meal preceding it, should consist mostly of carbohydrates, with some protein and only a small amount of fats. *Carbohydrates* are easy to digest, and they replace the glycogen supply better than other foods, thus providing quick energy. *Protein* foods are digested reasonably fast and are valuable in performance, but their metabolism results in the production of acids, large quantities

of which cause undesirable acidosis, and sometimes cramps. The acid products of protein are excreted only in the urine. During heavy work, the functioning of the kidneys is greatly restricted, and this contributes to the accumulation of the acids. *Fats* are digested slowly and, therefore, retard gastric emptying. However, fats should not be totally omitted because they tend to satisfy hunger readily, and in long-duration performances they become increasingly valuable as a source of energy.

3. Irritating foods, such as roughage and highly spiced foods, should be avoided. Also, gas-forming foods such as cabbage, beans, apples and onions should not be eaten.

4. Liquids are essential in the precompetition meal, because the digestion, absorption, and assimilation of foods depend upon an adequate supply of liquid. Coffee and tea are often used because they tend to give the athlete a "pickup." But this lasts only a short while, and the effects often vanish before time for competition. Milk, which has been taboo on training tables in the past, is now considered acceptable in reasonable amounts in both the regular diet and in the precompetition meal. It is a valuable source of emulsified fats that are ready and available to the body, as well as a calcium source which acts as a catalyst in increasing the O_2 capacity of the blood. Recent research indicates that no harmful effects result from drinking a moderate amount of milk 3 to 4 hours prior to competition.

5. The precompetition meal that has traditionally been recommended is similar to the following: 8-ounce broiled steak with fat removed, baked potato, green vegetable (cooked), toast and honey, fresh fruit, and two to three glasses of fluid. This is not a bad precompetition meal. The main criticism is that it probably is too heavy in protein (meat) and too light in carbohydrates.

Macaraeg studied the relative effectiveness of a precompetition meal composed of a high-carbohydrate, high-protein, low-fat liquid meal as opposed to the usual steak dinner.[11] He found that with the liquid meal practically all nausea and abdominal cramps were eliminated and dryness of the mouth was less frequent. It was found that with the liquid meal the stomach was emptied after 2 hours and complete absorption of the food occurred within 4 hours. Blood sugar levels at 1, 2 and 3 hours after the liquid meal were all significantly higher than those after a steak meal. It was concluded that the liquid meal was preferred because it was quicker and easier to digest, and it increased the level of sugar stores in the blood. Other studies have been conducted which generally support these findings about digestion. However, evidence indicating whether athletes perform better after a liquid meal or a steak dinner has not been produced. Many coaches and athletes believe that the steak menu provides a psychological benefit that outweighs any possible physiological disadvantage.

During Competition

During long-duration competition, such as basketball and soccer, athletes should be permitted to drink moderate amounts of water periodically in order to help replenish body fluids lost through sweating and to contribute to comfort. Large amounts of water should be avoided because this causes a loaded feeling in the stomach. A few athletes choose to eat bits of candy or other quick-energy foods periodically during performance. Probably there is no harm in doing this; however, the value of it is certainly doubtful.

After Competition

After a long-duration performance, the athlete is usually thirsty and hungry. If profuse sweating has occurred, an immediate concern is the replenishment of body fluids. This is done best by consuming moderate amounts of water every 15 to 20 min until the feeling of thirst and dehydration is satisfied. The consumption of too much fluid at once will result in overfilling of the stomach and cause temporary discomfort. Consumption of large amounts of ice-cold fluids during or immediately after vigorous work is considered bad practice.

Following the performance, the athlete should eat a well-balanced meal of nutritious, satisfying foods. It should include protein to replenish the body's supply of building material. It should exclude (1) large amounts of slow-digesting foods such as fats, (2) foods that tend to cause digestive disturbances, and (3) foods that are unfamiliar to the individual. The meal should contain enough bulk to satisfy the feeling of hunger, but not so much as to cause discomfort from overfilling. Once the athlete has recovered from the immediate effects of the competition, an ample rest will prepare him for return to his usual living routine.

WARM-UP

The question is often asked, "How important is warm-up to performance and the prevention of injury, and if it is important, which kind of warm-up is best?" Several points of argument in favor of warm-up have been advocated by experts on athletic performance:

1. Warm-up increases the speed and force of muscle contraction.
2. Warm-up related to the particular activity improves the necessary coordination.
3. Warm-up helps to prevent injuries to muscles, tendons, and ligaments.

4. In endurance activities, warm-up brings on second wind more readily.

The research results on warm-up are conflicting. We found 11 reports that support the values of warm-up, and 7 reports showed no evidence that warm-up is effective. Much of the conflict seems to be based on the definition of warm-up. For example, is any form of exercise preliminary to performance called a warm-up, or must it be vigorous and extensive enough to cause increased body temperature? Not all of the research was based on a common definition; therefore, contradictory results would be expected.

Astrand and Rodahl claim warm-up to be beneficial because increased temperature resulting from warm-up allows for a higher metabolic process in the cells.[2] They claim that for each degree of increased temperature, the metabolic rate of the cells increases by about 13%. At higher temperatures, the exchange of oxygen from the blood to the tissue is more rapid. The nerve impulses also travel faster at high body temperature. Mellerowica and Hansen found that through the use of warm-up, damage to the locomotive system can be reduced.[13] They pointed out that the elasticity of the muscles is dependent upon their blood saturation, and cold muscles (below normal body temperature) have low blood saturation and tend to be more susceptible to tears and ruptures than warm muscles (higher than normal body temperature).

Martin and associates studied the effects of warm-up on metabolic responses in strenuous exercise, and found that:[12]

1. Warm-up contributes to greater oxygen consumption, and thereby reduces the performance dependence upon the anaerobic process.
2. Warm-up contributes to a lower content of lactic acid following strenuous exercise. Further, vigorous muscular exercise of the kind included in a true warm-up causes a shift in the pattern of blood flow, and one aspect of the shift is increased flow in the vascular beds of the working muscles and decreased flow in the skin and viscera. This would cause greater exchange of gases at the working tissues.

Barnard studied the effects of warm-up on heart function and found that healthy adult men who participated in strenuous activity without warm-up had abnormal changes on electrocardiograms immediately after the exercise.[3] When 2 min or more of steady jogging preceded the vigorous exercise, changes on electrocardiograms were either eliminated or significantly reduced. He also found that when strenuous activity was performed without warm-up, arterial blood pressure increased abnormally. This greatly increased the oxygen demands of the heart and again produced abnormal changes on electrocardiograms. When strenuous exercise was preceded by a moderate to heavy warm-up (15 to 20 min of exercise followed by a short rest), the abnormal increase in arterial blood pressure was significantly reduced and the changes on electrocardiograms were abolished. He concluded that these findings provided a physiological basis for warm-up as a method of reducing or eliminating abnormal changes in cardiac functions and blood pressure associated with strenuous activity.

A. V. Hill found that increasing the temperature of muscle improved both contractile force and contractile speed.[9] DeVries reasoned that warm-up which results in increased temperature of the blood and muscles would improve performance because (1) muscles would contract and relax faster, (2) muscles would contract with greater efficiency because of lower viscous resistance, (3) hemoglobin would give up more oxygen and also dissociate rapidly, (4) myoglobin would show effects similar to those of hemoglobin, (5) metabolic processes would increase, and (6) resistance of the vascular bed would decrease.[7] Conversely, laboratory studies show that cooling of the body below normal body temperature causes a loss of reaction time and contractile time and reduces excitability of the muscles.

It is believed, and rightfully so, that performance of the specific skills involved in the activity will sharpen the competitor's coordination and timing. However, the degree to which the sharpening of skills actually occurs is not clearly established.

Intensity and Duration of Warm-up

Optimal combinations of intensity and duration are needed to bring about the desired warm-up effects. Too little work does not achieve optimal levels of temperature, and too much work can result in impaired performance owing to fatigue. The intensity and duration of warm-up must be adjusted to the individual. As a rule, one may look for signs of increased body temperature such as perspiration. For those who wish to be more scientific, an increase in internal temperature (core temperature measured rectally) of 1 to 2 degrees is desirable.

Effects on Injury

Several experts have claimed that failure to warm-up may lead to tearing of muscle tissue. Often a pulled muscle occurs in the relaxed fibers, those antagonistic to the contracting muscles. This happens because the opposing (relaxed) muscles do not yield to the pull suddenly placed on them by the rapidly contracting muscles. Morehouse and Miller support this idea by stating that the muscles most frequently torn because of inadequate warm-up are those antagonistic to the strong contracting muscles.[14] When not prepared, these antagonistic muscles relax slowly and incompletely, thus retarding free movement and hindering accurate coordinations. Further, it is generally accepted that the danger of injury is lessened when an athlete is prepared to react and move quickly. Warm-up seems to contribute to one's readiness to respond.

Effects on Performance Factors

Much of the research done on warm-up has been related to specific performance factors such as strength, speed, endurance, and the like.

Evidence from two studies wherein total body warm-up through exercise was used showed that warm-up will increase *strength*. Conversely, in three studies involving only local artificial heating, no increase in strength resulted. In one of the studies, strength decreased. The evidence supports the idea that if warm-up is to influence strength favorably the warm-up must work the muscles not heat them artificially.

Several researchers have found that local artificial heating of a body part does not improve *endurance*. Further, there is evidence that local cooling, which reduces skin temperature, may result in better performance of the underlying muscles. The rationale behind this is that cooling of the surface area results in less circulation near the surface and a better supply of blood in the muscles beneath the surface. Conversely, there is a good amount of support for the idea that total body warm-up through exercise has a favorable influence on endurance.

There is good evidence that warm-up will improve *power* as measured by the vertical jump or throwing speed. This is logical, because power is made up of the components of strength and muscle speed, both of which can be increased by warm-up. Several studies support the idea that warm-up improves swimming speed and running speed, and this further supports the claim that warm-up improves power, because swimming speed and running speed depend greatly upon power.

The research shows that either a swimming warm-up or passive warming in a hot shower can improve *swimming speed*, as can formal, related warm-up drills on the deck. But unrelated warm-up exercises apparently have little or no influence on swimming performance.

Kinds of Warm-up

Coaches and athletes should be acquainted with the different approaches to warm-up.

RELATED vs. UNRELATED WARM-UP.   Related warm-up involves movements included in the activity itself, whereas unrelated warm-up is a procedure to bring about warming without participating in the particular skill. There is no research in this area, but it can be reasoned that if the desired body temperature can be achieved by related warm-up this would be preferred, because of its potential positive effects on coordination and timing in the specific skills of the performance.

PASSIVE vs. ACTIVE WARM-UP.   There is adequate evidence that any method of exercise that results in an increase in body temperature can have a favorable influence on performance. This has been demonstrated through the use of active warm-up procedues such as running, calisthenics, and the like. But there is insufficient evidence that passive heating such as a hot bath, hot shower, turkish bath, or diathermy is effective for improving performance.

Most coaches and athletes seem to believe that warm-up is valuable, and we agree with this position. But it must be recognized that indiscriminate warm-up may waste energy while producing limited results. Some important guidelines are:

1. Warm-up should be intense enough to increase body temperature and cause perspiration, but not so intense that it causes partial fatigue.
2. Warm-up should include some stretching and loosening exercises along with some heavy work.
3. Warm-up should include movements that are common to the performance, that is runners should run, shot-putters should practice putting, and basketball players should do basketball skills. This helps to prepare the specific muscle groups involved in the performance. Maximal efforts should be avoided during the warm-up.
4. The warm-up should begin to taper off 10 to 15 min prior to the performance and end about 5 min before performance. This will allow recovery from temporary fatigue without loss of the effects of the warm-up.

MAKING WEIGHT IN ATHLETICS

In sports such as wrestling and boxing where competition is organized into divisions by body weight, the advantages of competing in the lowest possible weight class are obvious, provided the competitor does not pay too big a price in terms of his state of condition to adhere to the lighter weight class. Also, weight loss is often emphasized in early practice sessions of each football season for those who report for training in an overweight condition.

For mature athletes, "making weight" need not be a health hazard, owing to experience which has set a precedent as to their normal weight. However, many cases have been revealed of excessive short-term weight losses of immature high school and junior high school boys. Such weight losses can be obtained only by drastic changes in fluid metabolism (sweating it off) plus water and food restrictions, and this causes changes in kidney and cardiovascular functions. In young and physically immature athletes, a 5% weight loss in preparation for weigh-in is the outside limit of prudence, and it is likely that even this amount is too great for some youngsters.

The American Medical Association's Committee on Medical Aspects of Sports has stated that there are frequent excuses for weight loss in such sports as wrestling, in order to balance the squad's representation in all weight classes and to gain an advantage by getting a boy pitted against a lighter opponent. The Committee states that the desired modification of weight should be accomplished over an extended period of time, so the change is in body composition and not in excessive dehydration. It is possible to add muscle and lose fat and keep one's weight constant or to lose fat without adding muscle and thereby lose body weight. Weight loss by cutting calories is defensible if the athlete has enough nutrients and energy reserves to meet requirements during practice and competition.

The AMA Committee suggests periodical medical examinations and a year-round general conditioning program. It also recommends 4 to 6 weeks of intensive conditioning before competition. The athlete's final competitive weight should be his minimal "normal" weight. All during the preparation in competitive seasons athletes should keep themselves in a state of nutritional readiness.

Many coaches cause athletes to bring about the desired short-term losses by profuse sweating and abstaining from food and liquids for several hours before weighing in. Weight losses up to 10 pounds by this method (representing 5% of the body weight) have occurred in college wrestlers without negative effects. This abnormal loss of weight is partially regained after weighing in by eating and drinking moderate amounts in preparation for competition. More than 5 pounds may be gained in a few hours.

Research studies involving college wrestlers have shown that physically mature athletes may lose up to 7% of their body weight without adversely affecting *strength* (as measured by cable tensiometer tests), cardiovascular *endurance* (as measured by the Harvard step test), and *general performance* (as measured by the "sit out maneuver"). But this does not mean that 7% weight loss is advisable in view of its possible detrimental effects on health.

It should be clearly recognized that there are two important problems associated with dramatic short-term losses in weight. (1) The athlete might be weakened considerably as a result of lack of nutrition, and this could more than offset the advantage of competing in a lighter weight class. (2) Excessive abstinence from the consumption of liquids combined with profuse sweating can result in dehydration, and this can adversely affect several body functions and may result in illness, or even death. These problems are less serious in mature athletes than in teenagers. Thus coaches should be extremely cautious in the weight loss practices they encourage among young athletes.

Artificial vs. Real Changes in Body Weight

An interesting question is what causes *real* body weight changes, as opposed to temporary fluctuations owing to changes in fluid content. There are two simple facts that should be emphasized. (1) Body weight will fluctuate on an immediate but temporary basis as a result of perspiring but this does not result in a loss of *real weight*. It is only a loss of body fluids which will be replaced shortly through normal body processes. (2) *Real body weight* is lost or gained through a differential in the number of kilocalories consumed and the number utilized.

A pound of fat is equivalent to approximately 3,500 Kcal. This means that if 3300 Kcal of food are eaten each day and 2800 Kcal of energy are expended, the net gain would be 500 Kcal. In 7 days 3500 extra Kcal would be accumulated which would equal approximately 1 pound of body fat. Of course, the reverse would happen if 500 less cal/day were consumed than were expended. Body fat is gained and lost almost in direct relationship with the differential between the number of calories consumed and the number expended, and is the basis for gaining and losing *real weight*.

Coaches who require athletes to wear rubberized suits or heavy clothing to induce abnormal perspiration for the purpose of losing *real weight* demonstrate their ignorance about the physiological processes involved in weight reduction. Unfortunately, such lack of information frequently results in too much dehydration and too little ventilation, and this in turn causes heat injuries.

Aside from desired dehydration to cause temporary (or artificial) weight losses, the only physiologically sound reason for use of extra clothing during exercise is for warmth. It is clearly established that a person will perform better in vigorous activities if the ventilation processes work effectively and if the body is kept cool (only slightly above normal temperature). Excessive heating and perspiring as a result of too much clothing is a distinct disadvantage and presents a health hazard that ought to be avoided.

Under normal living conditions, *real body weight* tends to be highly stable. The great majority of persons who are overweight become so over an extended period time, usually several years, owing to a small but consistent differential of caloric intake and expenditure in favor of gaining weight. Under normal conditions, weight is not gained quickly or easily and neither is it lost quickly or easily. The best way for any individual to lose weight is to reverse the trend which caused the gain in weight. This means adjusting one's lifestyle in terms of diet and activity level. In other words, if you want to lose weight, change your eating practices to include less calories and, at the same time, design your life to include more physical exercise. Under these conditions, weight loss will not be dramatic, but it will be consistent. It is the healthiest and most sensible approach. It is an approach that every overweight person, both athlete and nonathlete, ought to adopt.

DEHYDRATION AND HEAT INJURIES

Long distance running, football practice sessions, and other long-duration vigorous activities place great demands on the circulatory system, particularly the heart and the body temperature regulatory process. Numerous studies have reported core temperatures in excess of 105° F in athletes after races of 6 to 26 miles, and each fall during preseason and early season football practices, many athletes suffer heat-related ailments of varying degrees of seriousness. Wrestling is also a sport in which potential heat injury deserves special attention. During the recent history of sports, numerous participants have died from heat stroke or severe dehydration, and each year many are temporarily incapacitated and their training programs disrupted.

Attempting to counterbalance body overheating, athletes sometimes incur large sweat losses of as much as a liter/hour. The resulting body fluid deficit may total 6% to 10% of the athlete's body weight. Dehydration of such proportion severely limits subsequent sweating, places dangerous demands on circulation, reduces exercise capacity, and exposes the athlete to the health hazards associated with hyperthermia (heat stroke, heat exhaustion, and muscle cramps).

The consequences of heat injuries are compounded by the current popularity of distance running and other forms of hard exercise among aging men and women, who may possess significantly less heat tolerance than their younger counterparts. This is not meant to discourage such participation, but only to add a word of caution.

Because of the hazards associated with long-duration heavy exercise under conditions of heat stress, the American College of Sports Medicine has issued position statements on the prevention of heat injuries. The statements were written for distance running, but they also apply to other situations involving long sessions of heavy exercise under conditions of heat stress. It is the position of the American College of Sports Medicine that:

1. Distance races of long duration should not be conducted when the humidity is high and temperature exceeds 85° F. Under such conditions, the event should be conducted prior to 9 am or after 4 pm.
2. It is the responsibility of the race sponsor to provide fluid which contains small amounts of sugar (less than 2.5 gm of glucose per

100 mg of water) and electrolytes (minute amounts of sodium and potassium in water).

3. Competitors should be encouraged to ingest moderate amounts of fluids frequently during competition, and to consume 13 to 17 ounces of fluid 10 to 15 min before competition.

4. In light of the high sweat rate and high body temperature during distance running in the heat, race sponsors should provide water stations every 2 to 3 miles for races exceeding 10 miles.

5. Runners should be instructed on how to recognize early symptoms of heat injury. Early recognition of symptoms, immediate cessation of exercise, and proper treatment can prevent serious injury.

6. Early warning symptoms include chilling, throbbing pressure in the head, unsteadiness, nausea, dry skin, and loss of orientation.

7. Race sponsors should make prior arrangements with medical personnel for the care of heat injury cases, and organizational personnel should reserve the right to stop runners who demonstrate clear signs of heat stroke or heat exhaustion.

Cooter has listed several other useful suggestions.[4]

1. Small amounts of liquids should be taken frequently during heavy exercise to replenish liquid loss, and salt tablets should be taken at the rate of one tablet for each pint of water.

2. Under conditions of heat stress, a large amount of skin should be exposed to the air because it will permit faster heat dissipation.

3. The use of rubber suits, plastic suits, and heavy sweat suits should be avoided when potential overheating is a factor. Loose clothing, short sleeves, and removal of headgear during rest periods will facilitate dissipation of heat.

4. Since most serious heat injuries occur during the early part of the season, it is good to remember the importance of starting practice sessions at a reasonable level and gradually increasing the intensity so the body has time to adjust.

5. Coaches of strenuous sports should be thoroughly familiar with heat injury symptoms and first-aid procedures.

6. A good precautionary measure under conditions of heat stress is application of a cold towel (35° F) to the abdominal region and head during rest periods. This will reduce core temperature and sweat loss by enhancing the body's ability to dissipate heat.

7. After a heavy work session, a warm shower with a cool shower following several minutes later should be required of the athlete or have the performer cool down by walking. A cold shower is

not recommended because it immediately cools the surface area and hinders heat dissipation.

In response to item seven, Falls and Humphrey found evidence that application of a cold towel to the abdomen and head periodically during exercise aided in cooling the body and helped to conduct the heat from the body surface.[8] They also found that taking a cold shower prior to the exercise period set up a situation wherein the periodic applications of the cold towel were more effective. Based on their study, they recommend that under conditions of heat stress, athletes take a pre-exercise cold shower for several minutes and receive periodic applications of cold towels to the abdomen and head.

Paolone reviewed the literature on thermoregulatory body adjustment to high temperature, and from the review he makes these important conclusions:[15]

1. Prior physical conditioning has a positive effect on the body's tolerance to increased heat in association with exercise.
2. A period of acclimatization to exercise under conditions of high temperature is important to safety. The physiological changes that occur as a result of acclimatization are (a) increased circulatory stability characterized by increased circulating blood volume and a reduction of heart rate, (b) increased sensitivity of the sweat mechanism, (c) increased efficiency of evaporative cooling, and (d) a prolonged gradual increase in sweat production.

Johnson did a study to measure the physiological effects of dehydration on male college athletes, and the evidence led to the following conclusions:[10]

1. The moderate consumption of liquids during strenuous exercise helps maintain higher levels of oxygen consumption than when no liquids are ingested.
2. The consumption of water seems to be as effective as the ingestion of commercially prepared liquids.
3. The quantity of liquids that an athlete drinks during exercise should approach the amount of dehydration that he experiences.
4. A psychological benefit may be gained from consumption of a moderate amount of liquid early in an athletic contest prior to any significant loss of body fluid.

MUSCLE SORENESS

Even though we have learned to deal with muscle soreness much more effectively in recent years, it still plagues athletes and coaches and it often interferes with training programs and reduces the effectiveness of performances.

Two forms of muscle soreness can occur after exercise: (1) immediate, pain which occurs shortly after exercise and passes quickly, and (2) delayed, localized soreness which appears 12 to 24 hours after exercise.

In *immediate soreness* one of the most popular theories holds that the pain is caused by the outward passage of potassium across the muscle cell membrane into the tissue space. Another explanation is the accumulation of waste products (mostly lactic acid) following heavy muscular work. In either case, the pain occurs soon after exercise and the athlete recovers from it rather quickly.

Delayed muscle soreness is not so transient as immediate soreness, and the pain sometimes persists for several days. Three popular theories exist for this affliction: (1) the accumulation of metabolites, (2) the rupture of muscle fibers, and (3) the onset of fatigue of muscle tissue.

It is a fact that the harder muscles are worked, the more likely will be the excessive *accumulation of metabolites*. However, there is a point against this theory in that muscle soreness has been found to be greater after exercise consisting of eccentric (lengthening) contractions than after a comparable amount of concentric (shortening) contractions. However, a greater quantity of metabolites result after concentric contraction. Thus, the theory of accumulation of metabolites does not correspond with all of the facts.

Aside from violent muscle contraction and excessive stretching, *rupturing of muscle fibers* does not occur as a result of muscle use. Thus, rupturing of muscle fibers is not an acceptable explanation for muscle soreness. This is particularly evident when one considers that muscle fibers should not rupture during normal action since their structure is adapted for that very purpose. However, there is evidence to show that excessive pull or stretch traumatizes muscle fibers and swelling develops. The credibility of this idea is further substantiated by the fact that greater muscle soreness occurs after extensive eccentric contraction than after concentric contraction.

It is possible that the onset of muscle soreness is caused by *muscle tissue fatigue*. As the muscle tissue fatigues, incomplete relaxation occurs and partial muscle spasms result.

Each of these theories can partially explain delayed muscle soreness, and it seems likely that all three factors contribute to the problem.

Relief of soreness can be enhanced by three techniques.

1. Mild, smooth exercise that does not contribute to additional soreness but does improve circulation in the muscle tissues.
2. Holding the muscles in a mildly extended, semirelaxed position for brief periods of time.
3. Mild massage or whirlpool bath, which helps to remove waste

products faster than normal and helps the muscles to feel loose and relaxed.

Prevention of muscle soreness involves focusing attention on a few simple precautions.

1. Do preliminary warm-up exercises before entering vigorous activities. Include in the preliminary routine some stretching, some loosening exercises, and some moderately heavy work.
2. Incorporate progression in the training program to increase the load and duration of exercise gradually. Do not make abrupt changes in exercise intensity.
3. Avoid bouncing or bobbing exercises and jerky muscle contractions which place excessive tension on muscle fibers and connective tissues.
4. Cool down after vigorous activity to enhance the dissipation of waste products from the muscles.

Apparently, not all forms of exercise lead to the same degree of residual soreness. Research indicates that eccentric exercise results in more residual pain than isometric or concentric exercise, concentric exercise resulting in the least amount of pain. The soreness from eccentric exercise peaks about 48 hours after exercise. This also is true of the soreness curve resulting from isometrics, although the amount of pain is usually much less. The soreness curve resulting from concentric exercise is relatively low, and it peaks about 24 hours after exercise.

In most cases, athletes will be ahead in their training programs and will feel better if they cautiously avoid the development of excessive muscle soreness. When soreness does occur, it requires a recovery period and treatment, and this is disruptive to training and often discouraging to athletes.

OFF-SEASON CONDITIONING

One of the important principles of modern sports training is that athletes must keep in reasonably good physical condition throughout the year in order to reach their peak during the performance season. Even a short period of inactivity can produce deterioration in cardiovascular endurance, muscular strength and endurance, flexibility, and timing. The athlete also can experience a decrease in lean body weight from a loss of muscle tissue and an increase in fat. Once the new season begins, the athlete who had been sedentary during the off-season is slow to regain a high performance level and will likely not reach his peak.

The off-season conditioning program can take a variety of forms, and to some extent it must be tailored to suit the individual. Here are some important guides: (1) Include enough vigorous total body activity to prevent substantial deterioration of the muscular system and the supporting systems. (2) Perform some activities that include the specific skills of the in-season performance. (3) Avoid a large deviation from optimal performance weight. (4) Follow a training routine that is less demanding and different from the in-season conditioning routine to prevent staleness and boredom. Variety is important.

SELECTED REFERENCES

1. Astrand, P.-O.: Something old and something new—very new. *Nutrition Today*, 4:9, 1968.
2. Astrand, P.-O., and Rodahl, K.: *Textbook of Work Physiology*, 2nd ed. New York: McGraw-Hill Book Co., 1970.
3. Barnard, R. J.: The heart needs warm-up time. *The Physician and Sports Medicine*, 4:40–41, 1976.
4. Cooter, R.: Heat control in athletes. *Athletic Training*, 10:56–57, 1975.
5. Counsilman, J.: *The Science of Swimming*. Englewood Cliffs, N.J.: Prentice-Hall, Inc., 1968.
6. Cureton, T. K.: What about the wheat germ? *Scholastic Coach*, November 1959, pp. 24, 30.
7. DeVries, H. A.: *Physiology of Exercise for Physical Education and Athletics*, 2nd ed. Dubuque: Wm C. Brown Co., 1974.
8. Falls, H. B., and Humphrey, D. L.: Cold water application effects on responses to peak stress during exercise. *Res. Q.*, 42:1, 1971.
9. Hill, A. V.: The design of muscles. *Br. Med. Bull.*, 12:165, 1956.
10. Johnson, D. J.: The psychological and physiological effect of hydration on male college athletes. *J. Sports Med.*, 15:138–146, 1975.
11. Macaraeg, P.: High carbohydrate, low fat liquid meal for athletes. *J. Sports Med.*, 14:259–262, 1974.
12. Martin, B. J., Robinson, S., Wiegman, D. L., and Aulick, L. H.: Effect of warm-up on metabolic responses to strenuous exercise. Medicine in Science and Sports, Vol. VII, No. 2, pp. 146–149, 1975.
13. Mellerowica, H., and Hansen, G.: Conditioning. In *Encyclopedia of Sports Science and Medicine*. L. A. Larsen (Ed.). New York, Macmillan, 1971.
14. Morehouse, L. E., and Miller, A. T.: *Physiology of Exercise*, 7th ed. St. Louis: C. V. Mosby Co., 1976.
15. Paolone, A. M.: Thermal regulatory adjustments to exercise at high temperatures. *The Journal of Physical Education*, 72:87–90, 1975.
16. Singer, R. N., and Weiss, S. A.: Effects of weight reduction on selected anthropometric, physical and performance measures of wrestlers. *Res. Q.*, 39:361, 1968.

Chapter 16

Exercise in Low and High Pressure

The choice of Mexico City as the site of the 1968 Olympics aroused a tremendous interest in the effects of altitude on athletic performance. It stimulated much discussion among physiologists and athletic coaches and caused considerable research on problems related to performance at high altitude. After all the medals had been distributed to the victors, it became obvious that the effects of altitude, although apparent, were not as severe as many experts had predicted.

The increased popularity of scuba and other water activities has made the study of the effect of high pressure on performance important. The purpose of this chapter is to investigate the effects of low and high pressure on the body during exercise.

EFFECTS OF LOW PRESSURE

As man ascends to higher and higher altitudes, the total pressure of the atmosphere decreases because of the decreased weight of the column of air above him. Since the percentage of each of the gases in the atmosphere remains the same regardless of altitude, the partial pressure of each of the gases decreases in proportion to the decrease in total pressure. Of course, when the partial pressure of oxygen is reduced, aerobic work capacity also is decreased. This decrease can be demonstrated by comparing the performance in the 1968 Olympics at

Mexico City with previous Olympic and world records. No new records were set in events requiring individual efforts of over 1 minute's duration.

	800 meter	1500 meter	5000 meter	10,000 meter
World record	1:44.3	3:33.1	13:16.1	27:39.4
Olympic record before 1968	1:45.1	3:35.1	13:39.6	28:24.4
1968 Olympic performance	1:44.3	3:34.9	14:05.0	29:27.4

From these figures it is apparent that altitude has its greatest effect upon endurance (aerobic) events, and the longer endurance events are affected more than the shorter ones. (The world 800-meter run record was equaled at Mexico City, but the 10,000-meter run was about 2 min slower than the world record.)

The cause of the reduced performance in endurance events is that the reduced oxygen pressure at high altitude reduces the arterial saturation of the blood, which in turn decreases the amount of oxygen available to the cells to be used for the production of energy. At sea level, the alveolar oxygen pressure is 104 mm Hg. At an elevation of 10,000 feet, it is reduced to 63 mm Hg; at 20,000 feet, to less than 40 mm Hg.

Luckily, the arterial oxygen saturation does not decrease at the same rate as the alveolar partial pressure because of the flattening of the oxygen dissociation curve at moderate altitude partial pressure (see Fig. 5–6). Even though the partial pressure of oxygen (PO_2) in the alveoli drops rapidly with increasing altitude, the saturation level of the blood remains fairly high to about 10,000 feet (97% saturated at sea level; 94% at 7000 feet; and 90% at 10,000 feet). Above this point, the saturation falls rapidly to 70% at 20,000 feet, 50% at 23,000 feet, and only about 20% at 30,000 feet. Because unconsciousness usually occurs between 25% and 50% saturation, pilots and mountain climbers are required to use oxygen at altitudes over 20,000 feet, if activity is carried on for a long period of time. Oxygen is often used at altitudes much lower than 20,000 feet because of the effects of hypoxia (oxygen lack) on the body. These effects include drowsiness, mental fatigue, and headaches. All adjustments made by the body upon exposure to altitude are for the purpose of increasing the amount of oxygen delivered to the cells as the alveolar O_2 pressure drops.

Not all the effects of altitude are detrimental to athletic performance, however. The reduced density of the air decreases the resistance of the airways to the flow of air into and out of the lungs. This allows larger volumes of air to be breathed during work with no significant increase in ventilation cost. Of course, this does not make up for the reduced partial pressure of oxygen, but it does allow the body to adjust

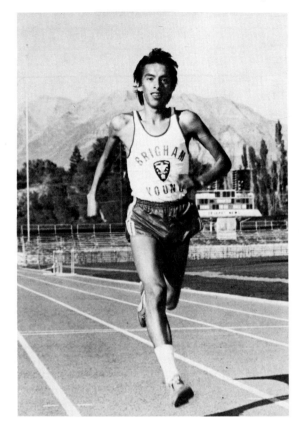

Figure 16–1.   High altitude takes a great toll in events requiring long periods of heavy work.

somewhat to the requirement for more oxygen during heavy work. The positive effects of decreased air resistance also are noticeable on sprinting activities, jumping events, and other high-velocity events which do not require extensive aerobic involvement. Performances in these activities are sometimes phenomenal. Take, for example, the long jump record of 29 feet 2¼ inches set by Bob Beamon in Mexico City at the 1968 Olympics. This performance might not have been achieved at a lower altitude.

Air is usually cooler and dryer at high altitude. Cooler temperatures can aid performances involving prolonged heavy work, but at the same time, the dryer air can increase the water loss from the respiratory system, causing discomfort to the performer.

There is no doubt that aerobic capacity is reduced with increased altitude.[9] This was clearly demonstrated in the Pan-American Games at

Mexico City in 1955. At 7370 feet, running times were about 10% longer than at sea level for distances over 1500 meters.[5] There seemed to be no effect on the events under 400 meters. These findings are logical in terms of our understanding of the anaerobic energy schemes discussed in Chapter 8. The body is able to provide energy for short periods of time without large quantities of oxygen. Any activity that can be completed before the depletion of readily available energy stores in the body will not be affected by the decreased oxygen pressure at high altitude. Events requiring energy from the oxidative systems are affected significantly.

Physiological Adjustment to Altitude

Several changes occur to the physiological systems which help them adjust to the decreased atmospheric pressure at high altitude. Some of these changes take place immediately, and others require several weeks. Each of the changes occurs for the purpose of overcoming the negative effects caused by the decrease in oxygen pressure.

The chemoreceptors in the aortic arch and carotid sinus are sensitive to either decreased O_2 pressure or increased CO_2 production. They stimulate ventilation rate and depth upon exposure to reduced oxygen pressure at high altitude in an attempt to provide sufficient O_2 to the alveoli. However, the increased ventilation tends to "blow off" CO_2, causing the blood to become more alkaline (higher pH), and lowers the partial pressure of carbon dioxide (P_{CO_2}). During normal work, the P_{CO_2} of the blood increases and causes an increase in respiration. At altitude, the decreased P_{CO_2} inhibits rather than aids the stimulus for increased ventilation from the lowered oxygen pressure, and only a small net increase in ventilation occurs initially.

Another factor related to the decreased P_{CO_2} is the O_2 dissociation curve. The oxygen dissociation curve shifts with changes in acidity or alkalinity of the blood. The shift in the curve for alkalinity is favorable for increasing the oxygen saturation of the blood.

Within a week or two the respiratory center becomes less sensitive to the decreased P_{CO_2}, and the kidneys readjust the blood pH to a normal range by reducing the blood bicarbonate level. This latter adjustment could decrease the buffering power of the blood and may negatively affect anaerobic capacity. However, the respiratory center then can respond fully to the reduced P_{O_2}, and pulmonary ventilation may increase by as much as 100%.

The large increase in respiratory rate increases alveolar oxygen pressure, which increases the diffusion of oxygen to the blood from the alveoli. However, blood O_2 saturation levels never reach those experienced at lower altitudes.

When an athlete moves from sea level to an intermediate altitude, there is a significant initial increase in heart rate at rest and during submaximal work. This is followed by a steady decline over a 10-week period to normal sea level rates. The heart rate pattern is followed closely by the cardiac output, except that sea level values usually will not be reached, even after a 10-week adjustment period. These adjustments are necessary to maintain cellular oxygen levels with the decreased alveolar oxygen tension.[7]

The cardiac output and heart rate will be greater at altitude for any given submaximal work load than for corresponding work at sea level. Although the initial adjustment in cardiac output is brought about primarily by heart rate, stroke volume takes on a greater portion of the cardiac output as the intensity of the work increases.[10]

Maximal cardiac output, stroke volume, and heart rate are affected little at intermediate altitudes (13,000 feet), but the maximal heart rate is reached at a lower work level. Maximal oxygen uptake is reduced by about the same value as the reduction in the arterial saturation. With a cardiac output which was 100% of sea level values, oxygen uptake during maximal work was reduced to 72% when the arterial oxygen content was reduced to 74%.[1]

At *extremely high altitude*, the cardiac output may be reduced significantly, with the decrease due primarily to decreased heart rate. Pugh and associates reported decreases in cardiac output from 22 to 25 l/minute at sea level to 16 to 17 l at 19,000 feet.[9] This reduction occurred because of a reduction in heart rate from 192 to 135 beats/ minute and a small reduction in stroke volume. This decrease in heart rate is probably associated with a lack of O_2 to the myocardium.

After only a few days at moderate altitude, the hemoglobin concentration increases owing to a decrease in plasma volume. Later, a real increase occurs in both hemoglobin and hematocrit, which increases the amount of oxygen the blood is able to carry per unit of volume.[3] Of course, the increased red blood cell percentage (hematocrit) also increases the viscosity of the blood which, in turn, increases the cardiac work at a given heart rate.

There also seems to be an increase in capillaries during acclimatization to altitude, along with vasodilation in those areas where gas exchange is needed for optimal functioning. This provides a source of oxygen closer to each cell even with a relatively lower oxygen tension.

In a summary statement at an altitude symposium, Dr. Bruno Balke mentioned the following compensating mechanisms which are used by the body to restore "normal" aerobic capacity: (1) an increase in pulmonary ventilation for any given level of work; (2) an increase of cardiac output for any submaximal work load brought about primarily by increased heart rate; (3) reduced maximal oxygen uptake, usually related to the reduction in arterial oxygen content; (4) initial hemoconcentration because of reduction in plasma volume; (5) a gradual increase in red blood cell count and hemoglobin content in the blood; (6) an increase in myoglobin, the oxygen-carrying pigment in the muscle; (7) a vasodilation in the areas where oxygen is needed for optimal performance; and (8) an increase in the number of capillaries per unit of tissue.[2]

Training Guidelines

The following guidelines can be used when working with athletes involved in aerobic (endurance) events at high altitude. No acclimatization is necessary for athletes involved in anaerobic events, such as short races, jumping, and throwing events.

1. There seems to be no evidence that performance is improved by training at a higher altitude for a performance at a lower altitude, with the possible exception that the anaerobic processes of the body may be improved slightly by high-altitude training.
2. Athletes who live and train at high altitude do not perform better at high altitude than athletes who train at sea level and then acclimatize themselves to the high altitude. Athletes who train at high altitude do not perform better at sea level than athletes who train at sea level.[5]
3. There may be individual differences in ability to acclimatize. Some athletes may be more vulnerable to the effects of high altitude than others. Some athletes will require longer periods of time to adjust.
4. The time necessary to acclimatize is related to the preceding training state of the individual athlete; a well-trained athlete will acclimatize more quickly than an untrained person. As a general rule, however, the acclimatization period should probably start 2 to 3 weeks prior to the competition in aerobic (endurance) events.[11]
5. Training programs similar to those used at sea level can be used for training at high altitude. However, the coach and athlete should be aware that fatigue will set in earlier. Less intense workouts of shorter duration will stress the system maximally at high altitude.
6. Man has the ability to adjust to higher altitudes and can perform more successfully after a period of acclimatization. Pugh states that man can probably acclimatize to altitudes in excess of 28,000 feet if sufficient time and proper procedures are used.[8] However, performance of aerobic activities will always suffer at high altitude no matter how well acclimatized the athlete becomes.

EFFECTS OF HIGH PRESSURE

With the interest in water sports and scuba diving, the principles of exercise in high pressures need to be explored.

Pressure Under Water

Each 33 feet (10 meters) of water causes an increased pressure of 1 atmosphere. This means that a person diving to 66 feet has 2 atmospheres of water pressure, plus the 1 atmosphere of air pressure above the water acting upon his body. Since standard atmospheric pressure at sea level is 760 mm Hg, the total pressure would be 2280 mm Hg at 66 feet. This pressure is enough to cause some strange things to happen physiologically and to require special care if a person exercises underwater.

Maintaining Pressure Equilibrium

The body can tolerate high pressures as long as the pressure is the same inside the body as it is outside the body. This principle is apparent when flying or driving up mountainous terrain. As the air pressure decreases on the outside of the body, a person must allow pressure to escape from the ears through the eustachian canals or suffer great pain. The potential pressure differences are much greater when diving, and can become a problem at only a meter or so when snorkeling. If the lungs are connected to a snorkel tube above the water, the difference in pressure between the water and the lungs will become so great at 1 meter, that the muscles of inspiration will be unable to overcome it, and normal breathing will be impossible.

A much greater problem exists as a person goes deeper. If he were to take a large breath of air from a scuba tank and try to hold it while ascending, the alveoli may explode. Remember that gas expands as pressure decreases. The volume of air in the lungs at 33 feet would double at sea level.[4] Even at 5 or 6 feet of water, a full breath held until the surface of the water is reached will overdistend the lungs and may lead to pulmonary hemorrhage. That is why air must be released by the diver any time he ascends from under the water.

Effects of Nitrogen

The deeper a diver goes, the more pressure is exerted by each gas he breathes. Nitrogen diffuses into the various tissues of the body slowly, and once in the tissues, also diffuses out slowly. When too much nitrogen is forced into the tissues, it affects the central nervous system, and causes symptoms much like those of drinking alcoholic beverages. This phenomenon is called *nitrogen narcosis*. The effects are related to the depth and duration of the dive. As a general rule, scuba diving

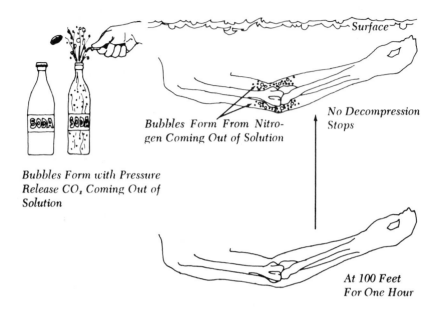

Bubbles Form From Nitro-
gen Coming Out of Solution

No Decompression
Stops

Bubbles Form with Pressure
Release CO₂ Coming Out of
Solution

At 100 Feet
For One Hour

Figure 16–2.   The bends. (Harper, D. D.: *Skin and Scuba Diving.* Columbus,
Ohio: Charles E. Merrill Publishing Co., 1968, page 36.)

should be limited to depths of less than 200 feet, with a practical depth
of around 100 feet to decrease the effects of nitrogen narcosis.

Nitrogen also causes problems if a diver surfaces rapidly after being
under water for some time. In this situation, the nitrogen which
diffused into the tissues is released as insoluble gas bubbles, much like
the CO_2 in bottled carbonated drinks when the lid is first removed.
These bubbles congregate in the small blood vessels, where they
obstruct the flow of blood and cause pain, or they may even become
trapped in the brain and cause paralysis. Pain is felt in the joints,
ligaments, and tendons first, usually within about 4 hours, and cause
what is commonly known as the *bends.*

Bends can be prevented by surfacing slowly so that the tissues can
get rid of the excess nitrogen without the formation of bubbles. Another
way to prevent the bends is to breathe a helium-oxygen mixture of gas.
Helium is less easily dissolved in the body tissues than oxygen, and
once dissolved, can diffuse out of the tissues more easily when normal
pressures are restored.[4] Breathing a helium and oxygen mixture decreases the likelihood of having the bends and decreases the chance of
nitrogen narcosis.

Once a diver has the bends, the only treatment is to subject the body
to the high pressure again to force the bubbles back into solution. The

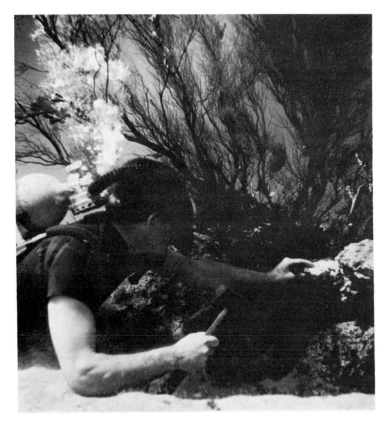

Figure 16–3.   A scuba diver must understand the effects of high pressure.

diver is then brought back to normal pressure slowly, allowing the nitrogen to come out of solution normally.

Oxygen

Prolonged breathing of 100% oxygen at sea level is not a good idea. However, in high pressures, it can be extremely dangerous. When pure oxygen is breathed under high pressure, the amount of oxygen in solution is increased so high that carbon dioxide cannot be accepted by the red blood cells, causing a buildup of CO_2 in body tissues, which disturbs cerebral blood flow and results in the symptoms of oxygen poisoning (tingling of appendages, visual problems, noise in the ears, confusion, muscle twitching, and convulsions).

Oxygen toxicity may occur at any depth greater than 10 meters, but there is a great range of individual sensitivity to oxygen under pressure. The onset of problems are hastened by physical activity.

SELECTED REFERENCES

1. Astrand, P.-O., and Rodahl, K.: *Textbook of Work Physiology*. New York: McGraw-Hill Book Co., 1970.
2. Balke, B.: Summary of scientific sessions of the International Symposium on the Effects of Altitude on Physical Performance. In *The International Symposium on the Effects of Altitude on Physical Performance*. R. F. Goddard (Ed.), Chicago: The Athletic Institute, 1967.
3. Faulkner, J. A.: Training for maximum performance at altitude. In *The International Symposium on the Effects of Altitude on Physical Performance*. R. F. Goddard (Ed.). Chicago: The Athletic Institute, 1967.
4. Folk, G. E., Jr.; *Textbook of Environmental Physiology*, 2nd ed. Philadelphia: Lea & Febiger, 1974.
5. Grover, R. F.: Exercise performance of athletes at sea level and 3,100 meters altitude. In *The International Symposium on the Effects of Altitude on Physical Performance*. R. F. Goddard (Ed.). Chicago: The Athletic Institute, 1967.
6. Guyton, A. C.: *Textbook of Medical Physiology*, 4th ed. Philadelphia: W. B. Saunders Co., 1971.
7. Hannon, J. P.: High altitude acclimatization in women. In *The International Symposium on the Effects of Altitude on Physical Performance*. R. F. Goddard (Ed.). Chicago: The Athletic Institute, 1967.
8. Pugh, L. G.: Animals in high altitude: Man above 5,000 meters-mountain exploration. In *Handbook of Physiology, Adaptation to the Environment*. D. B. Dill (Ed.). Washington: American Physiological Society, 1964.
9. Pugh, L. G., et al.: Muscular exercise at great altitudes. *J. Appl. Physiol.*, 19:431, 1964.
10. Vogel, J. A.: Cardiovascular function during exercise at high altitude. In *The International Symposium on the Effects of Altitude on Physical Performance*. R. F. Goddard (Ed.) Chicago: The Athletic Institute, 1967.
11. Weihe, W. H.: Time course of acclimatization to high altitude. In *The International Symposium on the Effects of Altitude on Physical Performance*. R. F. Goddard (Ed.). Chicago: The Athletic Institute, 1967.

Chapter 17
Psychological Aspects

The maximal ability of a person to perform in any athletic event is obviously limited by his physical characteristics. But beyond these broad restrictions psychological factors often play a decisive role. Many coaches and physiologists believe that, in the future, top performances and record-breaking efforts will be greatly enhanced by giving more attention to the psychological aspects of the athlete, and the psychological interactions between the coach and athlete.

An interesting song for all who are interested in competition and preparation for competition is entitled "Stout-Hearted Men." The more popular lines read:

"Give me some men who are stout-hearted men,
And I'll soon give you ten thousand more."

But there are other lines in the song that more correctly describe the importance of psychology:

"Hearts can inspire other hearts with their fire,
And the strong will obey when a strong man shows them the way."

Throughout the ages, some individuals have inspired others through the example of their own lives. In coaching, this approach is especially important. Someone once said, "A champion is a person whose heart can be educated." It is important when working with athletes to get them inspired—to make them *hot in the heart* for competition.

MOTIVATION

Motivation is possibly the most important word in athletics, because it is well established that performances consistently improve when athletes are properly motivated. They must be "up" for the game or "ready" for the competition. Further, they must be motivated to continue with long and hard training sessions over an extended period of time if they are to approach their potential in athletic performance. Often motivation makes the difference between ordinary and great performances.

In order for a coach to motivate his athletes, it is usually helpful to know (1) how the athletes think, feel, and respond to various circumstances; (2) their backgrounds and experiences; and (3) the circumstances of their homes and their relationships with their parents and friends. The more the coach knows about each athlete, the better equipped he will be to motivate the athlete properly for competition.

The word *motivate* means to move, impel, induce, and stimulate. A highly motivated and motivating coach can stimulate athletes to the point where they can perform near their maximal ability. Some of the methods that coaches use to motivate athletes are: group psychology, individual conferences, pep talks, a system of rewards, yells and battle cries, rules of discipline and squad rules, peer-group approval, special names for positions and groups, signs, point systems, grading, and seasonal goals. Coaches also may use psychological controls to suppress situations or attitudes that might interfere with maximal performance. Whatever approaches the coach uses to motivate, they all point to the desired level of "readiness" at the time of performance.

Sports competition seems to possess, because of its very nature, intrinsic interest for young people; however, many persons are inspired to work far beyond what would be considered mere love of the game. They are highly motivated by such things as the desire for social approval and prestige and by psychological and economic rewards. Psychologists claim that the various motives and incentives which make sports competition so highly desired by so many are:

1. Excess energy, play drive, and competitive urge.
2. Desire for prestige, approval of others, escape from inferiority feelings, and experience of success.
3. Desire to prove abilities to self and to others, to improve self-confidence, self-respect, and self-realization.
4. Escape from anxieties, frustrations, worries, monotony, and boredom of the daily routine.
5. Attempt to release aggressions and excess energy in socially approved ways.
6. Greater attention from opposite sex.

7. Tendency to emulate admired adults and to excel in activities of which they approve.

Some athletes need little psychological prodding in order to operate at maximal efficiency. These athletes are called *self-starters* and are often highly sought at recruiting time.

The self-starter has goals which seem to arise within himself. He seems to be able to find sufficient self-motivation to be psychologically prepared. He has good concentration and usually has a high degree of self-discipline and a mature attitude.

The research about the psychology of sports has uncovered some interesting information relating to motivation and psychological preparation:

1. Noise tends to produce great efforts.
2. External stimuli such as "yells" help the athlete to overcome internal inhibitions.
3. Elimination of stress factors before competition is usually beneficial to performance.
4. Introverts generally respond to praise, whereas extroverts often perform better under criticism.
5. Emotional excitement tends to be an aid in extending physical exertion beyond normal levels.
6. Extreme emotional stimulus may produce too much tenseness or "buck fever," and this can have negative effects on both learning and performance.
7. Fans, bands, cheerleaders, and home courts usually have a positive effect on performance.
8. The *fear* of losing tends to contribute to motivation.
9. Too many emotional peaks in any one season may contribute to staleness.
10. An *optimal* amount of competitive tension is the desirable result of motivation.

EMOTIONS

Humans are emotional beings, and emotions can be the causative factor in both victory and defeat. The experienced and informed coach is aware of this fact and conducts himself accordingly. He is able to design situations which cause players' emotions to act as assets to them rather than as liabilities. There are times in sporting events when the performer must be calm and tranquil. This feeling enables him to perform his assigned tasks in a more successful manner than usual. There are other times when he is better off if his emotions are at a fever pitch. The coach has to know which kind of emotional involvement is preferred and be able to influence it adequately.

Having the contestant "ready" at *contest time* is one of the important challenges. It makes relatively little difference how the athlete feels on Monday or Wednesday when the contest is on Saturday. The idea is to have him ready when the contest starts. To do this the coach must control the emotional climate.

Some coaches influence the emotions of the squad by explaining that if they play the way he has taught them to play, they will have the glory and credit if they win, while he will assume the blame if they lose. This, in effect, "takes the monkey off their back," and helps them relax and play the game the way they have been taught. Other coaches agree that the athletes and coach should always share in the glory of winning and the disappointment of defeat.

Bryant strongly believes that emotion is one of the prime ingredients of a winner.[1] He states:

> From the time I played at Alabama until a few years ago, I believed that if you weren't a winner, if the game didn't mean enough to you, you'd probably wind up quitting. So I've laid it on the line to a lot of boys. I've shook 'em, hugged 'em, kicked 'em, and embarrassed them in front of the squad. I've got down in the dirt with them, and if they didn't give as well as they took I'd tell them they were insults to their upbringing, and I've cleaned out their lockers for them and piled their clothes out in the hall, thinking I'd make them prove what they had in their veins, one way or the other, and praying they would come through.[1]

Most situations where good morale exists are found when the team is winning. Good morale can be thought of either as the reason for the team's success or as a by-product of success. However, once in a while, good morale exists in a losing situation. A group of athletes and the coach can band together in a harmonious and closely knit unit if they believe in themselves and believe that their plan will work—it might take a little while, but they believe that eventually they will win and they work toward that desired goal. As long as they feel a reasonable hope for success, morale can remain high.

Some coaches attribute much of their success to the fact that their teams are always characterized by outstanding morale. The following guidelines often are used to achieve exceptional team morale;

1. When the team is losing, it usually needs encouragement and not destructive criticism and sarcasm.
2. The coach should require group loyalty, and strictly prohibit criticism, wrangling, and jealousy within the squad.
3. The coach must be loyal to his team at all times, and he should treat all players fairly. He should be friendly with all his players, but not too familiar with any of them.
4. The coach should prevent inferiority complexes on the part of

second-string players. He should help them feel important and useful.

5. In dealing with each disciplinary situation, the following procedure is suggested: do not speak until there is absolute silence, then talk with a low tone of voice; do not say too much; be sure a penalty can be enforced before it is announced; and do not hold any malice afterward—treat the incident as closed.

THE WILL TO WIN

One of the most important aspects of coaching is the ability of the coach to recognize a *winner* and to get him in the game. The term *winner* is used here to mean an athlete whose attitude, determination, and fortitude, combined with his physical ability, will consistently contribute to success. Through the years, sports pages have been filled with the exploits of great performers who were not outstanding athletes but were winners. It is easy to recognize winners who have great performance ability, but some winners do not have unusual ability and are much more difficult to identify. One of America's great coaches expressed a useful idea related to this characteristic when he said, "Once I'm convinced that a boy is not a *winner,* I don't care if he runs a 100 yards in 9.3 and is eight feet tall, I'm forgetting him. He's not a winner and I'm not interested in all that other stuff." Obviously, "all that other stuff" can be important, but its usefulness is greatly enhanced by a *winner's* personality.

If a *winner* does lose, and if you were to say to him, "Why did you lose?" he might well reply, "We didn't plan to lose. We didn't practice to lose. We didn't play to lose. We used every ounce of our energy and every spark of our spirit all the way from the beginning to the end. Even though the scoreboard says we got beat, we didn't get beat in the heart. We are still undefeated where it really counts, and we'll be bouncing back on that scoreboard soon." Well, you can bet on it, because every fiber of this kind of athlete vibrates with a powerful, positive punch which pounds toward victory. It has become natural for him to win; it is part of his personality.

How can a coach make an athlete into a winner? It is not easy, because you are dealing with the forming and reforming of personality traits, and these traits are not easily influenced. But they can be changed as a result of effective teaching and exposure to the right experiences. It is within the ability of a good coach to inspire and motivate an athlete to want to be a winner, and the coach can teach courage, initiative, and good conduct, all of which are characteristics of a winner. Through his efforts, the coach will be able to make winners out of some athletes who otherwise would never achieve such distinction.

PERSONALITY OF THE COACH

The history of sport is replete with the names of unsuccessful coaches who taught techniques well but mishandled their players psychologically. It has become increasingly apparent that coaches must have personality traits that inspire athletes and cause them to respect the coach and feel confidence in him. The coaches who succeed the best are those who cause their athletes to "want to go to war for them."

Athletes look up to the coach who knows his field well—so well, that to work with him is to learn constantly. But most athletes also want a teacher whom they admire as a person. The mature coach with an attractive personality, a wholesome outlook on life, and a good measure of idealism seems to have great appeal to young persons.

The successful coach must be a practical psychologist as well as a sound technician. He must study his athletes to know how their minds work and to understand their dispositions and personalities, in order to get the best results from them. There is no foolproof method or standard approach. What works in the case of one athlete may be a poor approach for another. A coach who endeavors to treat all his athletes alike and handles all in the same manner is destined to encounter needless problems which contribute to lack of success.

Ogilvie and Tutko researched the personalities of successful coaches and found that they consistently possessed the following positive and negative traits:[13]

Positive traits

1. Success-driven with an outstanding need to be on top.
2. Highly orderly and well organized.
3. Outgoing and friendly.
4. Having developed consciences and much in tune with the appropriate values of the culture.
5. Unusually well equipped to handle emotional and stress problems.
6. Open and trusting and not excessively defensive in their relationships with others.
7. Exhibiting an abundance of leadership qualities.
8. Showing dominant, "take-charge" attitudes and actively seeking roles of leadership.
9. More prone to blame themselves than others when things go wrong.
10. Exhibiting a high degree of psychological endurance.
11. Emotionally mature and tending to face reality in a direct manner.

Negative traits

1. Exhibiting a low tendency to be interested in the dependency needs of the athlete, such as listening to personal problems,

protection when in trouble, emotional support. Their response was "I'm no social worker. My job is teaching them how to win."

2. Inflexibility or rigidity in terms of new learning techniques to increase performance. This is indicative of egocentric individuals.

PERSONALITY OF THE ATHLETE

Even though there are numerous theories concerning the personalities of athletes, only a limited amount of research has been done to gain information to support the theories. Neuman[12] and Seist[15] both suggest that participation in high level athletic competition provides an important addition to one's personality. They claim that harmonious development comes about through sports participation. In their research they found that athletes were more sociable, more aggressive in their approach to problems, more self-confident, more critical of themselves, and more extroverted than nonathletes. Conversely, Ogilvie and Tutko claim that athletic participation does not consistently contribute to character improvement.[14] Whether it does or does not depends greatly upon the leadership (coach) and how the leader deals with opportunities for character development.

In his study of a group of Austria's best athletes, Seist found that male athletes were less neurotic than male nonathletes.[15] Male athletes were more stable under stress than female athletes, and females tend to be more susceptible to depression than male athletes.

Research and practical experience indicate that only certain personality types have the ability to undergo the social and physical stress of participation in high-level competitive sports. As an athlete continues participation, he experiences both negative and positive personality changes as a result of his athletic involvement.

Athletes as a group cannot be labeled as either more or less intelligent than the population as a whole. Like other young people of today, contemporary athletes tend to be well informed, and they expect to be treated accordingly. Thus, it has been found helpful to prepare contemporary athletes intellectually as well as physically and emotionally for the demands of competition. This preparation takes the form of discussions, lectures, readings about the psychological, physiological, and biochemical demands of the sport, viewing of films of opponents and other performers, and analyzing their own performances on film and video tape.

STRESS

Generally, as stress increases beyond a normal level, reasoning, problem-solving ability, and efficiency progressively decrease. It appears that as an individual adapts to one kind of stress he loses his ability to tolerate other stresses. The organism is apparently limited by its defensive resources, so that if the resources are mobilized against one stress they are not able to cope with other stresses as effectively. This helps to explain how sustained bodily disease can lower resistance to psychological stress.

Many persons believe that after undergoing severe stress, rest can completely restore them. Generally, this has been an assumption among coaches and athletes. Selye presents evidence that this is not true.[16] With sustained and severe stress, there may be a considerable amount of irreversible wear and tear. Experiments with laboratory animals have shown that such stress leaves incurable scars, in that it uses up reserves of adaptability that cannot be replaced. Since we continually go through periods of stress and rest during life, just a little deficit of adaptation every day adds up to what we call *aging*.

According to Selye, as the stress level in athletic competition increases to a high point, analytical ability and judgment go down, and so do the biological adaptations of the body. Coaches and athletes must be aware of these factors and help to equalize heavy emotional stress, or in some cases, to eliminate it so that repetition of competition does not leave an indelible scar. Obviously, stress will not affect all individuals to the same degree. Each athlete will react to stressful situations in his own way, according to his past experiences and his emotional stability.

STALENESS

Staleness implies general fatigue as a result of overtraining, monotony, or sustained emotional stress. This problem, which is apt to occur in the latter part of the competitive season, must be perceived in the initial stages if there is to be a quick cure.

Frequent symptoms of staleness are slowness of reflexes, lack of enthusiasm, lack of interest, gradual loss of weight over an extended period, tiredness, a lack of staying power in a vigorous contest, and irritability. Contributors to staleness include inadequate sleep and lack of rest after hard work, too much routine and too little diversion, academic loads that require irregular and excessive study time, home worries, and poor diet. However, frequent and excessive emotional tension is believed to be the major factor contributing to staleness.

The stale athlete tries to improve but seems to get worse. He seems unable to drive himself to do better, and often the harder he tries the poorer are the results. The best cure for staleness is a combination of rest and diversion. If the stale athlete is allowed to attend practice, his workouts should be kept to a minimum and should contain variety and diversion until his energy and enthusiasm return to normal.

If it appears that the athlete is stale because of too much hard physical exertion, the antidote is rest or rest combined with exercise done in a playful manner. If the staleness seems to be associated with emotional stress, then the emphasis should be placed upon freeing the athlete from his worries and anxieties. A few athletes place themselves under too much stress. They need to be taught to worry less about losing. They need to emphasize the positive aspects of self-improvement and enjoyment of the game, and to worry a little less about the outcome.

According to Ogilvie and Tutko,[13] J. H. Schultz has devised a method of alleviating precompetition stress, known as *Das Autogenne Training* (the self-training method). He recommends the method for individuals whose precompetition tension is too high. The following procedure is recommended by Schultz: After assuming a comfortable position, usually on the back, the athlete breathes deeply several times and concentrates on his breathing. He then tightens all of his muscles maximally for several seconds and then relaxes as completely as possible. He pretends that his body is extremely heavy and concentrates on each segment until he is completely relaxed. Then the athlete tries to sleep. At this point the athlete repeats the procedure one or more times. It is hypothesized that after successive relaxation and reactivation the athlete will return with a more positive mind and be ready for effective performance. Schultz estimates that 40% to 45% of all athletes can profit from this procedure, but that the remainder may find the procedure of little or no value.

Some have suggested that hypnosis should be used to help athletes cope with heavy psychological stress. But experience shows hypnosis to be generally ineffective in helping athletes overcome stress.

PSYCHOLOGICAL AIDS

Psychological aids, or "crutches," can alter performance in direct and specific ways. Certain crutches such as drugs, alcohol, cigarettes, and extreme dietary alterations usually hinder an individual's performance, according to how frequently and excessively he leans on the crutches. The most important consideration is whether or not the athlete's feelings of inadequacies, frustrations, or anxiety are so great that his crutches become psychologically addictive. In some instances, an athlete will use another person as a psychological aid. He might be directly dependent upon his coach, his father, or some other individual to prepare him psychologically for competition. In the absence of this person, the athlete will tend to falter. Every athlete should be encouraged to avoid too much dependency on any kind of psychological crutch and should be encouraged to find psychological strength within himself.

RESULTS OF RECENT RESEARCH

Recent research studies have revealed a number of interesting facts pertaining to the general topic of psychology as it relates to athletics and physical fitness. Dowell and his associates reported a positive relationship between physical prowess and self-concept, along with positive relationships between both strength and athletic achievement and self-concept, and finally a positive relationship between physical fitness and physical self-acceptance.[3] In a follow-up study of earlier research, Dowell and others again reported a positive relationship between selected physical attributes and self-concept.[4]

Ismail and Trachtman found that when middle-aged men embarked on a regular exercise program, they became more self-sufficient, resolute, stable, and imaginative.[7] Murphy and his associates investigated the relationship between physical fitness and the reduction of certain aspects of emotional discomfort in alcoholics.[11] Results indicate that as alcoholics improve in physical fitness, they tend to report less depression and anxiety. Sharp and Reilly found a positive relationship between the development of aerobic fitness and the increase of selected positive personality traits in adults.[17]

Ogilvie and Tutko stated that their research over 8 years indicated that there was no empirical support for the traditional belief that sports and fitness developed character.[14] They did clarify, however, that the particular leadership could have significant influence on the outcome of character development. If the research results are true, this indicates that athletic coaches need to give considerably more attention to providing positive experiences for athletes and giving them leadership which will result in character improvement. Undoubtedly, athletic competition affords the opportunity for such development, but the leadership available to the youngsters is crucial to the outcome. Also, in many instances, parents should do more to cause positive character development through athletics or at least they ought to strive to contribute less to the opposite.

Cureton stated that Cattell had reviewed a number of studies on the relationship of mental efficiency and personality characteristics to physical fitness, and he concluded that motor fitness significantly correlated with desirable psychological attributes.[2] Husman summarized most of the existing research which related fitness and sports and their role in development of personality integration.[6] His findings were as follows: (1) team sport athletes seem to be more personable and social than individual sport athletes, and (2) 100 top-rated soccer players who were extremely fit indicated a high degree of personality integration.

Folkins and co-workers studied psychological fitness as a function of physical fitness, and found that the greater the improvement in time of the 1.75-mile run, the more likely it is that the subject will become less depressed, more confident, more personally adjusted, more efficient at work, and experience more restful sleep.[5] He found that as the heart becomes more efficient (heart rate decreases) the subject becomes less anxious. McGown and his associates found that there was an increase in self-concept from pre-test to post-test for the experimental group involved in a high-level endurance training program.[9] The control group showed no such improvement.

We have learned much during the past two decades about the relationship of athletics and physical fitness to the psychological and mental aspects of individuals, but much new knowledge will have to be derived from extensive research before we can approach our potential effectiveness for (1) utilizing sports and conditioning for improvement of psychological traits, and (2) utilizing psychological preparation to enhance athletic performances.

SELECTED REFERENCES

1. Bryant, P.: Philosophy of Coaching. Proceedings of the American Football Coaches Association Annual Meeting. Washington, D.C., Jan. 11–13, 1966.
2. Cureton, T. K.: Physical fitness and dynamic health. *Journal of Physical Education,* 69;117–125, 1972.
3. Dowell, L. J., Badgett, J. L., Jr. and Landiss, C. W.: A study of the relationship between selected physical attributes and self-concept. In *Contemporary Psychology of Sport.* G. S. Kenyon (Ed.). Chicago: Athletic Institute, 1970, pp. 657–672.
4. Dowell, L. J., Kandiss, C. W., and Mamaliga, E.: A twenty-year study of the physical fitness of entering freshmen at Texas A & M University. *Physical Fitness Research Quarterly,* 42:220, 1971.
5. Folkins, C. H., Lynch, S., and Gardner, M. M.: Psychological fitness as a function of physical fitness. *Arch. Phys. Med. Rehabil.,* 53:503–508, 1972.
6. Husman, B. F.: Sports and Personality Dynamics. 72nd Proceedings of the Annual Meeting of the National College Physical Education Association for Men. Durham, N. C., 1969, p. 56.
7. Ismail, A. H., and Trachtman, L. E.: Jogging the imagination. *Psychology Today,* 6:78–82, 1973.
8. Lawther, J. D.: *Psychology of Coaching,* 2nd ed. Englewood Cliffs, N.J.: Prentice-Hall, Inc., 1965.
9. McGown, R. W., Jarman, B. O., and Pedersen, C. M.: Effects of a competitive endurance training program on self-concept and peer approval. *J. Psychol.,* 86:57–60, 1974.
10. Moore, R. A.: *Sports and Mental Health.* Springfield, Ill.: Charles C Thomas, 1966.
11. Murphy, J. B., Bennett, R. N., Hagen, J. M., and Russell, M. W.: Some suggestive data regarding the relationship of physical fitness to emotional difficulties. *Newsletter Research Psychology,* 14:15–17, 1972.
12. Neumann, O.: Sport und Personlichkeit. Versuch einer Psychologischen Diagnostik mit Deutung der Personlichkeit des Sportlers. (Sport Activity

and Personality. The Use of Psychological Assessment to Evaluate the Personality of Athletes.) Munich, 1957.

13. Ogilvie, B. C., and Tutko, T. A.: *Problem Athletes and How to Handle Them.* London: Pelham Books, 1966.
14. Ogilvie, B. C. and Tutko, T. A.: If you want to build character, try something else. *Psychology Today*, 3:56, 1969.
15. Seist, H.: Die psychische Eigenart der Spitzensportler. *Zeitschrift der Diagnostischen Psychologie und Personlichkeitforschung* (Journal of Diagnostic Psychology and Personality), Vienna: 1965.
16. Selye, H.: *The Stress of Life.* New York: McGraw-Hill Book Co., 1956.
17. Sharp, M. W., and Reilley, R. R.: The relationship of aerobic physical fitness to selected personality traits. *J. Clin. Psychol.*, 31:428–430, 1975.
18. Singer, R. N.: *Motor Learning and Human Performance.* New York: The Macmillan Co., 1968.
19. Vanek, M., and Cratty, B. J.: *Psychology and the Superior Athlete.* New York: The Macmillan Co., 1968.

PART IV
PRACTICAL APPLICATION
OF CONTENT

After the facts and concepts of athletic conditioning have been studied, it is important to turn toward the practical application of the information. It is not feasible to discuss all possible applications of the material in this book because there is such great variety of activities to which it can be applied. However, it is possible to furnish some meaningful samples.

Chapter 18 includes important points of information about the training programs for specific sports, although it does not include all the information about training for any particular sport. The chapter content is meant to furnish only ideas about application. Chapter 19 deals with the measurement of athletic characteristics. Much useful information is contained here in a few pages, but additional valuable information on this topic is available in the various text books on tests and measurements in physical education and athletics.

Chapter 18

Sample Programs for Specific Activities

In preparing for the various athletic sports, emphasis is needed on the development of personal traits and factors that influence performance. Some performances depend heavily upon strength, others depend more upon endurance, and still others depend upon agility and speed. For this reason, training programs for the different sports vary, and each program is designed to emphasize the traits and factors most important in the performance of that sport.

Athletic sports can be logically grouped into court games, field games, track and field, aquatics, gymnastics, and combatives. Although different in many respects, the several activities in each group tend to require similar traits and so require similar methods of conditioning. This chapter contains descriptions of the essential characteristics of conditioning programs for several of the more popular sports. Each section deals with one of the major groups of activities. Only certain sports are discussed because it is not feasible to present training programs for all sports. The information presented here will serve as basic guidelines for an informed teacher or coach to design effective training programs for a variety of sports.

COURT GAMES

Court games are unique in the sense that they are played in a relatively small area and involve the handling of a ball or similar object and often an implement. Court games typically require a high degree of running maneuverability and total body agility in order for the player to be able to gain good court position and compete with his opponent on both offensive and defensive maneuvers. Fast starting, stopping, dodging, and darting are fundamental to good court play. Also, court play requires fast acceleration in order to be able to sprint to advantageous positions and to get away from opponents. Jumping is of great importance; thus leg power is a necessary attribute. Since court games often involve continuous bouts of play at a vigorous rate, a high level of anaerobic endurance must be developed.

Even though court games are primarily anaerobic in nature, a high level of cardiovascular, or aerobic, endurance should also be developed for several reasons: (1) aerobic conditioning makes preseason anaerobic conditioning easier, (2) aerobic conditioning allows the performer to recover more quickly between bouts of exercise, and (3) there is some evidence that aerobic conditioning decreases the number of injuries sustained in anaerobic activities.

In addition to the fundamental characteristics named previously, all of which can be improved to some degree through training, each court game requires a group of skills specific to that game. For example, a basketball player must be highly skilled in dribbling, passing, catching, shooting, and rebounding. Handball, tennis, and volleyball require a different set of specific skills. Thus, it is apparent that a training program for any court game must aim toward improving the several characteristics which are fundamental to all court games, and in addition, it must dwell on the development of the skills specific to the game.

The following training guidelines are for basketball. They are meant only to provide ideas which will aid in developing a training program for a particular situation. It is not possible to describe a program which would be acceptable under all circumstances, because training programs are influenced by the style of play the coach emphasizes and by the condition and maturity of the athletes.

Basketball Training Program

Basketball is one of the more vigorous court games, and it requires a great variety of athletic traits. In order to be successful, a player must develop the essential traits to a high level and achieve a high state of conditioning.

OFF-SEASON.   Off-season training should consist of activities that maintain a relatively high level of both cardiovascular and muscular fitness. Many coaches require the basketball player to participate in track during the spring and prescribe a running program for the summer. This program normally includes (1) distance running, especially over natural and uneven terrain; (2) long-interval training during which distances of a half-mile or more are used with short breaks of walking or jogging between; or (3) fartlek training, which includes continuous running at various speeds over a variety of terrains.

The off-season program also might include general weight training which develops a combination of muscular strength and endurance. Exercises for the leg extensors and arm muscles should be emphasized.

Players should be encouraged to participate in other athletic activities which they enjoy, such as baseball, soccer, tennis, or handball. Also, most coaches will encourage (or require) their athletes to play a limited amount of basketball during the off-season in order to improve their shooting and ball-handling skills.

PRESEASON.   Preseason training will be more intense than the off-season program. It is during this period that most athletes develop the high level of fitness and muscle conditioning necessary for the competitive season. The program normally starts soon after the beginning of the school year and continues until nearly the time of the first game. Preseason conditioning should include calisthenics, running, and weight training, plus a variety of vigorous basketball drills.

An interesting calisthenic program is called the "pain barrier." It consists of alternating pushups, sit-ups, and half-knee bends, starting at a low level of 20 or less and increasing to about 50 repetitions two times a day. The players can then be taken to a stadium where they jump or run up flights of steps.

Anaerobic conditioning should be emphasized in the preseason running program, with the number of work bouts and the length of each bout varied to stress locomotive muscles and anaerobic power sources. Some coaches use cross-country running on alternate days and give rewards for the best time to encourage improved performance.

The weight-training exercises used during the off-season should be continued during the preseason, but they should be intensified. These exercises can be done on the athletes' own time, and a record kept of weight used and repetitions performed. Here again, a general body-conditioning program should be followed, and special emphasis should be placed on the leg extensor muscles.

COMPETITIVE SEASON.   During the competitive season, drills and scrimmages will maintain the fitness level of the athlete without much formal conditioning work. However, in early season, practices can be followed by conditioning drills such as the shuttle relay, which consists of each player running to a line at fore court, back to the starting line, then to the mid-court line, back to the starting line, then to a three-quarter line, back to the starting line, to the end line, and back to the starting line. Relay teams may be formed for competitive purposes. This drill contributes to agility as well as to endurance. After mid-

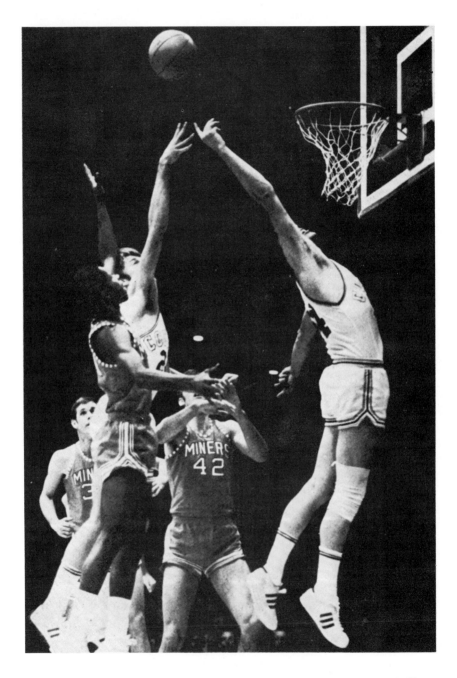

Figure 18–1.   Leg power is the key to jumping height in basketball.

season, many coaches discontinue this type of drill to avoid overtraining of the athletes.

Many drills have been used by outstanding coaches to help condition basketball players for improved performance. Only a few drills will be described here. Others can be developed to fit the particular needs of the athletes and to emphasize the playing style preferred by the coach.

1. Quarter-eagle drill. The players assume the defensive stance with their hands out and body in a low crouch position. Then they run in place rapidly for 30 to 60 sec. The players then move to a jump-spread eagle position, jumping eight to ten times, then back to the original drill. The procedure can be repeated as many times as desired.

2. Basic defensive drill. The athlete assumes a low defensive stance, then moves left or right or forward or backward as directed by the coach each time he blows the whistle and points in the direction of movement.

3. Passing drill. The players are organized into groups of four to six players. Formed into either a circle or two lines facing each other, the players pass the ball as many times as possible within a time limit. The losing team might be required to run laps.

4. Free-throw shooting. The players can be divided into small groups for competitive purposes, and the group that loses might be required to run laps.

5. Three-on-three drill. The athletes play a game of 21 points. They are encouraged to use the screens and defensive and offensive maneuvers taught during the practice.

6. Defensive-offensive drills. The players work one on one. The player with the ball attempts to work into a good position and then shoots. After five repetitions, the two players change positions. Again, the losing players (those making the least number of baskets) might be required to run laps.

7. Three-on-three rebound drill. One of the teams of three assumes the offensive position and the other team, the defensive position. The coach throws the ball against the backboard and the two teams scramble for the rebound. After five to ten repetitions, the two teams change positions.

FIELD GAMES

One of the unique features of field games is that they are ordinarily played on large areas and therefore involve a considerable amount of running. Most field games require the use of a ball or similar object, and often a club, racket, or some other implement. In order for a player to be able to gain and maintain good field position and to compete effectively with his opponent on both offensive and defensive maneuvers, various kinds of running skills are required. The player must accelerate rapidly, run fast at top speed, and have a great amount of running maneuverability. Since field games often involve short bouts of play at a vigorous rate, a high level of anaerobic endurance is essential. Fast reactions and fast movements are also important.

In addition to the fundamental characteristics which tend to be common to a variety of field games, each game requires a group of specific skills unique to that game. Baseball requires a set of skills that are quite different from those of football, and football requires a set of skills that are different from those for soccer and rugby. Thus, the training program for any field game must involve activities that will improve the several characteristics that are fundamental to all field games, and in addition it must dwell on the skills that are specific to the particular game. The following guidelines are for a football training program. These guidelines can provide ideas for a training program which will suit the purpose of a particular situation. It is not possible to describe a training program which can be used in all situations because training programs are influenced by the style of play and the condition and maturity of the athletes.

Football Training Program

The different positions in football require different emphasis on the fundamental characteristics of the players. For example, characteristics required in a lineman are somewhat different from those required in a running back. However, some characteristics tend to be common to all good football players. Among these characteristics are high levels of strength and power, fast reactions, acceleration speed, running maneuverability, and total-body agility. On the other hand, ball-handling ability is relatively unimportant in interior linemen, but it is a key to success among backfield players, especially the quarterback. Kicking skills are important only for a few players on the team.

OFF-SEASON.   Off-season training differs somewhat between high school and college, because at the college level the off-season includes spring practice, whereas in high school, football players are typically involved in other sports during the spring season. Among college athletes the off-season extends from about the first of December until the beginning of spring practice, and then from the end of spring practice until the first of July. July and August are typically considered to be part of the preseason period.

During the off-season it is recommended that football players condition themselves in a variety of vigorous activities which they find enjoyable, such as basketball, swimming, play-type running, and so forth. These activities should be supplemented with a weight-training program designed to maintain a high level of muscular strength and

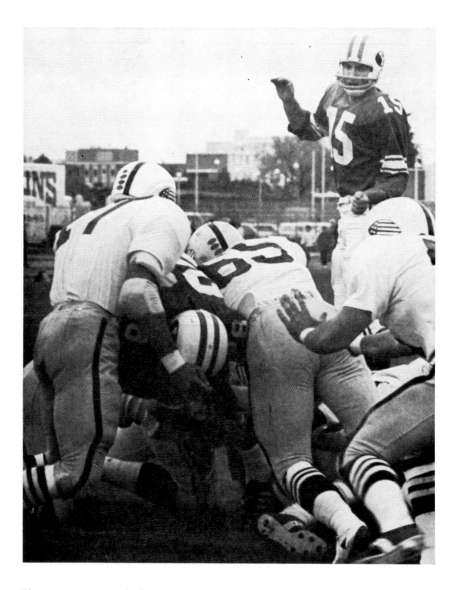

Figure 18–2.   Football is a game that requires an unusual amount of power, total-body agility, and running maneuverability.

endurance. The program should exercise all major muscle groups, with emphasis on the leg extensors (especially the quadriceps), the back extensors, and muscles of the arms and shoulders. Also, the athlete should do a considerable amount of running with emphasis upon running short distances at 80% to 100% of maximal speed. In addition, the running program should include agility running in which the athlete practices dodging, darting, zigzagging, and running back and forth between two lines 10 to 15 feet apart.

Those playing the end and backfield positions should place greater emphasis on the running phase of the off-season training, whereas those playing in the interior line should place greater emphasis on the development of strength. However, all football players should be somewhat concerned about both of these phases of conditioning. Also, it is important for the quarterbacks, running backs, and ends to do a considerable amount of handling of the football in order to improve their ball-handling skills. It is important that during the off-season football players not let their body weight deviate too much from their optimal playing weight, because extensive weight adjustments during the preseason and early season are both difficult and detrimental. Development of aerobic capacity during the off-season is important because it provides a basis for the anaerobic development later on, allows faster recovery between plays, and helps prevent injury from fatigue late in the game.

PRESEASON. Typically, the football player gets serious about preseason conditioning about the first of July. His individual conditioning program gradually increases in intensity from then to the time he reports to practice, after which a highly accelerated conditioning program is conducted by the coaches. During the 6 to 8 weeks of individual training before reporting for the first practice, the player involves himself in a great variety of vigorous conditioning activities. Each training session should include stretching exercises, vigorous calisthenics, strength and endurance training, running of various types, and a tapering-off procedure. The main objective is to develop the following characteristics: (1) running speed with emphasis on acceleration, (2) running maneuverability, (3) total-body agility, (4) cardiovascular endurance, and (5) muscle strength and endurance.

Once the athlete has reported for fall practice, the conditioning routines include a great variety of vigorous calisthenic exercises selected to work the major muscle groups of the body, sprint work with enough volume to improve both speed and cardiovascular endurance, a great variety of agility drills to improve both total-body agility and running maneuverability, and weight-training exercises to develop optimal levels of strength, with emphasis on the leg extensors, back extensors, and arm and shoulder muscles.

COMPETITIVE SEASON.   During the competitive season, extensive conditioning routines are difficult for two reasons. First, the players are involved in school and have only a limited amount of time for football, and second, most of the practice time must be devoted to running plays, learning strategy, and developing the team into a precision, smooth-functioning unit. Thus, it is obvious that the athletes must be highly conditioned prior to the beginning of competition.

Conditioning routines during the competitive season should be aimed at maintaining rather than at increasing the state of conditioning. During this period, weight training is included only once or twice a week, with the heavy work occurring during the early part of the week. The emphasis of this program should be on increasing the strength of identified weak areas of the body and thus filling the needs of the individual players. However, if time permits, emphasis should still be placed on the major contributing muscle groups which were identified previously.

The conditioning routines conducted on the football practice field during this season are typically divided into two phases, those done by the total team in one large group and those done in small groups and designed specifically for the players' positions. The conditioning routine involving the total group consists of warm-up and stretching exercises along with some vigorous calisthenics, which are of value to all players regardless of the positions they play. In recent years, there has been a definite trend toward decreasing the time spent on warm-up and general calisthenics and increasing the amount of time spent on drills specific to the skills required in the different positions of play.

Conditioning for Linemen.   The field drills for linemen include a variety of contact drills such as sled pushing, leg-driving drills, two-man resistance drills, tackling and blocking one-on-one and two-on-two drills, start and sprint drills, and other similar drills designed especially to increase blocking and tackling power and quickness. The weight-training exercises done by the linemen should emphasize strength and power and the building of muscle bulk. Among the more popular exercises are squat lifts, leg presses, knee and ankle extensor exercises, military and bench presses, curls, and rowing. The training should be done with high resistance and few repetitions.

Conditioning for Backfield Players.   The field drills for backfield players should resemble game situations as much as possible. They typically include agility drills, such as carioca, backward running, grab-grass run, and toe dance. But the primary source of field conditioning for this group should be involved with the basic play execution. Play patterns are normally run on a skeleton basis using only those players involved in the particular pattern. Other players are added to the skeleton team as needed to complete the total-team pattern. The weight-training program used for backs should include many of the same exercises as those used by linemen, but with a higher number of repetitions and slightly lighter weight.

Conditioning for Receivers.   The conditioning for running speed and agility is developed through actual execution of patterns. By running hard 20 to 30 yards downfield on each pattern, a player can maintain or improve his state of conditioning for this type of activity. In addition, drills typically included are net drills, the carioca, cross-over stepping, zigzag running, and so forth. The drills simulate game situations and usually involve receiving the ball. Many coaches run drills such as the dog-fight drill in which a receiver runs his pattern against defensive opposition. The defensive man hangs on, throws an arm in the face, pushes, and in other ways puts great stress on the receiver so that he gets a feeling of the actual game situation. Weight training by receivers should be identical to that done by backfield players.

TRACK-AND-FIELD ACTIVITIES

One of the unique features of track-and-field activities is that they are maximal effort events. In addition to competing against opponents, track-and-field athletes measure their achievements in terms of times and distances. In races, the athlete makes an all-out effort to cover the distance in the shortest time possible. He taxes himself to his maximum in either speed or endurance, or both. In throwing and jumping events, the athlete strives for maximal distance, and sometimes an inch can make the difference between success and failure.

The shorter races are tests of running speed. As discussed in Chapter 9, there are different types of running speed, such as acceleration speed, maneuverability speed, and top speed. Running maneuverability is not involved in track events, since the athlete always runs a straight or curved course. The relative importance of acceleration speed and top speed depends on the length of the race. In short sprints such as the 60-yard dash, acceleration speed is a major factor because it takes approximately half the distance of the race to reach top speed. As the race becomes longer, top speed becomes more important, whereas acceleration rate becomes less critical. Both acceleration speed and top running speed are greatly dependent upon power and coordination, in addition to correct running technique.

Success in distance running depends primarily upon running stamina, where the main limitation is cardiovascular endurance. Running efficiency has a major influence on stamina, because those who use less energy for a given distance will place less load on their body systems. Speed also is a factor in stamina, because a fast runner can coast and still keep ahead of a slower runner who may be working hard to keep up with his faster opponent.

The throwing events—shot put, discus, javelin, and hammer throw—are primarily power activities. They depend upon the athlete's ability to apply great force rapidly. Therefore, in addition to improving his technique, everything the athlete does is geared to increasing his ability to apply great force more rapidly in order to project the implement with greater speed. The two components of power, strength and speed of contraction, have different relative importance in the throwing events, with strength being the dominant factor in throwing heavy objects, such as the shot and hammer, and speed being proportionately more important with lighter objects, such as the discus and the javelin.

The four jumping events—high jump, long jump, triple jump, and pole vault—are also greatly dependent upon power, because they are tests of the ability to project the body through space. In these events, running speed, which in itself is greatly dependent upon power, will often make the difference between winning and losing (possibly with the exception of the high jump) because running speed at the moment of take-off determines the horizontal component which carries the body over the given distance. In addition to running speed, a powerful vertical thrust at the moment of take-off is fundamental to success in jumping events.

The following information about training techniques for each of the four kinds of track-and-field events provides ideas and guidelines which will aid in establishing effective conditioning programs. It is not possible to describe a conditioning program that would be acceptable under all circumstances, because of the differences in the state of conditioning and the maturity of athletes.

Sprint Races

Sprinting is primarily a power event because it is a series of projections done alternately with the right and left legs. In order to increase sprint speed, an athlete must increase either the length of stride or the speed of leg movement, or both. Research has shown that the length of stride is the main limiting factor, whereas leg speed is usually not a serious limitation. Length of stride depends upon the ability to contract the muscles rapidly with great force (power). Leg speed depends upon coordination and contractile speed of the muscles. The training program of the sprinter should consist primarily of three factors: (1) perfecting the techniques involved in starting and sprinting (improving the mechanics), (2) doing a considerable amount of sprint running because this will help to improve leg speed and leg power, and

(3) weight-training exercises to improve power, with emphasis on the leg extensor muscles.

OFF-SEASON AND PRESEASON TRAINING. Typically, the off-season extends from June to December, and the preseason includes January and February. During the off-season the athlete should maintain a relatively high level of general conditioning by participating regularly in vigorous activities which he enjoys. Emphasis should be on activities involving short bursts of fast running, such as soccer, football, basketball, and play-type running. This should be supplemented by an exercise program that emphasizes the development of strength and speed in the muscle groups used the most in sprinting.

During the preseason the sprinter should continue with the conditioning exercises, but with increased intensity in order to build a new maximal level of power in the key muscle groups. Along with this he should do a considerable amount of sprint running to develop power, and to improve his leg speed running mechanics and coordination. Also, he should practice starting and accelerating in order to perfect these phases of the race.

COMPETITIVE SEASON. During this time the workout involves essentially the same techniques and procedures used during the preseason, except the volume of work gradually increases because the athlete will be better conditioned by this time and will be working toward a peak by the end of the season. Also, during the competitive season, greater emphasis should be placed on the fine points of correct technique. In this respect, emphasis should be on three factors: (1) the start, (2) the acceleration phase, and (3) the top-speed phase of the race. The increased amount of work during this season will result in greater anaerobic endurance, a contributing factor in sprint racing which becomes more significant as the race gets longer.

During the late season the sprinter will ordinarily do the same kind of training as during the early part of the competitive season, except the amount of work will normally increase at a gradual rate. How much the amount is increased must be decided by the coach and athlete in the light of the conditions of the athlete and whether he shows signs of staleness. During the last 2 or 3 weeks, increased emphasis should be placed on the fine points of correct technique and form.

Endurance Running

Distance races, including middle distance, depend upon a combination of endurance and speed. The shorter the distance race, the more significant is speed; whereas the longer the race, the greater it depends upon endurance alone. The kind of speed that contributes to endurance running is different from sprint speed. It is speed at a relaxed pace and is usually called coasting speed. A person who can run fast and

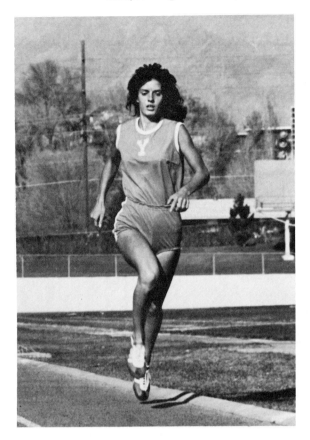

Figure 18–3. Woman middle-distance runner in action.

efficiently at an easy pace has a great advantage in distance running. The technique for developing this kind of speed is to do a large amount of running at nearly top speed and consciously relax while doing so in order to increase efficiency.

From the standpoint of endurance, it has been found that one of the main limiting factors is the oxygen supply to the working muscles. This supply, in turn, is directly dependent upon the efficiency of the cardiovascular system. Thus, the distance runner must have great cardiovascular endurance.

OFF-SEASON AND PRESEASON TRAINING. During the off-season (June through December), the distance runner should engage extensively in vigorous activities which are enjoyable to him and which involve an extensive amount of running, such as soccer, basketball, and play-type running. In addition, some athletes choose to use conditioning exercises to maintain a high level of muscular endurance in the leg muscles with emphasis on the leg extensors. Conversely, many good distance runners do not become involved in such exercises during the off-season.

During the fall and early winter, the distance runner should be extensively involved in cross-country running. This is a competitive event by itself, but also is an excellent off-season and preseason conditioner for distance runners.

During the preseason, the athlete should continue with an extensive amount of cross-country running, but at the same time should move toward more systematic training schedules. The amount of work should increase, and the emphasis should shift more toward interval training, but should include some cross-country work. The interval training should be of the type that emphasizes aerobic development. Such a program should consist of a series of work bouts 3 to 5 min in length with short rest periods between bouts. For more detail about the recommended procedure, see the section on aerobic endurance in Chapter 8.

COMPETITIVE SEASON. During the competitive season, a combination of cross-country running and interval training should continue, with increased attention given to interval training, more particularly to speed work. The amount of work should gradually increase as the athlete becomes better conditioned. The program should gradually and systematically progress in such a way that it brings the athlete along at the most rapid rate possible, but not so rapidly that he peaks prior to the end of the season.

During the season, the athlete typically does some long-distance running at the beginning of his workout; this should be followed by an optional amount of interval training and a tapering-off period of jogging and light exercises. It is important that the length and intensity of the work bouts be designed to fit the particular athlete's ability. Also, it is important that the athlete be consistently overloaded in terms of endurance so that his endurance will improve consistently throughout the season. Again, it should be mentioned that the emphasis should be on overloading the cardiovascular system in order to improve oxygen delivery to the tissues and to improve the aerobic processes.

During the late season, the athlete continues with approximately the same training routine, except the amount of work continues to increase as the athlete is ready to take more work. During this phase of the season, great care must be taken to peak the athlete for the final races of the year without bringing on staleness, which may be caused by overwork or monotonous routines.

Throwing Events

Success in the throwing events depends primarily upon power and correct technique, power being a combination of strength and speed, and correct technique depending primarily upon mechanics and coordination.

OFF-SEASON AND PRESEASON TRAINING. During the off-season, the athlete should participate in a variety of vigorous and enjoyable activities. He should emphasize activities that tend to keep the total muscular system well conditioned. This should be supplemented by conditioning exercises which maintain a high level of strength in the muscle groups used in throwing. Also, the athlete should do a considerable amount of throwing at less than maximal effort in order to improve his coordination and throwing mechanics.

During the preseason, the intensity of the exercise program should increase to develop a high level of strength prior to the beginning of competition. During this season, the exercises should shift more toward power development which combines strength and speed training. The relative emphasis placed on strength and speed will be influenced strongly by the particular throwing event for which the athlete is training, as the heavier implements require more strength and the lighter implements require proportionately more speed and less strength. The particular muscles that should receive attention in a conditioning program can be determined easily by analyzing the movements involved in the throwing event. Then exercises involving these same movements or the muscles causing these movements should be selected. For more detailed information on the correct approach for developing strength, power, and speed, refer to Chapters 7 and 9.

COMPETITIVE SEASON. It is important that athletes in throwing events develop the highest possible level of strength prior to the beginning of the competitive season, because once this season begins the athlete can do little more than retain his strength level. It is recommended that he do strength training only during the early part of the week, preferably on Monday, and that he concentrate on other forms of training between Tuesday and the competition on Friday or Saturday. It is acceptable to do speed exercises on Tuesday or Wednesday because these exercises do not take as much out of the muscles, and they do not interfere as much with coordination as heavy-resistance strength training. In addition to doing the conditioning exercises designed for strength and speed, the athlete should spend a great deal of time on perfecting his technique and on throwing less than maximal distance. At certain times during the early and middle portion of the week, he will want to make a few maximal effort throws. He must spend much of his workout time on drills selected to help improve weaknesses in his technique. Also, he should do much repetitious throwing with emphasis on correct technique and coordination.

During his training routine, the athlete should constantly keep in mind that his primary objective is to increase the final velocity of the implement (velocity at time of release) as much as possible. This is what determines the distance the implement will travel, provided it is projected at the correct angle. In order to achieve maximal final velocity, the athlete must apply as much force as possible as rapidly as possible and over the greatest distance possible so that he can accelerate the implement to a maximal velocity. Whatever he does toward improving technique and increasing his state of conditioning should be geared toward this end.

During the late season, the athlete should pay even greater attention to the fine points of his technique and to the development of movement speed. For some athletes, it might be wise to pay renewed attention to the development of strength during the few weeks prior to the final competitive events. Perhaps at this point in the season some strength will have been lost, or perhaps the athlete will have reached a plateau where he cannot increase any further without additional strength. The amount of emphasis that should be placed on strength at this point in the season will need to be determined by the particular coach and athlete.

Jumping Events

Excellence in the jumping events depends primarily upon running speed and the ability to thrust the body into the air. The relative importance of these two factors, the vertical and horizontal components, depends on the nature of the jumping event, whether it is primarily vertical or horizontal.

OFF-SEASON AND PRESEASON TRAINING. During the off-season, the jumper should participate regularly in vigorous activities which include a considerable amount of running and jumping. This will help to maintain a high level of general conditioning with emphasis on the development of the leg muscles. This program should be supplemented with a program of specific exercises selected to improve the power of the muscles involved in jumping, with emphasis on the leg extensors.

During the preseason, the athlete should participate extensively in wind sprints and running over low hurdles to improve his speed and the consistency of his stride. Also during this period, he should increase the intensity of the conditioning exercises in order to improve

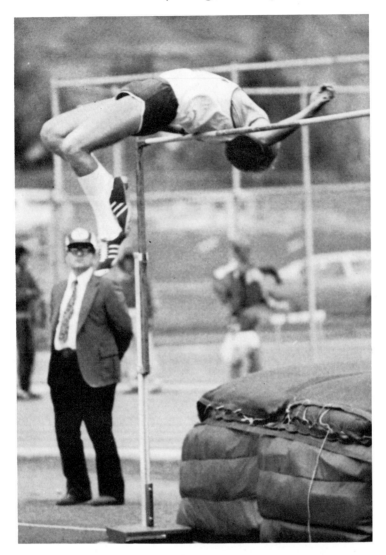

Figure 18–4. Jumping requires both leg power and good technique.

power. He should spend a considerable amount of time perfecting the approach run and jumping technique.

COMPETITIVE SEASON. During the competitive season, the jumper should continue with about the same routine as during the preseason, except he should place greater emphasis on running speed and on the fine points of jumping techniques. During this season, he should continue with conditioning exercises designed to develop power with emphasis on leg extension.

During the late part of the season, the athlete might want to increase the volume of work, depending on his state of conditioning and whether he shows any signs of staleness. Still the emphasis should be on (1) improving the fine points of his technique, (2) increasing the speed of the approach run, and (3) increasing leg power which will aid him in his upward thrust.

AQUATIC ACTIVITIES

Although aquatic activities are performed in the water, the characteristics required by an excellent swimmer are similar to those required by many other athletes, but the characteristics must be emphasized in different body parts. For example, power is important in court games and in swimming, but in court games the power must be primarily in the legs, whereas in swimming arm power is of paramount importance.

Swimming, like running, involves two general categories of events, sprint races and distance races. Obviously, the sprint events depend primarily upon swimming speed over a short distance, whereas distance races depend primarily upon swimming endurance. In the progression from short races, such as the 50-yard sprint, to longer races, speed becomes progressively less important and endurance becomes more important.

Speed in swimming is dependent primarily upon a combination of two factors: (1) application of as much propelling force as possible by means of the stroke and kick, and (2) the reduction of the resistive forces to a minimum. Correct technique (mechanics) results in the correct body position (that is, the position that will cause the least amount of resistance) and in the correct movement of the arms and legs. However, in addition to correct technique, power is fundamental to fast swimming. The swimmer must be able to apply great force rapidly with the arms and legs in order to propel the body through the water at high speed. This means that strong and fast muscle contraction are necessary. It can be said that in addition to correct technique, power and coordination are fundamental to success in speed swimming.

In the endurance events, speed is still a factor, because a fast swimmer can swim at a given pace with greater ease than a slower swimmer. Thus, he will tend to fatigue less readily. In addition to speed, the distance swimmer must have a large amount of endurance and must learn to swim as efficiently as possible in order to conserve his energy.

Training Program for Swimming

Expert swimmers usually participate in two competitive seasons—the winter season (December to March) and the summer season (June to August). Even though the winter season is considered the main one, most serious swimmers train rigorously during most of the year.

OFF-SEASON.   During the off-season, the swimmer should work on activities that maintain a moderate level of fitness and are somewhat enjoyable to him. These activities should include dry-land exercises along with running, bicycling, tennis, and other sports which maintain cardiovascular and muscular fitness. Training in the water during this season should concentrate mostly on skill development, with little pressure placed on the athlete to increase speed. Continuous heavy work during this period may contribute to staleness during the competitive season; however, a high level of general conditioning must be maintained.

PRESEASON.   The preseason program should begin 6 to 8 weeks prior to competition. During this time, lectures and movies can be used to improve skill and build enthusiasm. Dry-land exercises and weight training should receive increasing emphasis in order to improve strength, flexibility, and muscle endurance to the desired levels. The intensity of the work done in the water should increase and should include work on stroke mechanics, starts, and turns.

There are three important reasons for preseason training: (1) to improve the swimmer's strength and flexibility through dry-land exercises; (2) to improve the stroke mechanics, starts, and turns; and (3) to prepare or condition the body for the hard work that is to come in the next phase.

Care should be taken to be sure that the weight-training program does not develop the muscles to the point that their size becomes a handicap to movement. Weight-training exercises should be designed specifically to improve and strengthen endurance of the prime movers. Any increase in the size of other muscles can slow the swimmer by creating additional drag. With regard to strength development, a practical question is whether an increase in strength will more than offset the disadvantage of the growth in size that may accompany the strength. The object should be to attain a high level of strength with as little increase in muscle growth as possible.

The five prime-mover muscle groups which should receive emphasis in the weight-training program are:

1. Arm adductors and extensors (muscles that pull the arm through the stroking action)
2. Arm rotators

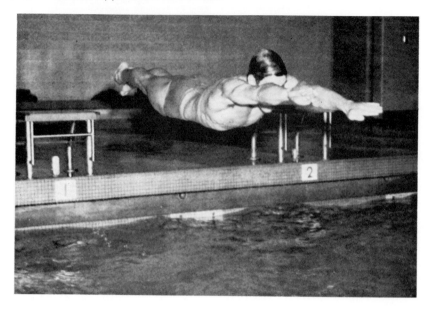

Figure 18–5.   Nearly perfect form midway through the racing dive.

3. Wrist and finger flexors
4. Elbow extensors
5. Leg and ankle extensors

Some attention also should be given to the trunk muscles because of their role in streamlining and stabilizing the body.

The cardiovascular development activities used during this period should be mostly aerobic in nature. Distance swimming, speed play (fartlek swimming), and long-interval swimming are recommended for building endurance. Sprint and short-repetition training are seldom used during preseason.

Adequate attention should be given to flexibility exercises, because swimmers need great flexibility, mainly in two areas, the ankles and the shoulders. Ankle flexibility is important in the free-style, butterfly, and backstroke events, because a large range of motion in the ankle results in more force against the water at more advantageous angles. Adequate shoulder flexibility is necessary in the free style, backstroke, and butterfly, because these strokes require the arms to move through long ranges of motion. To achieve the desired flexibility in the shoulder region, the interior deltoid and the pectoral muscles must be stretched.

COMPETITIVE SEASON.   During the competitive season, the stress-and-strain aspect related to endurance and general conditioning is more pronounced. During this season, many coaches prescribe double workouts, and some even recommend three sessions per day. Championship swimmers do a fantastic amount of work, the world-class swimmers covering as much as 15,000 yards per day, and some college and high school swimmers, between 6000 and 9000 yards per day. This great volume of work seems to be the key to excellence in swimming.

Because of the many hours devoted to training, it is important to vary the workout as much as possible and still accomplish the objectives. This can be done by utilizing the various training methods such as sprint training, overdistance, speed play, interval training, and time trials.

The training programs vary significantly between long-distance, middle-distance, and sprint swimming. However, the variation does not occur much in terms of total work accomplished but more in the way the work is designed. For example, if the training program calls for a total of 5000 yards in a given day, the sprinters might swim 1000 yards of easy swimming, fifteen 100-yard repetitions, thirty 50-yard repetitions, followed by 1000 yards of easy swimming. A middle-distance swimmer might swim three 500-yard repetitions, two 1000-yard repetitions, three 400-yard repetitions, and finish with three 100-yard repetitions. Physiologically, it is wise to taper off with at least 200 to 500 yards of easy swimming following a rigorous workout. Long-distance swimmers usually do much of their work with middle-distance and sprint swimmers but also do some additional work separate from these groups.

Swimming endurances seems to be developed best by long swims (3 to 5 min) with relatively short rest intervals. However, in addition to doing an extensive amount of this type of endurance work, all swimmers should do some speed work. Sprint swimmers should spend considerable time on repetitious short distances at 80% to 90% of maximal effort. This will help to increase their speed and will improve the anaerobic processes, which are important in short maximal-effort events.

Even though swimmers need much high-pressure work at regular intervals, they also need relief from this pressure at certain times. Low-pressure workouts at the correct times can afford the athletes an opportunity to gather themselves and once again prepare for high-pressure training. This helps to reduce the stress levels and tends to postpone the onset of staleness.

Because of the heavy work load during the season, swimmers should taper off during the peaking process near the end of the season. The amount of tapering that should be done depends on the athlete's condition and whether he has any signs of staleness. However, some amount of tapering should be used with all swimmers. During the tapering period, start and turn work can be practiced, along with further perfection of swimming technique. The important thing during the tapering period is not to work the swimmer to fatigue, but at the same time not to allow his state of conditioning to deteriorate. The purpose is to permit the athlete to become rested from the stress and strain of a long hard season and to permit him to concentrate on the fine points that result in better performance.

WRESTLING

Wrestling is the only combative activity discussed in this section because it is the only activity of that type commonly included in school athletic programs. Success in wrestling depends primarily upon strength, agility, and endurance, in addition to knowledge of the correct techniques. If a person is strong and agile, it is likely that he can develop into an excellent wrestler. To be able to continue at a high rate of performance throughout a match, the wrestler must have a large amount of endurance. Related to agility are reaction time and speed of movement, which also are important.

Wrestling requires rigorous training and personal sacrifice in order to achieve top condition and to keep the body weight as low as possible so as to gain the advantage of wrestling in a lighter class. The following information about conditioning will furnish some useful guidelines, but it must be recognized that the training program cannot be the same for all wrestlers because they vary greatly in ability and state of conditioning.

OFF-SEASON.   The serious-minded wrestler will keep himself in a high state of conditioning the year round, and he will not let himself become much overweight. During the off-season, the wrestler should participate in a variety of strenuous and enjoyable activities. Preferably, he should select activities that work the muscles of the upper part of the body and the cardiovascular system. Gymnastic activities, swimming, and calisthenics are good for keeping the muscular system in condition, and distance running and swimming are good activities for the cardiovascular system. In addition to participation in vigorous sports activities, the wrestler should carry on a moderate weight-training program designed to condition the total body, with emphasis on the upper portions. He should work against relatively light weight with many repetitions in order not to develop an extensive amount of muscle bulk.

PRESEASON.   Preseason training usually starts about 2 months before competition. The program should include:

1. Strenuous calisthenics, such as pull-ups, pushups, Japanese pushups, squat thrusts, sit-ups, and so forth.

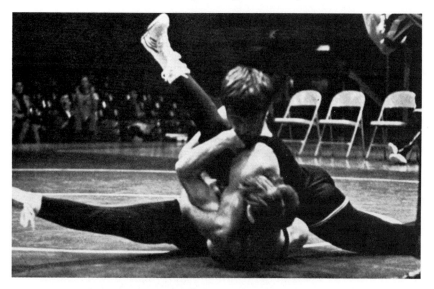

Figure 18—6.   Wrestling depends greatly upon reaction time, total-body agility, strength, and endurance.

2. Weight-training exercises selected only for those muscle groups in which maximal strength is needed in wrestling, such as the leg extensor muscles, back extensors, and arm flexors. It is doubtful that total-body weight training for strength should be included in the program, because this will result in too much increase in weight.
3. Distance running, mostly of the cross-country type, to develop basic cardiovascular endurance. When the competitive season draws near, the running of sprints and stadium stairs would prove beneficial.
4. Wrestling maneuvers and drills for approximately 30 min a day. Included in these maneuvers should be scrimmages of 1 min on top, 1 min on bottom, and 1 min from the standing position (1—1—1). These scrimmages can be increased to 2—2—2 and then to 3—3—3.

COMPETITIVE SEASON. During the competitive season, the conditioning program should include most of the same activities included in the preseason program, but the emphasis is different. During this season, the major part of the workout should involve wrestling situations. The workout can include positional wrestling, where the athlete is placed into various positions and required to wrestle himself out, or it can include a series of wrestling periods where the athlete wrestles for 1 min from the bottom position, 1 min from the top position, and 1 min from his feet, with short rest periods between. This pattern can then be expanded to 2-min wrestling periods from each position, and then to 3-min periods. Some coaches prefer that their wrestlers work a longer period of 8 to 12 min of wrestling with 2- to 3-min rest periods between for as many repetitions as seems desirable. It is obvious that several approaches can be used, but the important thing is that the wrestler should get 20 to 40 min of intensive wrestling during every workout.

Vigorous wrestling workouts over an extended period make a major contribution to muscular strength and endurance, and these workouts minimize the need for supplementary strength and endurance exercises. Because of this, many coaches consider the actual wrestling phase of the workout to be the prime conditioner. However, it is still advisable to supplement the wrestling drills with other forms of conditioning. A good amount of running, including some sprinting, should continue as part of the training program throughout the season. Running is vital to cardiovascular endurance, and it helps to keep the body weight down. Some coaches agree that weight training on a limited basis should be used to maintain maximal strength levels in the key muscle groups. If weight training is used, it should be included in workouts only on Monday or Tuesday and not within 3 or 4 days of a match.

In summary, the following can be said about wrestling: (1) The athlete should do a good deal of endurance training of the kind that overloads the cardiovascular system. This can best be accomplished by running and strenuous wrestling for relatively long periods of time with 3- to 5-min rest intervals. (2) He should develop maximal strength and muscle endurance with emphasis on the muscles of the upper body portions. (3) He should keep himself as lean as he can in order to be able to wrestle in the lightest possible class.

GYMNASTICS

Gymnastic activities require precision performances which depend greatly upon high levels of strength and skill. Therefore, a good portion of the gymnast's formal training program emphasizes the development of these abilities. Muscular endurance in the upper portion of the body is also important, but this is for the most part a by-product of strength, or it is developed at the same time as is strength. The gymnast requires a reasonable level but not a large amount of cardiovascular endurance. A high degree of total-body flexibility is desirable, and unusual amounts of flexibility in certain body movements are necessary to maintain correct form.

OFF-SEASON.   Many gymnasts take several years to gain the strength necessary to perform certain routines. They can lose a good portion of that strength in a few months if training is discontinued. Because of the need to maintain a high level of strength, most serious gymnasts keep themselves in a high state of conditioning year round. During the off-season, the gymnast should be encouraged to participate in vigorous and enjoyable activities which work the upper part of the body. The two best possibilities for this are swimming and exercise programs. There is little need for the gymnast to participate in activities which involve mostly running and jumping, because development of the legs and the cardiovascular system makes only a limited contribution to gymnastics.

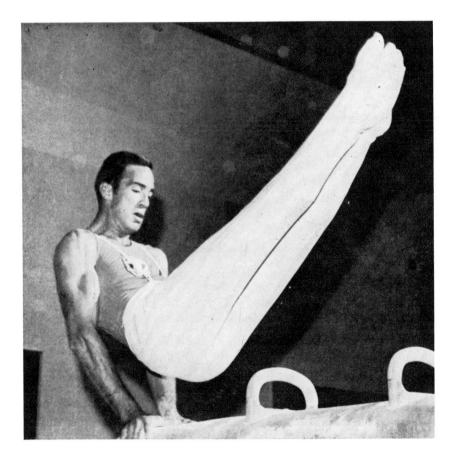

Figure 18–7.   Gymnastic maneuvers require a great amount of strength, coordination, and rhythm.

During the off-season, the desired level of strength and muscle endurance can be maintained best by use of weight-training activities. However, in designing a weight-training program for this purpose, two factors are important: (1) to select only those exercises which work the muscles used extensively in gymnastics, and (2) to do routines which develop a combination of strength and endurance with a minimum amount of muscle growth (10 to 15 repetitions using medium weight). Any unnecessary growth is undesirable because it adds weight to the body and tends to restrict maneuverability. However, some growth of selected muscle groups might be necessary in order to develop and maintain the desired strength levels, but obviously increases in size and weight of muscle groups that do not contribute to gymnastic performance would be undesirable. If a weight-training program is used, it should be supplemented with a well-rounded calisthenic routine.

In the absence of weight-training equipment, calisthenics can serve as a substitute, but it must be recognized that maximal strength levels cannot be developed with calisthenics because of the lack of sufficient resistance. The calisthenic progam should include exercises which emphasize strength, muscle endurance, and flexibility in the specific body regions where these traits are required. Many gymnasts participate in modern dance and ballet classes to increase their flexibility, sense of body position, and rhythm.

Regardless of what other activities the gymnast involves himself in during the off-season, he should do a reasonable amount of gymnastic work. This will assist in the maintenance of a high level of strength, endurance, and flexibility, and will allow him to maintain his coordination and timing.

PRESEASON.   During the preseason, the major emphasis should be on gymnastic work. Each workout should start with a period of light calisthenics with emphasis on stretching exercises to increase flexibility. This is typically followed by 1 to 2 hours of instruction, demonstrations, and actual practice of gymnastic routines, with the emphasis on practice. This should be followed by a session of vigorous calisthenics. During this season, it is desirable for some gymnasts to do a limited amount of weight training, the exercises being chosen carefully to increase the strength and endurance of selected muscle groups where additional strength and endurance are needed. For example, if a gymnast is having difficulty with the iron cross, a strength-development program for the latissimus dorsi and pectoralis muscles might be highly beneficial.

COMPETITIVE SEASON.   During the season, gymnasts involve themselves in about the same training program as during the preseason, with the major emphasis on repetitions of the various gymnastic routines. For example, a free-exercise gymnast might go through his compulsory routine six to ten times a day and through his optional program the same number. The volume of work that he does will increase progressively as he becomes better conditioned. Here again, the heavy part of the workout should be preceded by a variety of light calisthenic exercises especially selected to increase flexibility. The workout should end with a session of vigorous calisthenics supplemented by selected weight-training exercises if these seem desirable for the particular gymnast. Some gymnasts like to finish the workout with light jogging or light stretching exercises to help relax the muscles after the heavy workout.

Chapter 19
Measurement of Athletic Characteristics

On the surface, it seems that contests are won by the best times, the longest distances, or the highest scores, but it is more correct to think of victory and achievement as resulting from proper preparation and correct technique. An athlete who is knowledgeable and who is under the leadership of a knowledgeable coach has a far better chance of eventually standing on the victory stand than one who lacks these advantages.

Athletic conditioning comes alive when one is able to measure the results accurately. Of course, one important measurement is success in competition. In some activities, *time* and *distance* measurements describe the final result, whereas in other activities, the final result appears only in numbers on the scoreboard, and this often tells little about the specific achievements of individuals.

Useful tests have been prepared to measure such traits as strength, endurance, power, agility, and several other athletic characteristics. It is true that any characteristic can be measured with some degree of accuracy, but it is also true that some characteristics can be measured much more accurately than others. Only tests that are useful to coaches and athletes have been included in this section, and tests that lack accuracy and are cumbersome and impractical to administer have been avoided.

It is recognized that practically all college students majoring in physical education or athletic coaching take a class in tests and measurements, and the experience of taking such a course should add significant meaning to the present content. Knowing that the reader has had or will have this kind of course, the material presented here is in condensed form, including only carefully selected information and short descriptions. See the reference list for more information.

STRENGTH TESTS

As explained in Chapter 7, there are two kinds of strength: static and dynamic. Consequently, there are two kinds of strength tests. *Static strength* is easier to measure and it can be measured more accurately than dynamic strength, but the measurement of it is less valuable to athletes and coaches because *dynamic strength* is the kind of strength that is used predominantly in athletic performances.

The relationship between isometric strength measures and isotonic measures has been found to be rather low, indicating that the value of measuring isometric strength and predicting ability in dynamic motor activities is questionable. Results of several studies indicate that performances on strength tests are easily influenced by motivational situations; therefore, one's performance on strength tests may vary upward and downward in accordance with motivation.

Static Strength Tests

Static strength of different body parts can be measured accurately by use of a cable tensiometer, a back and leg lift dynamometer, or a hand grip dynamometer (Fig. 19–1). It must be remembered that owing to the strength curve of each movement, static strength varies at different points through the range of motion. Therefore, if comparisons are to be made, it is important that the strength be measured at exactly the same angle each time (see Fig. 7–9).

CABLE TENSIOMETER TESTS.   The cable tensiometer can be used to measure accurately the static strength of almost any body segment, provided the tests are administered correctly. Coaches and teachers who have been well prepared will have sufficient insight into muscular reactions to be able to identify the muscle groups they want to test.

The person being tested assumes the desired testing position. One end of the tensiometer cable is attached to the body segment and the other end to a fixed object. The tensiometer is placed on the cable and the amount of force applied by the segment is measured. For measures of this kind to be accurate, the body must be in a stable position to allow for the application of maximal force by the body segment. As with all other tests, consistency in the application technique is of utmost importance because inconsistency can greatly detract from the reliability of the test results.

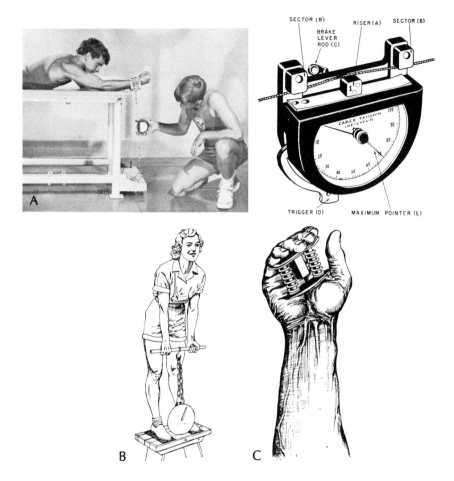

Figure 19–1.   Strength testing instruments. A, Cable tensiometer. B, Back and leg lift dynamometer. C, Hand grip dynamometer. (*A, left,* from *Measurement and Statistics in Physical Education* by N.P. Nielson and C.R. Jensen. © 1972 by Wadsworth Publishing Co., Inc., Belmont, Calif. 94002. Reprinted by permission of the publisher. *B,* from Mathews, D.K., and Fox, E.L.: *Physiological Basis of Physical Education and Athletics.* ed. 2. Philadelphia, W.B. Saunders, 1976. *A, right,* and *C,* from Mathews, D.K.: *Measurement in Physical Education.* ed. 4. Philadelphia, W.B. Saunders, 1973.)

BACK AND LEG LIFT DYNAMOMETER TESTS.   For the leg lift test, the person stands on the dynamometer platform and crouches to the desired leg bend position while he is strapped around the waist to the dynamometer. At a prescribed time he exerts a maximal force straight upward by *extending his legs.* He keeps his back straight, head erect, and chest high. Here again, a small amount of inconsistency can detract significantly from the reliability of the results.

When the dynamometer is used for the *back lift* test the length of the chain is properly adjusted and then the person bends forward and grasps the bar firmly with one palm upward and one palm downward, keeping his legs straight, feet flat on the platform, head up, and eyes straight forward. At the signal he lifts upward with maximal force by *straightening his trunk*, legs locked in the straight position.

HAND GRIP TEST.   In performing the *hand grip* test, the grip dynamometer is placed in the palm of the hand with the dial toward the palm so that the convex edge is between the first and second joints of the fingers and the concave edge is against the base of the hand. The grip is started with the elbow slightly bent and the arm raised upward. The arm moves forward and downward while the hand grips with maximal force.

Dynamic Strength Tests

Maximal lifts with different kinds of weight-training equipment provide some of the best measures of dynamic strength. A certain amount of experimentation is necessary to determine the maximal weight that can be lifted for one repetition, but when this is finally determined, it represents the dynamic strength for that particular movement. The two most commonly used tests of this kind among athletes are the bench press, and the squat or half-squat lift (Fig. 19–2). However, any of the exercise movements done with weights provides the opportunity for measuring dynamic strength for that particular movement. Strength can be measured by use of (1) free lifting equipment, (2) weight-lifting machines such as Nautilus or Universal gyms, and (3) isokinetic exercise devices such as the Cybex equipment.

DYNAMIC STRENGTH–ENDURANCE TESTS.   Often movements against one's body weight such as pull-ups or pushups have been used to measure dynamic strength. However, such tests actually measure a combination of strength and muscular endurance. A pure strength test involves only a single maximal muscle contraction; a second maximal contraction in succession would be weaker than the first, and a third contraction would be even weaker than the second. The degree to which either strength or endurance is the primary factor in a particular strength–endurance test depends on the number of times a person can repeat the movement. If an athlete is able to perform only one pull-up, then strength rather than endurance is measured. A failure to do even one pull-up results from insufficient strength, not lack of endurance. On the other hand, if an athlete performs 25 pull-ups, then the test is primarily one of endurance rather than of pure strength, although he would have to be unusually strong to do 25 pull-ups.

Many of the muscular strength–endurance tests are simple to administer, require limited space, and involve no unusual equipment.

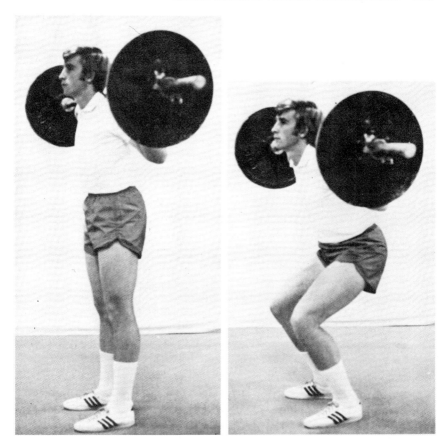

Figure 19–2. Athlete doing a half squat with heavy weight, a form of a dynamic strength test. (Robinson, C. F., Jensen, C. R., James, S. W., and Hirschi, W. M.: *Modern Techniques of Track and Field.* Philadelphia: Lea & Febiger, 1974, page 318.)

Among the more commonly used tests of this kind are *floor pushups, pull-ups* (or chin-ups), *dips* on the parallel bars, *sit-ups* (or body curls), and *squat jumps.*

Here again, precision and consistency in test administration are of the utmost importance, because if two people do slight variations of the same exercise, pull-ups for example, this can influence the results by 10% to 20%. Thus, the results cannot be compared meaningfully. (For women athletes, modified tests such as bench pushups or knee push-ups, and modified low bar or diagonal pull-ups may be administered, if preferred.)

CYBEX TESTS.   The Cybex exercise system consists of a group of commercially produced machines, examples of which are illustrated in Figures 7–7 and 19–3. The machines are designed for muscular development, but they can also be used effectively for muscle testing. By properly setting the adjustments on the machines, they can be used to measure *isometric strength, isotonic strength,* or *muscular power.* For the basic principles underlying the use of the machines, read the section entitled Isokinetic Strength Training in Chapter 7. These machines are designed for isokinetic programs.

Isometric strength can be measured at any particular angle within the range of motion by adjusting the machine for the angle and then setting the dial on zero. Under these conditions, the machine will not permit movement, and the force of the isometric contraction will be recorded.

Dynamic strength can be measured by adjusting the dial to a slow contractile velocity (30 degrees/second is recommended). The performer contracts with maximal force, and the machine permits movement through the range of motion at the rate of 30 degrees/second. The amount of force applied throughout the range of motion is recorded.

Power can be measured in a manner similar to dynamic strength except a meaningful power test would involve a faster rate of contraction. It is recommended that the dial be set on 180 degrees/second. The performer applies the maximal force through the range of motion at the speed of 180 degrees/second, and the amount of force is recorded.

Recall that in the discussion on power in Chapter 9, it was pointed out that power, which is a combination of strength and speed, varies in kind depending on whether strength or speed is the predominant factor. In performances against light resistance, such as pitching a baseball, speed is the dominant factor, whereas when heavy resistance is involved, as in putting the 16-pound shot, strength is the dominant factor. Either variety of power can be measured on Cybex machines by setting the dial for relatively fast speed (180 degrees/second) or relatively slow speed (120 degrees/second). The strength component will be emphasized at the slower speed.

CARDIOVASCULAR ENDURANCE TESTS

The best test of cardiovascular endurance is the maximal oxygen uptake test described in Chapter 4. This test measures the actual oxidative capacity of the individual and should be used whenever a high level of accuracy is desired. Several other tests can be used to *estimate* endurance. These tests usually involve speed and distance relationships, or heart rate response to various work loads measured either during the work or in recovery. The following tests have been included because they give a fairly accurate estimate of fitness, and are administered easily.

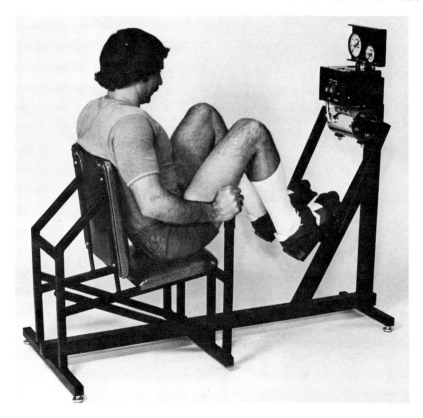

Figure 19–3. Dynamic strength test being performed on a Cybex machine.

COOPER'S TEST. One of the simplest ways to check cardiovascular endurance is to have a subject run a given distance for time or to run a given time to see how much distance he can cover. Table 19–1 shows the fitness categories for men and women who run various distances in 12 min.[2] Table 19–2 presents fitness categories for the time it takes men to run 1.5 miles.These tables are based upon thousands of tests where time and distance information were compared to measure maximal oxygen consumption. The advantages of this kind of test are that (1) it is easy to administer to large groups, and (2) no specialized equipment is needed.

ASTRAND—RHYMING TEST. This test requires the use of an accurate bicycle ergometer and metronome. A submaximal work load is performed at a level which will elicit a heart rate between 120 and 170 beats/minute. This range has been shown to be the most linear range of heart rate response.[1]

TABLE 19-1
12-Minute Walking/Running Test
Distance (Miles) Covered in 12 Minutes

Fitness Category		Age (Years)					
		13-19	20-29	30-39	40-49	50-59	60+
I. Very poor	(men)	<1.30*	<1.22	<1.18	<1.14	<1.03	<.87
	(women)	<1.0	<.96	<.94	<.88	<.84	<.78
II. Poor	(men)	1.30-1.37	1.22-1.31	1.18-1.30	1.14-1.24	1.03-1.16	.87-1.02
	(women)	1.00-1.18	.96-1.11	.95-1.05	.88-.98	.84-.93	.78-.86
III. Fair	(men)	1.38-1.56	1.32-1.49	1.31-1.45	1.25-1.39	1.17-1.30	1.03-1.20
	(women)	1.19-1.29	1.12-1.22	1.06-1.18	.99-1.11	.94-1.05	.87-.98
IV. Good	(men)	1.57-1.72	1.50-1.64	1.46-1.56	1.40-1.53	1.31-1.44	1.21-1.32
	(women)	1.30-1.43	1.23-1.34	1.19-1.29	1.12-1.24	1.06-1.18	.99-1.09
V. Excellent	(men)	1.73-1.86	1.65-1.76	1.57-1.69	1.54-1.65	1.45-1.58	1.33-1.55
	(women)	1.44-1.51	1.35-1.45	1.30-1.39	1.25-1.34	1.19-1.30	1.10-1.18
VI. Superior	(men)	>1.87	>1.77	>1.70	>1.66	>1.59	>1.56
	(women)	>1.52	>1.46	>1.40	>1.35	>1.31	>1.19

* < Means "less than"; > means "more than."

From The Aerobics Way by Kenneth Cooper, M.D., M.P.H. Copyright © 1977 by Kenneth Cooper. Reprinted by permission of the publisher, M. Evans and Company, Inc., New York.

TABLE 19–2
1.5-Mile Run Test
Time (Minutes)

Fitness Category		Age (Years)					
		13–19	20–29	30–39	40–49	50–59	60+
I. Very poor	(men)	>15:31*	>16:01	>16:31	>17:31	>19:01	>20:01
	(women)	>18:31	>19:01	>19:31	>20:01	>20:31	>21:01
II. Poor	(men)	12:11–15:30	14:01–16:00	14:44–16:30	15:36–17:30	17:01–19:00	19:01–20:00
	(women)	18:30–16:55	19:00–18:31	19:30–19:01	20:00–19:31	20:30–20:01	21:00–21:31
III. Fair	(men)	10:49–12:10	12:01–14:00	12:31–14:45	13:01–15:35	14:31–17:00	16:16–19:00
	(women)	16:54–14:31	18:30–15:55	19:00–16:31	19:30–17:31	20:00–19:01	20:30–19:31
IV. Good	(men)	9:41–10:48	10:46–12:00	11:01–12:30	11:31–13:00	12:31–14:30	14:00–16:15
	(women)	14:30–12:30	15:54–13:31	16:30–14:31	17:30–15:56	19:00–16:31	19:30–17:31
V. Excellent	(men)	8:37– 9:40	9:45–10:45	10:00–11:00	10:30–11:30	11:00–12:30	11:15–13:59
	(women)	12:29–11:50	13:30–12:30	14:30–13:00	15:55–13:45	16:30–14:30	17:30–16:30
VI. Superior	(men)	<8:37	<9:45	<10:00	<10:30	<11:00	<11:15
	(women)	<11:50	<12:30	<13:00	<13:45	<14:30	<16:30

*< Means "less than"; > means "more than."
From *The Aerobics Way* by Kenneth Cooper, M.D., M.P.H. Copyright © 1977 by Kenneth Cooper. Reprinted by permission of the publishers, M. Evans and Company, Inc., New York.

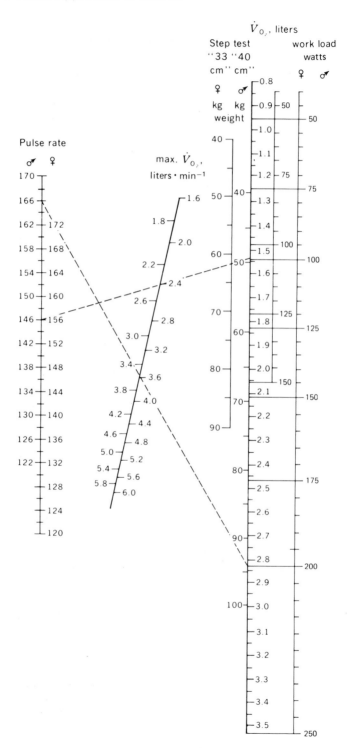

TABLE 19–3
Factor to be Used for Correction of
Predicted Maximal Oxygen Uptake

Age	Factor	Max Heart Rate	Factor
15	1.10	210	1.12
25	1.00	200	1.00
35	0.87	190	0.93
40	0.83	180	0.83
45	0.78	170	0.75
50	0.75	160	0.69
55	0.71	150	0.64
60	0.68		
65	0.65		

From *Textbook of Work Physiology*, 2nd ed., by Astrand and Rodahl, page 352. Copyright © 1977 by McGraw-Hill, Inc. Used with permission of McGraw-Hill Book Company.

The bicycle is carefully adjusted to the subject, and the metronome set at 100 beats/minute (50 revolutions/minute of either leg). Initial load settings for inactive females are usually between 300 and 450 kg-m/minute, and for inactive males, between 600 and 750 kg-m/minute. A work load that is too high will not allow a submaximal adjustment by the heart. Figure 19–4 is a nomogram which can be used to determine the predicted VO_2 max of a subject, in view of heart rate response to any given work load. Table 19–3 gives the age adjustment factor to use for subjects of different ages.

VO_2 max in milliliters/kilograms/minute can be computed easily by multiplying 1/minute (from the nomogram) by 1000 (to yield milliliters) and dividing by body weight in kilograms.

FOX'S TEST. A modification of the Astrand-Rhyming test was made by Fox who devised an equation using the heart rate during the fifth minute of a bicycle ergometer ride using 900 kg-m/minute work load.[3] There might be a problem with untrained subjects who would reach maximal heart rate before 5 min at this work load. The equation is:

$$\text{Pred. max } VO_2 = 6.3 - (0.0193 \times \text{5th min heart rate})$$

←

Figure 19–4. Nomogram to determine the predictive maximal oxygen uptake. (From *Textbook of Work Physiology* by Astrand and Rodahl, page 356. Copyright © 1970 by McGraw-Hill, Inc. Used with permission of McGraw-Hill Book Company.)

TABLE 19–4
Fitness Index for Men

	Body Weight												
	120	130	140	150	160	170	180	190	200	210	220	230	240
180	33.0	32.8	32.8	32.6	32.6	32.3	32.3	32.3	32.3	32.1	32.1	31.9	31.9
175	34.8	33.9	33.9	33.7	33.4	33.4	33.4	33.0	33.0	33.0	32.8	32.8	32.8
170	35.4	34.8	34.8	34.8	34.3	34.3	34.3	34.3	34.1	34.1	34.1	34.1	34.1
165	36.7	36.7	35.9	35.6	35.6	35.6	35.2	35.2	35.2	35.2	35.0	34.8	34.8
160	37.2	37.2	37.2	37.2	37.0	36.7	36.7	36.7	36.5	36.5	36.5	35.9	35.9
155	38.7	38.5	38.3	38.1	37.8	37.8	37.8	37.8	37.8	37.8	37.6	37.4	37.4
150	40.3	39.8	39.8	39.6	38.9	38.9	38.9	38.9	38.7	38.7	38.7	38.7	38.5
145	41.6	40.9	40.7	40.3	40.3	40.3	40.0	40.0	40.0	40.0	40.0	40.0	40.0
140	42.9	42.7	42.0	41.8	41.8	41.8	41.6	41.6	41.6	41.6	41.6	41.6	41.6
135	44.4	44.0	43.3	43.1	43.1	43.1	43.1	43.1	43.1	42.9	42.9	42.7	42.5
130	46.2	45.8	45.5	45.3	45.1	44.9	44.9	44.9	44.7	44.7	44.7	44.2	44.2
125	48.0	47.3	47.1	46.9	46.6	46.6	46.6	46.6	46.4	46.4	46.4	46.4	46.4
120	49.7	49.3	49.1	48.8	48.6	48.6	48.4	48.4	48.4	48.4	48.4	48.4	48.4
115	51.7	51.7	51.5	51.0	51.0	51.0	51.0	51.0	50.6	50.6	50.6	50.4	49.5
110	53.7	53.7	53.5	53.2	53.2	53.0	52.8	52.8	52.8	52.6	52.6	51.7	51.3
105	56.1	56.1	56.1	55.7	55.4	55.2	55.2	55.0	55.0	55.0	53.9	53.5	53.0
100	59.0	58.7	58.3	58.1	58.1	58.1	57.4	57.4	57.6	56.5	56.1	55.3	
95	64.2	61.8	61.2	61.2	61.2	60.9	60.7	60.7	59.4	58.7	57.2		
90	67.3	65.1	64.7	64.7	64.5	64.2	64.0	62.5	61.6	60.1			
85	69.3	69.3	68.2	67.8	67.8	67.8	65.8	64.9	63.7				
80	72.8	72.6	71.9	71.9	71.9	69.5	68.4	67.2					
	120	130	140	150	160	170	180	190	200	210	220	230	240

Post Exercise Pulse (left-side vertical label)

Men's Fitness Rating as Calculated from the Above Table

NEAREST AGE	SUPERIOR	EXCELLENT	VERY GOOD	GOOD	FAIR	POOR	VERY POOR
25	55	50	45	40	35	30	25
35	53	48	43	38	33	28	23
45	51	46	41	36	31	26	21
55	49	44	39	34	29	24	19
65	47	42	37	32	27	22	17

Sharky, B.J.: *Physiological Fitness and Weight Control.* Missoula: Mountain Press Publishing Co., 1978, page 109.

TABLE 19–5
Fitness Index for Women

Post Exercise Pulse	Body Weight												
	80	90	100	110	120	130	140	150	160	170	180	190	
175											31.2		175
170				31.9	31.9	32.1	32.1	32.1	32.1	32.1	32.1	32.3	170
165			32.3	32.6	33.0	33.0	33.2	33.2	33.2	33.2	33.2		165
160			33.4	33.7	33.9	34.1	34.3	34.3	34.3	34.3	34.3	34.3	160
155		34.5	34.8	35.2	35.4	35.4	35.4	35.4	35.4	35.4	35.4		155
150		35.6	36.1	36.3	36.3	36.7	36.7	36.7	36.7	36.7	36.7		150
145		37.2	37.4	38.1	38.1	38.1	38.1	38.1	38.3	38.3	38.9	38.9	145
140		38.7	39.4	39.4	39.6	39.6	39.6	39.6	39.6	39.6	39.6		140
135	39.6	39.8	40.0	40.3	40.3	40.9	40.9	41.1	41.1	41.4	41.6	41.6	135
130	40.5	41.1	41.8	42.0	42.2	42.9	42.9	43.1	43.3	43.3	43.6	43.6	130
125	41.4	43.6	43.8	44.0	44.0	44.4	44.7	44.9	44.9	45.3	45.3	45.3	125
120	42.5	45.3	45.8	46.0	46.0	46.4	46.9	47.1	47.1	47.3	47.5	47.5	120
115	44.4	47.7	48.0	48.0	48.0	48.0	49.3	49.3	49.3	49.3	49.3	49.3	115
110	48.0	50.2	51.5	51.7	51.7	51.7	51.9	52.4	52.4	52.8			110
105	51.7	53.7	53.7	53.9	54.1	54.6	55.4	55.7	55.7				105
100	55.2	56.8	57.0	57.6	58.3	58.3	59.4						100
95	58.1	60.7	61.2	61.6	62.3	62.3							95
90	62.7	64.7	65.6	67.5	67.5	68.6							90
	80	90	100	110	120	130	140	150	160	170	180	190	

Women's Fitness Rating as Calculated from the Above Table

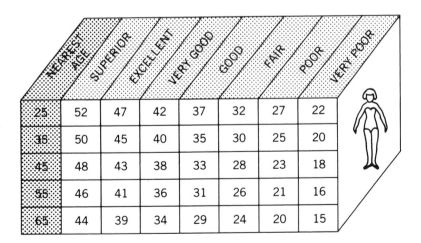

NEAREST AGE	SUPERIOR	EXCELLENT	VERY GOOD	GOOD	FAIR	POOR	VERY POOR
25	52	47	42	37	32	27	22
35	50	45	40	35	30	25	20
45	48	43	38	33	28	23	18
55	46	41	36	31	26	21	16
65	44	39	34	29	24	20	15

Sharky, B.J.: *Physiological Fitness and Weight Control*. Missoula: Mountain Press Publishing Co., 1978, page 108.

SHARKEY'S STEP TEST.   Sharkey's step test is an excellent test of cardiovascular fitness. A 15¾-inch bench is used for men and a 13-inch bench, for women.[6] The subject steps up and down at 90 beats/minute (using a metronome) for exactly 5 min. The recovery pulse is counted for 15 sec starting exactly 15 sec from the end of the work bout. The 15-sec heart rate is multiplied by 4 and the result is entered into Table 19–4 or Table 19–5 using the nearest weight. The results are expressed as VO_2 in milliliters/kilograms/minute. The fitness ratings for men or women, based upon the results of the test, are shown under the tables. An age adjustment should be made when necessary (see Table 19–3).

This test can be administered to large grous of subjects, such as physical education classes or adult fitness groups, if they are first taught to count pulse rate.

FISHER'S TEST.   Using the prediction equations presented in Chapter 3, one can compute an estimated maximal oxygen uptake ($\dot{V}O_2$ max) from the average speed a person can maintain for a run of 2 miles or more.

For instance, a person who can run 5 miles in 40 min averages 8 minute-miles or 7.5 mph (7.5 mph is equal to 201.15 m/minute). From the prediction equation for running, the cost of running at this rate is 43.73 ml/kg/min ($201.15 \times 0.2 + 3.5$). Since most moderately trained subjects can work for an extended period of time at about 75% of their maximum, the computed cost of the work is equal to 75% of their maximal $\dot{V}O_2$. A simple mathematical maneuver ($43.75/75 = X/100$) shows that the person described needs a maximal $\dot{V}O_2$ of about 58 ml/kg/min to accomplish the work he does.

MEASURES OF POWER

Muscular power tests ordinarily take three forms: ability to project or accelerate one's body, ability to project an object, or ability to impart a striking force. The more useful tests of power are:

MARGARIA–KALAMEN POWER TEST.   Margaria and his associates first published the Margaria leg power test; then Kalamen revised the test.[4] The performer begins 6 meters from the bottom stair and runs up a flight of stairs as rapidly as possible, taking three steps at a time (Fig. 19–5). Switch mats are placed on the third and ninth steps. By stepping on the third stair, the performer activates a clock accurate to 1/100 sec; when he steps on the ninth stair, the clock is stopped. The time recorded by the clock represents the time required to move the body a height of 1.05 m. Power is calculated by the formula:

$$\text{Power} = \frac{\text{Body weight (kg)} \times 1.05 \text{ m}}{\text{Elapsed time}}$$

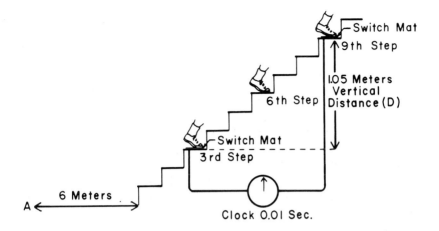

Figure 19–5. Margaria-Kalamen power test. Subject commences at point A and runs as rapidly as he can up the flight of stairs, taking them three at a time. The time it takes him to traverse the distance between stair 3 and stair 9 is recorded in 0.01 sec. The power generated is a product of the subject's weight and the vertical distance (D), divided by the time. (From Mathews, D.K., and Fox, E.L.: *The Physiological Basis of Physical Education and Athletics*. ed. 2. Philadelphia, W.B. Saunders, 1976.)

VERTICAL JUMP TEST (JUMP AND REACH OR SARGEANT JUMP). This test measures explosive power of the extensor muscles of the legs. However, other movements also contribute, such as the associated actions of the arms and shoulders. The athlete faces the wall with both feet flat on the floor and toes touching the wall, and then reaches as high as possible with either hand and makes a mark on the jump board (chalkboard). From the desired jump position with the preferred side to the wall, he jumps as high as possible, and at the peak of the jump makes another mark above the first one. The score is the difference in inches or centimeters between the two marks.

STANDING LONG JUMP. This test measures essentially the same characteristics as the vertical jump; however, it depends on upper body movement a little more and leg extension a little less. Also, the standing long jump is slightly less reliable than the vertical jump because it is a more difficult and less common skill, and it improves more easily with practice.

The athlete stands with his feet a comfortable distance apart and his toes just behind the takeoff mark. He crouches, leans forward, swings his arms backward, and then jumps as far as possible horizontally, leaving from both feet and landing on both feet simultaneously. His score is the distance from the back of the takeoff mark to the nearest point where any part of the body touches the floor at the completion of the jump. Obviously, the amount of friction between the feet and the jumping surface is important to success in this test.

BALL THROW FOR DISTANCE.   This test measures power of the total body with emphasis on the upper extremities. It can be done with one of several kinds of balls: softball, weighted softball, basketball, or medicine ball.

The athlete stands behind the restraining line, then using the desired approach, he projects the ball as far as possible using the overarm throwing technique and being careful not to cross the restraining line. The measurement is taken from behind the restraining line to the spot where the ball first strikes the surface.

SHOT PUT.   As a test of power for noncompetitive shot-putters, the 12-pound (high school) shot is ordinarily used (8-pound shot for junior high school students). Starting from the back of a 7-foot shot-putting ring or between two lines 7 feet apart, the athlete projects the shot by use of the usual shot-putting technique. The distance is measured from the back of the restraining line to the point where the shot first strikes the ground. This test involves a skill that is unfamiliar to many persons, and in such cases, this detracts from its reliability.

Running Acceleration Tests

The rate at which a person can accelerate is a measure of power with emphasis on the leg extensor muscles. Running is essentially a series of body projections from alternate legs. The rate at which a body is accelerated is directly proportional to the force causing it (muscular force in this case), according to Newton's second law of motion.

An electronic device is necessary to measure acceleration speed accurately over short distances up to 15 yards. Beyond 15 yards, measurements can be made fairly accurately with stopwatches. With proper equipment, acceleration tests of 5, 10, or 15 yards are meaningful measures of power, whereas tests of sprint speed for longer distances are less meaningful but still quite significant as measures of power.

It is true that most persons reach maximal sprint speed between 15 and 20 yards out of the blocks, and at this point, maximal running speed instead of acceleration speed becomes the dominant factor. Maximal running speed is dependent upon power but less so than acceleration speed.

In summary, measures of acceleration speed up to 15 yards timed with highly accurate equipment are good tests of power, and tests of sprint speed over longer distances (40 or 50 yards) are indicators of power. Many athletes in court and field games are measured by their coaches over the 40- or 50-yard distance. Football players especially are measured over the 40-yard distance. These measurements of acceleration speed combined with sprint speed are indicators of power but they are not pure power tests. However, such a test measures an important characteristic in this case, the ability to cover 40 yards in the shortest time possible from a stationary start.

AGILITY TESTS

Agility is the characteristic of being able to change direction and position of the body and its parts rapidly. In athletics, we are mostly concerned about two kinds of agility: *running agility* and *total body*

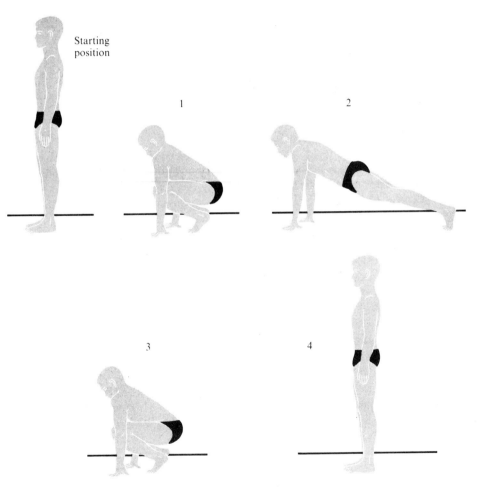

Figure 19–6. Squat thrust test. (From *Measurement and Statistics in Physical Education* by N. P. Nielson and C. R. Jensen, page 180. © 1972 by Wadsworth Publishing Company, Inc., Belmont, California. Reprinted by permission of the publisher.)

maneuverability. Running agility is tested by dodging and zigzag running, and total body maneuverability can be measured by the squat thrust test.

SQUAT THRUST TEST–10 SECONDS (BURPEE TEST). The performer stands erect at the start of the squat thrust test (Fig. 19–6). He then moves to the squat position with both hands on the floor, then thrusts his legs backward keeping his arms, back, and legs straight, then back to the squat position, and finally to the erect position. A complete cycle is counted as one squat thrust, and the test is scored to the last one fourth of one squat thrust. If a person does not reach an acceptable position in any of the four phases, one fourth of a point is deducted. The objective is to do as many squat thrusts as possible in 10 sec.

Even though the 10-sec test is the only agility test of this kind that has been standardized, many believe that for well-conditioned people, 10 sec is too short a time to get an accurate measurement, and that 20 sec gives a more correct indication of agility.

Incidentally, this same test held for 60 sec is sometimes used as a measure of anaerobic endurance. Even though this crude measure of endurance does produce some meaningful results, it should be recognized that there are more useful and precise endurance tests available.

SHUTTLE RUN. The standard shuttle run is done over a 30-foot course, however, it is possible to do it over a shorter course, and there is some argument that a shorter course provides a purer measure of agility with less emphasis on running speed. In order to do the standard

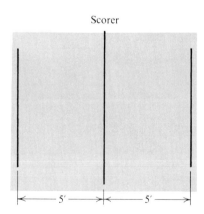

Figure 19–7. Sidestep test floor plan. (From *Measurement and Statistics in Physical Education* by N. P. Nielson and C. R. Jensen, page 184. © 1972 by Wadsworth Publishing Company, Inc., Belmont, California. Reprinted by permission of the publisher.)

agility test over a 30-foot course, two small blocks of wood are placed 30 feet from the starting line. At the signal the athlete starts from behind the starting line, retrieves one of the blocks and places it behind the starting line, then retrieves the second block and sprints back across the starting line. The run is measured to the nearest $1/10$ sec. Lines on the surface can be used instead of blocks, if this is preferred.

SIDESTEP TEST.   This test measures agility in lateral movements. Three lines are placed parallel on the surface of the floor, 5 feet apart (Fig. 19–7). The athlete straddles the middle line. On signal, he sidesteps to the right until one foot crosses the right-hand line. Then he sidesteps to the left until one foot crosses the left-hand line. He repeats these lateral movements as rapidly as possible for 20 sec. His final score is the number of times that he crossed an outside line.

RIGHT-BOOMERANG TEST.   This simple test has been popular for a long time and is still considered a good test of running agility. To

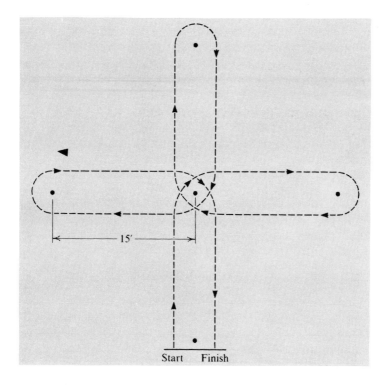

Start   Finish

Figure 19–8.   Right-boomerang course. (From *Measurement and Statistics in Physical Education* by N. P. Nielson and C. R. Jensen, page 183. © 1972 by Wadsworth Publishing Company, Inc., Belmont, California. Reprinted by permission of the publisher.)

establish the course, a jumping standard or similar object is placed at the center point with four smaller objects, such as Indian clubs, wastebaskets, and the like placed at the four outside points (Fig. 19–8). At the starting signal, the performer sprints toward the center point and then follows the course as indicated in the illustration. His time is recorded to the nearest $1/10$ sec.

MEASURES OF FLEXIBILITY

A large number of flexibility measures are possible because of the large number of specific movements that can occur in the body. Only three of the more commonly used tests are included here. They serve as examples of the kinds of flexibility measures that can be performed.

HIP AND TRUNK FLEXION TEST. The performer sits on a table or on the floor with his feet flat against the wall, hip width apart, and his legs straight and rigid. He bends his trunk forward and downward as far as possible extending his hands toward the heels of his feet. There are two important measurements that can be taken at this position: first, the distance the person's fingertips are from his heels, and second, the vertical distance from the top of his sternum to the surface of the table or floor. Lack of flexibility demonstrated in this test indicates tightness of the muscles and connective tissues that cross the back of the hip joints and the lower back.

UPWARD ARM MOVEMENT TEST. The person lies prone on a table with his chin touching the table and his arms stretched forward directly in front of his shoulders. He holds a stick horizontally in both hands. Keeping his elbows and wrists straight and his chin on the table, he raises his arms upward as far as possible. The examiner measures the vertical distance from the bottom of the stick to the table. Insufficient flexibility in this movement indicates tightness of the muscles and connective tissues in the front of the shoulders and chest region.

PLANTAR-DORSAL FLEXION TEST. The subject sits on a table or on the floor with his leg straight. Keeping heel and back of knee on the table, he plantar flexes one foot as far as possible (Fig. 19–9). With a pad of paper placed in a vertical position as a backdrop to the foot, the examiner places a dot on the paper at the end of the toenail of the great toe. The subject dorsally flexes his foot as far as possible and the examiner again places a dot on the paper at the end of the toenail of the great toe. Finally, the subject relaxes his ankle, and the examiner places a third dot on the paper where the ankle bends at the top of the instep. The pad is removed, and lines are drawn connecting the third dot to each of the other two. Using a protractor or a goniometer, the examiner determines the range of motion in degrees.

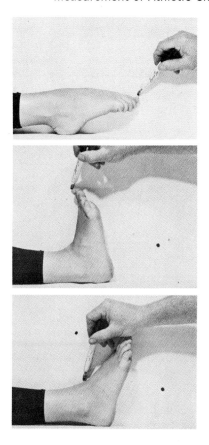

Figure 19–9.   Plantar-dorsal flexion test. (From *Measurement and Statistics in Physical Education* by N. P. Nielson and C. R. Jensen, page 189. © 1972 by Wadsworth Publishing Company, Inc., Belmont, California. Reprinted by permission of the publisher.)

REACTION TIME AND SPEED MEASUREMENTS

Reaction time can be measured best by a laboratory electronic device that automatically registers the time from the initiation of a stimulus to the completion of the given response (this is more correctly termed *response time.*) However, since there are no standardized devices available on the market for such tests outside of laboratory situations, less exact but more practical approaches must be taken. The best non-laboratory test to indicate reaction time is the alternate response test.

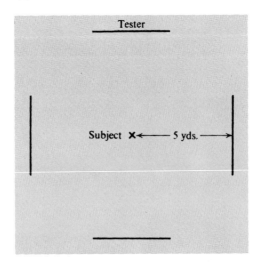

Figure 19–10.   Floor area for four-way alternate response test. (From *Measurement and Statistics in Physical Education* by N. P. Nielson and C.R. Jensen, page 201. © 1972 by Wadsworth Publishing Company, Inc., Belmont, California. Reprinted by permission of the publisher.)

FOUR-WAY ALTERNATE RESPONSE TIME.   The one being tested stands at point X on the floor (Fig. 19–10). On each of the four sides is a line 5 yards from point X. The one administering the test gives the hand signals from in front of the performer but behind the 5-yard line. The test administrator gives a distinct signal for the performer to move in one of the four directions and then times how long it takes the performer to cross the line. He administers the test numerous times (20 is recommended—5 in each direction, but in no particular order) and then computes the average time.

RUNNING SPEED TESTS.   Running speed can be measured best by sprint tests. The most commonly used distances for such measures are 40 yards and 50 yards, but any distance to 100 yards would be satisfactory. If pure running speed is to be measured, the subject should have a running start, so that *acceleration* speed is not a factor. Whereas if running speed over a given distance including acceleration speed is to be determined, the subject should be stationary at the start. The importance of consistency in the conduct of such tests is apparent. When there is a high level of consistency, the test results can be compared meaningfully among individuals or among performances of the same individual.

SELECTED REFERENCES

1. Astrand, P., and Rhyming, I.: A nomogram for calculation of aerobic capacity (physical fitness) from pulse rate during submaximal work. *J. Appl. Physiol.*, 7:218–221, 1954.
2. Cooper, K. H.: *Aerobics.* New York: Bantam Books, 1968.
3. Fox., E.: A simple, accurate technique for predicting maximal aerobic power. *J. Appl. Physiol.*, 35:914–916, 1973.
4. Margaria, R., Aghemo, I., and Rovelli, E.: Measurement of muscular power (anaerobic) in man. *J. Appl. Physiol.*, 21:1662–1664, 1966.
5. Neilson, N. P., and Jensen, C. R.: *Measurement and Statistics in Physical Education.* Belmont, Calif.: Wadsworth Publishing Co., Inc., 1972.
6. Sharkey, B. J.: *Physiological Fitness and Weight Control.* Missoula: Mountain Press Publishing Co., 1974.

Glossary

Acceleration: Rate of increase in velocity.

Acetylcholine: A chemical mediator in the body, normally associated with depolarization of neurons.

Actin: A muscle protein which, with myosin, is responsible for muscle contraction and relaxation.

Action potential: The electrical change that can be recorded during muscle contraction.

Active transport: The process of moving molecules against a concentration gradient.

ADP (adenosine diphosphate): A high-energy chemical compound with two phosphate radicals.

Adrenergic: Having to do with the release of epinephrine or norepinephrine.

Aerobic: Occurring in the presence of oxygen. Aerobic processes occur with oxygen present.

Aerobic training: A training technique specifically designed to improve the aerobic processes of the body and thereby increase aerobic endurance.

Afferent nervous system: The bodily system that directs impulses from sensory receptors toward the spinal cord and brain; also called *sensory nervous system.*

Agility: The ability to change directions of the body or its parts rapidly, demonstrated in such movements as dodging, zigzagging, stopping, starting, and reversing direction of movement.

Agonistic muscle: A muscle which contributes to the desired movement by its concentric contraction; a prime mover.

Alactacid: A process which provides energy without involving the glycolytic pathway.

Alveoli: The tiny air sacs in the lungs where gaseous exchange takes place.

Amylases: Enzymes which digest carbohydrates.

Anaerobic: Occurring in the absence of oxygen. Anaerobic processes occur with no oxygen present.

Anaerobic training: A training technique designed to increase the anaerobic processes of the body and thereby increase anaerobic endurance.

Anisotropic: Describing the movement of light through an opaque medium in which the velocity of the emerging light is not the same in all directions.

Annulospiral endings: Specialized sensory neurons which surround the nuclear bag and fire when the bag is stretched.

Antagonistic muscle: A muscle which causes a movement opposite the desired movement. Resistance to the desired movement would occur if it were to contract.

Apneustic center: A center in the brain which helps control breathing.

Appendicular skeleton: The bones of the arms, hands, legs, and feet.

Artery: A vessel that carries blood away from the heart.

Atherosclerosis: A condition in which plaques occur inside blood vessels.

ATP (adenosine triphosphate):   A chemical compound used by the body to supply energy to many physiological mechanisms.

Atrium: An upper heart chamber.

Attitude: Readiness to act in a particular way. Attitudes express different degrees of acceptance or rejection.

Autonomic nervous system: That portion of the nervous system which controls the involuntary processes of the body, such as the functioning of the internal organs.

a-$\bar{v}$ O$_2$ diff: The difference in the amount of oxygen carried by the arterial blood and that carried by the venous blood.

Axial skeleton: The bones of the head, neck, and trunk.

Axis: A fixed line around which a moving object revolves.

Axon: Appendage of the neuron that conducts impulses away from the cell body.

Balance: Ability to keep the center of gravity over the base of support and to maintain equilibrium.

Beta oxidation: A metabolic pathway for the breakdown of long-chain fatty acids.

Boyle's law: The law that states that the volume of gas is inversely proportional to the pressure exerted upon it when the temperature is constant.

Buffers: Substances which decrease the chemical reaction otherwise produced by acids or alkalies.

Calcium flux: The movement of calcium into the myocardium to cause contraction.

Calorie: A unit of heat used in metabolic studies.

Calorimeter: A machine to measure the number of calories used.

Capacity: The limits within which ability can be developed. Ability cannot extend beyond capacity.

Capillary: The smallest of the blood vessels.

Cardiac output: Volume of blood pumped from the left ventricle in one minute.

Cardiovascular endurance: The endurance of the circulatory system; the ability of this system to carry on its functions efficiently under conditions of heavy work.

Central nervous system (CNS):   That portion of the nervous system that includes the brain and spinal cord.

Chemoreceptors: Receptors sensitive to changes in certain chemicals in the body.

Cholinergic: Having to do with the release of acetylcholine.

Cholinesterase: An enzyme which is capable of destroying acetylcholine.

Chylomicrons: Lipoprotein molecules which carry fats to the blood stream through the lymph.

Closed-circuit calorimetry: The method of estimating metabolic rate of the body using a spirometer to measure air taken into and expelled from the lungs.

Concentric contraction: Shortening of a muscle due to nervous impulses.

Conditioned reflex: A reflex pattern which is learned, as opposed to one that is inborn.

Connective tissue: Body tissue whose primary purpose is to connect one body part to another, such as ligaments connect bone to bone and tendons connect muscle to bone. There are several kinds of connective tissue.

Contractile force: The amount of tension applied by a muscle or group of muscles during contraction.

Coordination: The act of various muscles working together in a smooth, concerted way; correct and precise timing of muscle contractions.

Coronary system: The body system which includes the blood vessels that service the heart muscle.

CP (creatine phosphate):   A high-energy chemical compound which transfers energy interchangeably with ATP.

Cristae: Shelflike infoldings of the inner membrane of a mitochondrion.

Cross training: The training effect that occurs in one side of the body as a result of exercising the opposite side of the body.

Dalton's law: The law that states that the total pressure of a mixture of gases is equal to the sum of the partial pressure of the component gases.

Deceleration: Rate of decrease in velocity.

Dendrite: The appendage of a neuron which directs impulses toward the cell body.

Depolarization: The condition of the cell membrane when it has reached threshold and the sodium ion has rushed to the inside of the cell.

Diastole: The relaxation phase of each heart beat.

Diastolic pressure: The blood pressure during the relaxation of the ventricles.

Dicrotic notch: A notch which occurs when recording the pressure after aortic valve closure in the cardiac cycle.

Diffusion: A movement of molecules through a membrane, from an area of high concentration to an area of low concentration.

Direct calorimetry: A method used to estimate the metabolic rate of the body by measuring the heat released by the body.

Dynamic contraction: See isotonic contraction.

Dynamic flexibility: Flexibility that can be exhibited as a result of contraction of the agonistic muscle and that does not result from the pull of gravity or from the body parts being moved by an outside force such as another person.

Dynamic strength: Strength exhibited in motion.

Eccentric contraction: Controlled lengthening of a muscle. The muscle becomes longer as it contracts because the resistance is greater than the contractile force.

Ectomorph: An individual who has a light or slender body build.

Edema: Swelling caused by abnormally increased amounts of fluid in tissue spaces.

Efferent system: The motor nervous system which directs impulses from the brain and spinal cord to muscles, glands, and organs.

Electrical potential: An electrical difference between the outside and the inside of a cell, caused by a difference in the ionic composition on each side.

Endocardium: A thin, smooth, shiny membrane covering the inside surfaces of the heart.

Endomorph: An individual who has a fat or heavy body build.

Endomysium: Connective tissue surrounding the muscle cell.

End plate: That portion of a motor neuron which attaches to a muscle fiber.

Endurance: Ability to resist fatigue and recover quickly from fatigue.

Epicardium: A thin, shiny membrane covering the outer surface of the heart.

Epimysium: Connective tissue surrounding the whole muscle.

Ergometer: A device to measure work.

Expiratory reserve volume: A volume of air in the lungs which can be used to increase tidal volume.

Facilitation: The movement of the cell membrane toward the threshold.

Fascicle: A small group of muscle or nerve fibers.

First-class lever: A lever arrangement with the fulcrum between the effort and the resistance.

Flexibility: Property of muscles and connective tissue that allows full range of motion.

Flower-spray receptors: Specialized sensory neurons attached to each end of the nuclear bag in the muscle spindle.

Functional residual capacity: The combination of residual volume and expiratory reserve volume.

Gamma motor system: A motor system which causes movement through gamma efferent motor activity to the intrafusal fibers of the muscle spindle.

Gay-Lussac's law: The law that states that the pressure of a gas increases directly in proportion to its absolute temperature if the volume remains constant.

Glycolysis: An anaerobic energy-producing pathway; the breaking down of sugars.

Grams percent: A method of expressing concentration in grams per hundred milliliters of a substance.

Gray matter: The tissue in the central nervous system made up of nerve cell bodies.

Heart rate: The number of times the heart beats during one minute.

Hemodynamics: The basic physical principles of circulation.

Hydrogen-electron transport system: An energy scheme in which hydrogen atoms are passed through a series of oxidizing enzymes and are ionized with the release of energy.

Hydrolysis: The breakdown of a food particle by adding water at certain bonds.

Hydrophilic: Water loving.

Hydrophobic: Water hating.

Hydroxyl ion: An OH molecule with an extra electron.

Hypertension: A condition of persistently high arterial blood pressure.

Hypertrophy: Substantial increase in the overall size of a tissue; significant enlargement.

Hyperventilation: The state caused by hard breathing in which too much air pressure results in dizziness and/or unconsciousness.

Hypoxia: Below normal levels of oxygen in air.

Indirect calorimetry: A method of estimating metabolic rate by measuring the amount of oxygen used by the body.

Inhibitory control: The control placed on muscle contractions as a result of inhibitory impulses which originate in the central nervous system.

Inotropic: An increase in the contractile condition of the myocardium.

Inspiratory capacity: The combination of tidal volume and inspiratory reserve volume.

Inspiratory reserve volume: A volume of air in the lungs which can be used to increase tidal volume.

Intercalated discs: Cell membranes which separate individual cardiac muscle cells and allow the action potential to spread to all fibers.

Internuncial neuron: A neuron in the spinal cord that serves as a connection between motor and sensory neurons.

Interval training: A training program which consists of short bouts of heavy work alternated with periods of rest or light work.

Intrafusal muscle fiber: Specialized muscle fibers within muscle spindles.

Isometric contraction: A contraction in which muscle tension increases, but the muscle does not shorten because it does not overcome the resistance.

Isotonic contraction: A contraction in which muscle fibers shorten as a result of stimulus.

Isotropic: Having like properties in all directions, as in movement of light through an opaque medium in which the velocity of the emerging light is the same in all directions.

Isovolumic: Occurring without an alteration in volume. This term is used to describe the isovolumic pressure line in the cardiac function curve.

Junctional fibers: Specialized transmission fibers of the heart between the atrium and ventricle which delay the entrance of an electrical impulse into the AV node.

Kilocalorie: One thousand calories; sometimes called *large calorie*.

Kinesthetic sense: A sense of awareness, without the use of the other senses, of muscle and joint positions and actions.

Krebs cycle: A sequence of chemical reactions in the metabolic pathways where the end products of glycolysis are degraded to carbon dioxide and hydrogen atoms; sometimes called the *tricarboxylic acid cycle* or *citric acid cycle.*

Laminar flow: The flow of blood through vessels in which the velocity of flow in the center of the vessel is far greater than that toward the outer edges.

Lever: A rigid bar (one or more bones) which revolves about a fulcrum (joint).

Ligament: Tough connective tissue which binds bones together, forming joints.

Lipases: Enzymes involved in the digestion of fats.

Lung capacities: Lung measurements made up of at least two lung volumes.

Lung volumes: Single measurements of primary lung subdivisions.

Maximal oxygen uptake: The maximal amount of oxygen which can be used by the body during heavy work.

Mesomorph: An individual who has a husky or muscular body build or a medium-type body build.

Mitochondria: Cellular organelles which produce energy for cellular metabolism.

Momentum: The property of a moving body that determines the force required to bring the body to rest. Momentum = mass × velocity.

Monosynaptic: Pertaining to or relayed through only one synapse.

Motor end plate: A connection between the nerve and muscle fiber.

Motor unit: A group of muscle fibers dispersed throughout a muscle and supplied by a single motor nerve fiber.

Movement time: The amount of time that it takes to accomplish the movement after the impulse to respond has been received.

Muscle-bound: Having a pathological condition brought on by improper training in which the joints lose some of their range of motion due to hypertrophied muscles.

Muscle spindle: A group of specialized muscle tissues which are sensitive to changes of muscle length.

Muscular endurance: Ability to continue muscular action.

Myocardium: Another name for the muscle tissue of the heart.

Myoneural junction: The intersection between the motor end plate of a nerve branch and the muscle fiber.

Myosin: A muscle protein which, with actin, is responsible for muscle contraction and relaxation.

Nerve: A cablelike bundle of many nerve fibers.

Neuromuscular coordination: Coordination which results from nerve impulses reaching the proper muscles with sufficient intensity at the correct time.

Neuron: A complete nerve cell, including the cell body and all its appendages.

Neutralizer muscle: A muscle that acts to equalize the action of another muscle.

Nuclear bag: A specialized area of the muscle tissue inside the muscle spindle, surrounded by annulospiral endings.

Open-circuit calorimetry: The process of estimating metabolic rate by collecting and analyzing expired air.

Overload: The process of demanding more performance from a system than is ordinarily required.

Oxidation: The loss of electrons from an atom or molecule.

Oxygen debt: A condition which results when the demand for oxygen is greater than the supply.

Oxygen dissociation curve: A curve which represents the percentage of saturation of the hemoglobin of the blood at various partial pressures of oxygen and blood CO_2 levels.

Pacemaker: A small section of the heart located in the upper right portion where the beat of the heart originates. The beat spreads from the pacemaker throughout the remainder of the heart.

Parasympathetic: Pertaining to a major subdivision of the autonomic nervous system.

Passive flexibility: Flexibility exhibited as a result of the pull of gravity or an outside force such as pressure by another person, as opposed to flexibility exhibited as a result of muscle contractions.

Perimysium: Connective tissue which surrounds fascicles of muscle fibers.

Peripheral nervous system: The body system which includes all those parts of the nervous system not included in the brain and spinal cord.

pH: The relative acidity or basicity of body fluids. More exactly, pH is the negative logarithm of the hydrogen ion concentration.

Pneumotaxic center: A center in the brain which helps control breathing.

Poiseuille's law: The principle which attempts to explain the factors of blood flow, especially the velocity in relation to the size of the vessel.

Postural muscles: The muscles used to maintain posture; also called *antigravity muscles.*

Power: The product of force and velocity; the ability to apply force at a rapid rate.

Progressive overload (see "overload"):   Progressive increase in work load in accordance with the athlete's ability to do work, resulting in continuous overload over an extended training period.

Progressive resistance: A muscle-training program in which the amount of resistance is systematically increased as the muscles gain in strength.

Ptyalin: An enzyme found in the mouth which hydrolizes starches.

Q̇:   A standard symbol indicating blood flow, normally cardiac output.

Range of motion: The amount of movement that can occur in a joint, expressed in degrees.

Reaction time: Time between the reception of a signal to respond and the beginning of the response.

Reciprocal inhibition: The automatic blocking of nerve impulses to those muscles in opposition (antagonistic) to a desired movement. This automatically occurs with all well-coordinated movement patterns. Lack of reciprocal inhibitions is a contributor to poor coordination.

Reflex: An immediate response to a situation in which the thought process is bypassed.

Reflex time: Time of nerve impulse travel in a reflex action.

Refractory period: A period of time when muscle tissue is unable to be restimulated.

Repolarization: The condition of the membrane after depolarization when the ionic balance on each side of the cell has been restored.

Reserve strength: Strength which cannot be exhibited voluntarily under normal conditions but which can be exhibited under conditions of extreme excitement or emergency.

Residual volume: Amount of air in the lungs which cannot be expired.

Respiration: The movement of air into and out of the lungs.

Response time: A combination of reaction time and movement time. The total time that elapses from the beginning of the external stimulus until the act or response is completed.

Resting potential: The electrical potential across a cell membrane during resting conditions.

Reverse potential: The electrical potential across a cell membrane at a given point following depolarization.

R. M. (repetition maximum):   In weight training, the maximum number of repetitions that can be accomplished against a given amount of resistance.

Saltatory conduction: The rapid, high speed conduction of myelinated fibers which occurs along the nodes of Ranvier.

Sarcolemma: Muscle-cell membrane.

Sarcomere: The functional unit of a muscle cell (from Z line to Z line).

Second-class lever: A lever arrangement with the resistance between the fulcrum and the effort.

Sinusoid: A hollow or cavity, a recess or pocket.

Skeletal muscle: A muscle which attaches to and causes movement of the skeleton; also called *striated, motor* and *voluntary* muscle.

Skill: The ability to coordinate effectively the actions of the different muscles used in a bodily movement (the term *intellectual skills* should not be used; *skill* should refer to neuromuscular functions).

Smooth muscle: A muscle located in the internal organs, with the exception of the heart; also called *visceral* and *involuntary* muscle.

Soma: Another name for a nerve cell body.

Somatotype: A category of body types or physique among humans.

Spatial summation: The movement of the membrane toward threshold as a result of two or more neurons firing in close proximity.

Sphygmomanometer: A device used to measure blood pressure.

Sphincter: An opening which can be closed.

Stabilizer muscle: A muscle which contracts at a particular time to hold a body portion firmly in position.

Static contraction: Same as tonic or isometric contraction.

Static strength: Strength exhibited without overt motion.

Steady state: A condition in which the supply of oxygen to the tissues is equal to the demand for oxygen.

Steroids: Organic compounds including bile acids, sterols, and sex hormones.

Strength: The ability of the muscles to exert force against resistance. Strength is lessened by inadequate nutrition or inadequate exercise.

Stretch reflex: An automatic reflex to contract in skeletal muscles, brought on by sudden stretching of the muscles.

Stroke volume: The volume of blood pumped out of the left ventricle with each contraction.

Summation: A sustained muscular contraction caused by rapid firing of nerve impulses.

Sympathetic nervous system: A major division of the autonomic nervous system.

Synapse: A weblike relay junction between neurons, which relays impulses in only one direction from axons to dendrites.

Synaptic trough: A small area beneath the motor end plate.

Syncytium: A mass of cytoplasm with numerous nuclei. This term is used to describe the functional relationship of heart muscle cells.

Systole: The contracting phase of each heart beat.

Systolic pressure: The blood pressure during the systolic phase of the heart beat.

Temporal summation: The movement of the membrane toward threshold caused by increased frequency of firing by a single neuron.

Tendon: A tough, fibrous tissue that connects muscles to bones.

Tetanization: The increased contractile condition of muscle when stimulated by high frequency stimulation.

Third-class lever: A lever arrangement with the effort between the fulcrum and the resistance.

Threshold: The resistance level of a fiber to nerve impulses. If the fiber is to be activated, the impulses must be strong enough to exceed the fiber's threshold.

Tidal volume: The normal breathing pattern of the lungs.

Triglyceride: A form of fat containing one glycerol molecule and three fatty acids.

Tropomyosin: A protein molecule in the actin filament of muscle.

Troponin: A protein molecule in the actin filament of muscle.

Turgor: The natural pressure from fluids inside a cell.

Utilization coefficient: The percentage of the total oxygen in the blood which is utilized by the tissues.

$\dot{V}_E$: Expiratory volume.

$\dot{V}_I$: Inspiratory volume.

$\dot{V}_{O_2}$: Oxygen consumption in liters per minute (l/min).

Valsalva's maneuver: The increase of pressures in the abdominal region associated with breath holding and extreme effort.

Vasomotor tone: The tone of the muscles that line the walls of the blood vessels.

Vein: A vessel that returns blood to the heart.

Velocity: The rate at which an object travels in a given direction.

Ventilation: The exchange of air in and out of the lungs. The process of inhaling and exhaling.

Ventricle: A lower chamber of the heart.

Viscosity (blood): The thickness of a fluid; the resistance to flow.

Vital capacity: The total amount of air that can be forced out of the lungs after a forced inhalation.

Volume percent: Method of expressing concentration in milliliters per hundred milliliters.

Voluntary nervous system: That part of the nervous system which is consciously controlled.

White matter: The tissue in the central nervous system made up of nerve fibers, not nerve cell bodies.

Wind-kessel vessel: A description of the aorta as it opens to receive blood and rebounds to push blood through the system.

Work: The result of muscle contractions. If the muscle contractions cause movement, the work is dynamic; if no movement occurs, the work is static.

Index